Your Natural Health Makeover

Dr. Lauri M. Aesoph

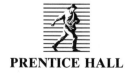

PRENTICE HALL

Library of Congress Cataloging-in-Publication Data

Aesoph, Lauri M., N.D.
    Your natural health makeover / Lauri M. Aesoph, N.D.
        p. cm.
    Includes index.
    ISBN 0-13-628652-6 (PPC)   0-13-6286607 (C/J)
    1. Health. 2. Diet therapy. 3. Naturopathy. I. Title.
RA776.5.A37   1998
613—dc21   97-36541
                                                                        CIP

Acquisitions Editor: *Doug Corcoran*
Production Editor: *Eve Mossman*
Formatting/Interior Design: *Robyn Beckerman*

Printed in the United States of America

10 9 8 7 6 5 4 3 2

ISBN 0-13-628652-6 (PPC)   ISBN 0-13-628660-7 (C/J)

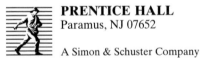

PRENTICE HALL
Paramus, NJ 07652

A Simon & Schuster Company

On the World Wide Web at http://www.phdirect.com

Prentice Hall International (UK) Limited, *London*
Prentice Hall of Australia Pty. Limited, *Sydney*
Prentice Hall Canada, Inc., *Toronto*
Prentice Hall Hispanoamericana, S.A., *Mexico*
Prentice Hall of India Private Limited, *New Delhi*
Prentice Hall of Japan, Inc., *Tokyo*
Simon & Schuster Asia Pte. Ltd., *Singapore*
Editora Prentice Hall do Brasil, Ltda., *Rio de Janeiro*

For Chris, Adam, and Will.

Thank you for all your love and support—and for disappearing when I needed to work.

Acknowledgements

I'd like to acknowledge all those individuals who helped me pull this book together: Deb Carlin and Barbara Papik from Lommen Health Sciences Library at the University of South Dakota School of Medicine—thank you for finding last-minute references and searching obscure topics for me. Warm gratitude to the staff at Sioux Valley Hospital Library for allowing me to monopolize your time, computers, and journals. Thank you to JoEllen Koerner, Hal Fletcher, MD, and Karen Fletcher and the other health care practitioners in and around Sioux Falls who have supported my work here.

Thanks to my many colleagues for their pearls of wisdom and encouragement. Thanks to Dr. Joe Pizzorno for his scientific vision of natural medicine, and to Dr. Steve Austin for making nutrition class so much fun and so informative. My gratitude to John Weeks for handing me opportunities and Paul Bergner for mentoring me during the early years.

Thank you, Doug Corcoran, for being a wonderful editor with a sense of humor.

Finally, thank you to my grandparents for making "natural" seem normal. (Kim and Steve, I can't forget you.) And a great big hug and thanks to my parents, Jim and Pat Baillie, for raising me right and getting me started on this path called natural medicine.

Contents

Chapter 3
Defend Your Body for Total Revitalization—21

Chapter 4
Revitalize Your Digestive System—39

Chapter 5
Better Inner Cleansing—63

Chapter 6
Maximize Your Immunity—75

Chapter 7
Lasting Stress Relief—91

Chapter 8
Improve Circulation and Live Longer—105

Chapter 9
Attain Tiptop Muscle Tone—121

Chapter 10
Regain Your Sexual Vitality—137

Chapter 11
Build Stronger Bones and Teeth—149

Chapter 12
Secrets of Beautiful Skin—167

Chapter 13
The Keys to Keener Vision—179

Chapter 14
Supercharge Your Brain—193

How Did You Do?
Complete the Before-and-After Chart—206

part two
Natural Remedies for Over
Thirty Common Ailments

Introduction

How many times have you picked up a natural health book and said: "There's no way I can do this! It's too weird. It's too strange. It's too natural!"

Well, I hope *Your Natural Health Makeover* is the book that changes your mind.

Rather than tell you what you're doing wrong, rather than insist you give up chocolate forever (Heaven forbid!), rather than demand you give up coffee today, I'm going to build on all those healthful things you're doing right now. (And you are.) I'm going to take you by the hand, and step-by-step, show you simple, natural, non-threatening ways to make over your entire body from head to toe.

Let's face it, while there is a minority of people who can maintain a perfect diet, exercise three hours each and every day, and do those other things we all should, the fact is most of us don't. I live in the real world. I know about those days when exercise is out of the question and the only answer for stress is a chocolate chip cookie. The person eating tofu next to you who runs 10 miles every day—rain or shine—is not better than you; taking healthful steps is not a moral issue. But I also want you to feel and look the very best you can. *Your Natural Health Makeover* is a very good idea, and something that you can incorporate into your daily schedule, and fall back on as health needs arise. For those sick times during and after your makeover, turn to Part Two for dozens of natural health ideas for common ailments.

Your Natural Health Makeover came about because I saw people struggling with making health changes all the time. Has your doctor ever said, "Eat better!" but didn't tell you how or why? Maybe you're not sick, but don't quite feel right—tired, tense, slightly achy—and don't know what to do. I wanted to take all those suggestions I've handed out to audiences, readers, and patients during the past decade, and compile them into a simple format: a Natural Health Makeover format.

To make this makeover a truly personal one, I give you the choice of what you want to change and offer you practical, easy ideas that you can "plug" into your current way of doing things. You'll find over one hundred Makeover Hints with specific, do-now tips. I also explain the principles behind natural health; for true health is more than popping a vitamin pill or drinking herbal tea. It's an attitude and a way of life.

Also included are hundreds of scientific studies backing up these very practical makeover steps interwoven with personal stories. I purposely put a lot of myself into this book—my stories, frustrations and triumphs—so you don't feel alone in making these difficult health revisions.

Don't feel ashamed if you can't carry out all the Natural Health Makeover recommendations in order and immediately. Just do your very best. Take a break. Then try a health touchup. Pursuing good health habits is a lifelong venture, and one worth striving for. It's fun and feels good (and yes, is sometimes frustrating). You might feel out of place occasionally, especially when you become the person eating tofu at the dinner table or insist on stretching your body every hour at work. But that's O.K. All of America (and the world) is turning to natural health for help; be a leader and include your family, friends, and colleagues in your Natural Health Makeover.

How to Use This Book

This book is laid out so you can either read it straight through (I suggest you do this the first time) or use it as a reference. Begin by reading all of Chapters 1 and 2; these will give you background on natural health and useful thoughts for a smooth makeover. Next proceed to Chapter 3, and onward through the rest of Part One, to begin your Natural Health Makeover journey. Try not to vary the order in which you use these makeover chapters, as they've been placed in sequence for a reason. The first six chapters set the stage for better digestion, elimination, circulation, immunity, and stress management, so that the rest of your Natural Health Makeover will be more effective. For example, Chapter 3 shows you how to protect your body from poisons. Detoxification, or poison control, is an important first step in building and maintaining health. Next is Chapter 4 on how to make over your gastrointestinal tract. Without well-functioning digestion and absorption, you are unable to use all those good foods you'll be eating.

How quickly or slowly you work through the Natural Health Makeover depends on you. If you're already practicing the suggestions in a particular step, then move on. If the information in a certain section is new, take a little time to practice and absorb it. It's been my observation and experience that if you give yourself some time to become accustomed to a new habit, you'll be more likely to stick with it.

A Full Body Makeover

For first-time customers, I recommend a head-to-toe body makeover beginning with Chapter 3 and working all the way through Chapter 14. Think of this as spring-cleaning your entire body—inside and out. Not only will you touch on all aspects of health, but you will learn about your body in the process. (See the sixth principle of natural health: education.) If you get stuck along the way, do your best, and move on. You can always go back and repeat a chapter.

Health Touch-ups

Taking care of your body is a lifetime commitment. If, after completing your Natural Health Makeover, you slip here or there (and we all do sometime), use this book to touch up your health habits. Think of this as a body tune-up. Good health habits aren't an ethical issue. Also, health care information and techniques are continuously evolving. Through your readings or practices, you may find a better or different way to clear your skin or treat your cold. If you do, let me know. (See Appendix E.)

How to Make Over Your Illness

Even those who live a natural and healthful existence sometimes get ill. There are factors beyond our control—stress, pollution, genetic weaknesses—that shape health. This is why I've included a section called Natural Remedies for Over Thirty Common Ailments (Part Two); you can apply the same natural health principles when you're sick as you did while well.

Often the medicines we use give only temporary relief for specific symptoms—itchy skin, a stuffy nose, constipation. They do nothing to enhance overall health or assist the body to heal. Side effects are a common problem with both over-the-counter and prescription conventional medicines. Aspirin and acetaminophen (Tylenol®) can cause liver damage when taken in large enough dosages. These same medicines when used to squelch pain or a fever during a cold, have been shown to suppress immune response, boost viral action, and make your runny nose even worse. Many drugs are known to cause nutritional havoc by changing nutrient absorption, metabolism, utilization, or excretion.

In addition to your Natural Health Makeover, start to use effective, safe natural health therapies when you're sick. Begin with suggestions in Part Two. Note what works for you, and learn from there. Read magazines and other books on natural health, talk to friends who use these methods, visit your local health food store, and for complex and hard-to-treat problems, consult with natural health practitioners in your area (see Appendix D).

Now sit back, take stock and enjoy a makeover like you've never experienced before. Grasp hold of those time-tested lifestyle steps that will grace you with a natural and healthy beauty.

Lauri M. Aesoph, ND

part one
Make Over Your Health

Chapter 1

What Is a Natural Health Makeover?

A beauty makeover may make you look more attractive, but only a Natural Health Makeover does the job in depth. Rather than brighten your outer body with curlers and cosmetics, a Natural Health Makeover reaches your core, resulting in health and beauty. And unlike a beauty makeover, this isn't a plan that will go out of date as hair styles or clothes do; good health is always in fashion.

A Natural Health Makeover also helps you fight chronic disease like arthritis, clogged arteries, and high blood pressure; it saves you money as well. Americans spend $600 billion annually—in the most expensive health care system in the world—fighting these and other illnesses.[1]

Save your money and your health. Rather than fight an uphill battle to health while racked with pain, why not take care of business now while you feel good enough to make over your health? Contrary to what you might think, you can take steps to enhance well-being. Diseases of old age are not inevitable; many illnesses are due to factors within your control.

A couple of years ago I had the good fortune to interview Dr. Ronald Klatz. Knowledgeable and effervescent about the topic of growing old, this president of the American Academy of Anti-Aging Medicine told me that the average American life span will eventually increase to 120 years and beyond. If this is true, I don't want to spend the last 40 or 50 years hurting or relying on false teeth to chew my food. Do you? How well you live in those latter years depends on how well you live now. Today's Natural Health Makeover can mean the difference between savings spent on medical treatment or exotic travel. Let's face it, it's cheaper to prevent illness than treat it.

The trick is how to avoid falling victim to heart disease and other lifestyle-linked ailments efficiently and effectively. How do you stay healthy for as long as possible? That's what I'm going to teach you. I've supervised, witnessed, and personally undergone many Natural Health Makeovers over the last 20 years. One of the first involved a young college student.

This young woman was studying for her pre-medical degree at the University of Victoria in British Columbia. Even so, she found herself reading more and more on nutrition and vitamins. It was 1976, and natural medicine was making a comeback. One day, while researching a paper, this student started talking with a fellow named Leonard who told her he ate no meat or sugar, and feasted only on natural foods. Thrilled to meet a real live vegetarian, the young woman quizzed Leonard about how he changed his diet. "No big deal," he replied, "I just decided to eat naturally. It wasn't hard at all."

The pre-med student couldn't believe her luck. Up to now, she'd read about the new natural ways of living, but had been afraid to try them. According to her new friend, there was nothing to it! The next day, the young woman began her life as a vegetarian. She quit caffeine, meat, and sugar, and gave her life over to tofu and brown rice. After a full day on this diet, the young lady felt terrible. Her head ached from coffee withdrawal. Her sweet-tooth cried out for a Kit Kat™. Plus, she had no idea how to cook tofu. What had gone wrong?

This is a perfect example of how not to begin your makeover. Perfect health cannot be achieved in a day, and health habits don't change overnight. I was that young college student, and it took me many years to learn that lesson. I'm sure there are other Leonards in the world who find switching to healthful living a breeze. But as you've read, I'm not one of them.

If you're like me, let me take you by the hand, and show you step-by-step how to gain better health using my Natural Health Makeover plan. You don't need to be a doctor to take care of yourself. In fact, the foundation upon which natural health care rests is lifestyle—what you select to eat and drink, how and if you exercise, the relationships you enter into and the work you do. Your doctor can suggest a diet, tell you to exercise, recommend you relax more, but the style of your life is ultimately your own choosing.

Unfortunately, changing your appearance with cosmetics and clothes is a lot easier than altering health habits. Real health can't be painted on or coiffured; a touch of rouge won't replace the rosy glow of health. A Natural Health Makeover is also more lasting than a beauty touch-up. If you're truly well, you'll still feel rosy even when the lipstick (or aftershave lotion) wears off.

Before we get started, let's look at the six principles that rule natural health. Reading and understanding these not only give you basic knowledge about this fascinating field, but will ensure a successful makeover.

Whole Health Means a Whole-Person Approach

This book is about how to stay whole and healthy using natural means. By doing this, you're practicing the first principle of natural medicine: prevention. Some of you probably already use techniques to stay well such as wearing a seat belt when you drive and having a yearly physical examination. While these are important, there's much more to preventive health care. True prevention involves taking steps that enhance overall health.

According to the Surgeon General's 1988 *Report on Nutrition and Health*, half of the top ten causes of death in America—heart disease, cancer, stroke, diabetes, and atherosclerosis—are linked to diet.[2] These chronic diseases are not only killing us, but stealing our money, too.

Principle number one: Practice an ounce of prevention to save dollars (and illness) down the road.

Body, Heal Thyself

The body is a wondrous entity. Under the right circumstances, it has tremendous healing abilities. Thus the second principle of natural medicine refers to the inherent healing power of nature. It's not the doctor or medicines or herbs that cure you when you're sick, it's your body. The immune system, a complex assemblage of cells, organs, and other factors, is your defense against germs, toxins and other foreign matter, and the equipment your body uses to recover from most illnesses or injuries. Natural health practitioners recognize this, so they do their utmost to support this system, and when that's done, get out of its way.

An example of which works better—drugs or the body—is illustrated with a classic study conducted 20 years ago by European researchers Marcus Diamant, M.D., and Bertil Diamant, M.D. They wanted to find out if antibiotics were really necessary for the treatment of ear infections, a condition that plagues many young children. After observing over 10,000 cases over a 14-year period, they discovered that 88 percent of their young patients didn't need antibiotics, due to what they termed "spontaneous healing." Even more surprising, the antibiotic-free kids had fewer recurrent infections than children treated with these drugs during the first week of illness.[3] The body's ability to heal, largely via the immune system, improves when given the chance to work unencumbered by drugs or other obstacles.

My youngest son, Will, came into this world with weak lungs. During his first Midwest winter—he was healthy in the summertime—he not only suffered from a continuous runny nose, but was finally struck down with pneumonia. Rather than give him antibiotics, I used various means to build his immunity. By his second winter, I noticed a slight improvement in his health. He was still susceptible to colds, but his symptoms were less severe and frequent. During his third winter, he was mostly well. I attribute this gradual health improvement to the natural building of his immune system. (Caution: Whenever treating young children with natural therapies, especially for severe ailments, seek the advice of a qualified physician.)

Principle number two: The body knows how to heal itself, given half a chance.

Natural Is Not a Four-Letter Word

Every doctor takes an oath to "do no harm." Naturopathic physicians take this promise very seriously by using the most natural, safe, and non-invasive therapies possible. This is the third principle of natural medicine: Do no harm by using safe treatments. According to Webster's dictionary, natural is defined as "pertaining to nature," "to be expected" (I like this one), "innate," and "reproducing the original state closely." So natural health simply refers to the way our bodies are meant to be—healthy. Even the word physician, based on the French word "physicien," means *natural* philosopher.

It pleases me to see more conventional medical institutions becoming interested in these therapies. Yet in truth, natural health care is no different from conventional medicine in its complexity—both deal with the human body. Still the former is often given short shrift because in many people's minds natural equals "simple" or "ineffective."

Now, don't get me wrong. I'm tremendously grateful for modern medicine and its technology. Without it, my grandfather, a robust 81-year-old who was advised by his naturopathic doctor a few years ago to have a hip replacement, would be sitting in a wheelchair. Antibiotics, used judiciously, are lifesavers for serious bacterial infections. However, I also recognize that straying too far from our original (natural) way of doing things is hard on our "natural" bodies. Life in the city exposes us to polluted air and water, excessive noise, sedentary jobs, and too little leisure time.

Principle number three: Use safe and natural therapies whenever possible.

Health Is More Than Skin Deep

The fourth principle of natural medicine says you must search out the root or cause of a health problem in order to heal completely. In a sense, naturopathic physicians are the anthropologists of the medical world. We piece together the information we unearth during an office visit in order to solve the mystery behind a patient's health. You can help your doctor, and yourself, on this healing expedition by paying attention to how your body feels under different conditions—after eating, when ill. In some cases, using natural therapies, like homeopathic medicines, requires you to pay attention to very subtle sensations that you may have ignored in the past or didn't realize were there.

For some this is difficult. In a society where fast food feeds us, correspondence travels by e-mail and instant financing is expected, it's hard to slow down. Taking time to listen to your body can be as difficult as asking an active three-year-old to sit still for half an hour. However, failure to do so can mean relying on drugs and medical procedures fraught with annoying, and sometimes harmful, side effects.

You only need to open a copy of the *Physician's Desk Reference* or other such drug guide to learn that most medications carry with them lists of adverse reactions and situations where they shouldn't be used. For example, some antibiotic acne creams can cause your skin to burn, peel, itch, feel tender, dry out, or turn red while clearing up pimples. Sleeping pills, like Nembutal® (pentobarbital), allow you to drop off—but at a cost. This addictive drug may bring on nausea, vomiting, constipation, headaches, liver damage, dizziness and, ironically, may create insomnia and nightmares.[4]

> *Principle number four: You can only solve a health problem by finding and curing the cause.*

■ *Makeover Hint #1—Body Scan*

Makeover artists begin their work by stepping back and surveying the outer appearance of their client's face, posture, and clothes. In order for you to be successful during your Natural Health Makeover, you must do the same—only you're scanning your body from the inside. Use this exercise to help you understand how your body reacts to different situations.

1. Select a situation. This could be after eating, upon waking, after sitting, after exercise, after or during work.
2. Close your eyes.
3. Take note of all bodily sensations. These could include pain, perspiration, breathing, muscle tightness, stomach upset, gas, bloating, itching, feelings, fatigue.

The Whole Person Makeover

The fifth principle of natural medicine is that one must address the whole person in order for treatment to be effective. Depending on whom you talk to, the word "whole" can mean many things. To say you're "whole" might mean you're healthy or uninjured. A whole-some body is one that is well. Wholeness indicates something that's complete—another way of stating health. "Whole" also refers to a state in which every part is accounted for, a process that natural health care and a Natural Health Makeover are very good at.

When you take care of the whole body, not just the part that hurts—like the head or big toe—other complaints often disappear as well. The billions of cells in your body are like individual members of an expansive community. Each operates independently, but can also work together to form, for example, an organ like the heart or stomach. And, like most communities, your body works best when each member or cell is getting along and pulling its own weight. When one or a group of cells gets sick or injured, others are affect-ed either directly or indirectly. While the big toe might be way down there and the head up here, they're both housed in the same skin covering. They both receive the same blood supply, are influenced by the same immune system, and are fed by the same foods. Thus chronic headaches and an aching toe (gout) could be clues there's a digestive problem going on.

Even though the Natural Health Makeover plan is laid out in twelve different stages for a dozen body systems, you will be addressing your whole health by following all these steps. This is evidenced by specific recommendations repeated throughout many sections. For example, the advice to eat whole foods is suggested in every makeover chapter. That's because consuming healthful foods has body-wide effects. The same goes for quitting smoking, avoid-ing drugs, and other makeover steps.

Principle number five: Keep the whole body healthy and every-thing else will work better.

The Motions of Emotions

I recently spoke at a half-day health care seminar to a group of counselors, psychologists, and psychiatrists about the relationship between the body and mind. I told this group that we talk about body-mind or psychosomatic medicine as if the body and mind are two distinct and separate factions. The doctor treats physical ail-ments, while the counselor cares for feelings. As health care practi-tioners, we need to remember that this separation is artificial, and that physical and emotional components often overlap and influence one another.

It's understood that chronic pain or other physical ailments can be emotionally upsetting. But, psychoneuroimmunology (PNI), the study of how emotions and thoughts influence physical symptoms and immunity, is a growing field. So now when you say your headache or other pain is from stress or worry, know that the scientific world is backing you up. Recent research has found that treating feelings can help a wide scope of physical ailments such as leukemia,[5] breast cancer,[6] psoriasis,[7] gum disease,[8] and colds.[9]

Let the Spirit Cure You

The spiritual side of healing is as old as shamans and faith healers, and as modern as the chapels found in many hospitals. However, including religious belief as part of conventional health care treatment has been taboo, or, at the very least, irrelevant in past decades. That is changing as spirituality slowly makes it way into medical discussions and research.[10] Mary Ann Miller, R.N., Ph.D., an associate professor at the College of Nursing, University of Delaware, writes: "If one believes that spirituality permeates all human experiences rather than being additional to them, one must accept it as integral to health or a sense of *wholeness* (my italics) or well-being." She points out that not only does this "belief in something greater than the self" give meaning, value, and direction to life—a wonderful stress reducer—but many religions advocate healthy living habits. Seventh-Day Adventists, for instance, discourage alcohol and cigarette use.[11]

Finding your own spiritual niche, be it attending church each Sunday, meditating silently each morning or going for a reflective walk in the evening, will help you complete your circle of health.

Educate Yourself to Health

The final and sixth rule of natural health is education. The more you know about your body and how to take care of it, the healthier you'll be. I'm constantly amazed by how many people are ill-informed about the state of their health. When I met Muriel, an 82-year-old California woman with excruciating back pain, I asked her what was wrong. She said: "I have osteoporosis." Then she paused a moment. "Or is it osteoarthritis? I'm not sure." I suggested she call her doctor for the correct diagnosis. "Oh no," she replied, "I couldn't do that. My doctor's far too busy. Besides, I trust that he'll take care of me."

Don't become a Muriel. Use this and other books and your doctor to learn about the state of your health. In fact, "doctor" is derived from the Latin word *docere,* which means "to teach." So a doctor is (or should be) your private instructor, ready to educate you about your illness and your health, and then guide you toward wellness. To make the most of this situation, be a good student. Ask a lot of questions, do your homework by reading up on what concerns you, and attend health classes that interest you. See Appendix C for books and magazines you can read.

Principle number six: The more you know, the healthier you'll be.

Chapter 2

Making the Most of Your Natural Health Makeover

The Importance of a Healthy Foundation

To be successful in business you must plan for the future. If you don't, your business can end up bankrupt. Health is much the same way. If you take care of business now, there's less chance your health will go bankrupt later on. This can be difficult to do when you feel fine. Practicing naturopathic medicine is my motivation to embrace healthy habits. Not only do I see how ill people can become from years of lifestyle indiscretions, but I get to witness how healthful living helps reverse disease.

If you need convincing in this regard, talk to your older relatives. With any luck, you'll have different people in your family living different lifestyles with the results to prove it.

The other plus to living the healthy life is that you have more room for moderation. In other words, if you make over your health now, your body will better tolerate the odd glass of wine or the occasional cookie. A healthy body has reserves, ready to handle stress. Very ill people who decide to pursue natural treatments are often required to make radical and immediate changes in order to get well. Limited reserves often require them to stick with these changes if they want to return to health. It's like the difference between maintaining your car with regular tune-ups or waiting until it breaks down and then having to replace expensive parts.

Turn Everyday Habits
Into Health Enhancers

Changing or even building upon your current lifestyle is a powerful way of boosting wellness and treating sickness. Most people have at least some habits that are healthful and can be used as a foundation during a Natural Health Makeover. Before you begin, make a list of all the health-enhancing factors in your life. These can include drinking water (any amount), eating fruits or vegetables, sleeping, or having fun. Save this sheet so you can list additional items or modify your current ones as they apply during your makeover plan.

Your Talkative Body Is Your
Makeover Guide

The body is constantly chattering about how it's doing and what it needs. Uncomfortable or intense needs, like pain or fever, are simplest to listen to. The quieter the need, the easier it is to ignore. How often have you put off going to the bathroom because you're busy? Or eaten past the point of satiety because the food tastes good? If you continue to discount these requests, your body will speak up. Dismissing thirst, for instance, may result in constipation or chronic urinary tract infections. Neglect these pleas and your body will eventually scream at the top of its lungs with even more serious ailments.

When I first started teaching people about natural health, I'd tell them to listen to their bodies, assuming they'd know what to do. While what I said was true, I often got blank stares from my audience because they didn't know what I was talking about. They didn't know how to listen; and even when they did hear their bodies talk, they didn't know how to respond.

Attentive body listening also clues you into, and helps you prevent, sickness that can take a foothold. In getting to know your body, you need to determine what your warning systems are, that is, what are the signs that you've pushed it too far, health-wise. Perhaps a stiff neck or upset stomach are signals that you need a Natural Health Makeover tune-up. Each of us also has an Achilles heel that falls victim most easily to stress or neglect. Identify yours, so you can concentrate on the section or sections in this book that address your frailest body system.

■ *Makeover Hint #2—How to Converse with Your Body*

Acquire body-listening skills by learning how to consciously listen to, not merely hear, what your body has to say. Merely find a quiet spot to sit, and pay close attention to how your entire body feels, starting with your head and slowly working down to your toes.

Twelve Practical Tips to Overcome Makeover Blocks

Your Natural Health Makeover needn't be difficult. Read on for practical tips to help you get started and stay motivated.

- Get ready, get set—make over. If you find it difficult getting started, pick a date when to begin. Circle that day on your calendar; tell friends and family if it helps. Then enjoy the anticipation of getting ready for the big day.
- Groom yourself for success. Setting forth on a makeover is like quitting smoking. It's only going to work if you want to do it.
- Use your imagination. Picture the results when you're done—a vibrant, energetic, healthier you. Know what you want, and then take steps to get there.
- Follow your passion. A Natural Health Makeover works best when you identify and follow those aspects that excite you the most.
- Accessorize your life. Although this book is laid out as a specific plan, feel free to insert your own ideas where you want, when you want, how you want. Think of a Natural Health Makeover as a powerful way of integrating your current lifestyle with healthy new ways of living.
- Take baby steps. Make one or two small, easy-to-swallow changes that you'll stick with at a time.
- Try it on for size before you say no. Before turning your nose up at tofu or flaxseeds, try them—you might like them.
- Let your taste buds guide you. Fortunately, Mother Nature gave us a vast variety of foods—as well as exercise, relaxation, and natural treatments—to choose from, to fit our many tastes.

- Learn to mix and match. Combining old lifestyle ways with new in a way you find comfortable is an important part of this health makeover plan.
- Make over your schedule. You must make room in your regular routine for exercise, sleep, and learning about new foods. If at first the scheduling-in of makeover steps feels forced, wait for a month or two. You'll soon adjust to—even yearn for—everyday exercise and wholesome meals.
- Rest up for the big makeover. Make sure you're sufficiently rested before you dive into your Natural Health Makeover plan. Fatigue can make lifestyle changes harder.
- Stay motivated. Last, but certainly not least, know that with each step you make, you'll feel better. This is your motivation to continue. Once people understand that a health makeover and maintenance is a lifelong endeavor, they are more inclined to make permanent changes and stay the course.

Before and After—Snapshots of Your Health

The Before-and-After Chart is not unlike the before-and-after pictures you see of a beauty makeover. Not only is it a good record of the progress you've made during your Natural Health Makeover, but because the results of a health makeover can be subtle—a few pounds lost here, slightly more energy there—it will serve as a reminder of where you started health-wise.

There are a couple of ways to rate symptoms: both by intensity and by frequency. For intensity, I use a 1 to 10 scale to assess a patient's health, where the number 1 indicates feeling poorly and 10 is perfect health. This works especially well for those vague, hard-to-define symptoms like fatigue and malaise. Under the frequency column, record whether a symptom occurs daily, weekly, monthly, or several times during the day, week, or month.

With that in mind, fill out the Before section of this chart. You'll complete the After part once you've finished your Natural Health Makeover. I've grouped symptoms according to the different body systems you'll be working on; some fit under many categories but I have listed each one only once.

Table 2.1
THE BEFORE-AND-AFTER CHART

	Before		After	
	Intensity (1–10)	*Frequency*	*Intensity (1–10)*	*Frequency*
LIVER				
Itching				
Bad breath				
Sensitive to chemical smells (paints, solvents, perfumes)				
Sensitive to cigarette smoke				
Food intolerances or allergies				
Foul-smelling stools				
Prone to infections				
"Toxic" feeling				
DIGESTION				
Weight (lbs)				
Abdominal bloating				
Excessive gas				
Excessive belching				
Heartburn/indigestion				
Nausea				
Constipation				
Diarrhea				
KIDNEYS AND URINARY TRACT				
Urinate frequently				
Urinate at night				
Pain/burning with urination				
Weak urine stream				
Difficulty starting urine stream				
Bladder doesn't feel empty after urination				
Retain water throughout body				
Dull mid-backache				
Side ache				
Weakness				
Loss of appetite				

Table 2.1, cont'd.

	Before		After	
	Intensity (1–10)	*Frequency*	*Intensity (1–10)*	*Frequency*
IMMUNE SYSTEM				
Difficulty recovering from illness				
Poor wound healing				
Chronic infections				
Recurring warts				
Cold sores				
Canker sores				
Genital herpes				
Yeast infections (anywhere)				
Nail fungus				
Athlete's foot				
ADRENAL GLANDS				
Fatigue				
Frequent colds/flus				
Headaches				
Upset stomach				
Insomnia				
Irritable				
PMS				
Many allergies (foods, pollens, animals, drugs etc.)				
Feel "stressed out"				
HEART AND CIRCULATION				
Shortness of breath when exerting self				
Bruise easily				
Cold arms/legs				
Irregular heartbeat				
MUSCLES				
Joint pain				
Joint stiffness				
Body aches				
Tight muscles				
Chronic backache				

Table 2.1, cont'd.

	Before		After	
	Intensity (1–10)	*Frequency*	*Intensity (1–10)*	*Frequency*
LOVE LIFE				
Low libido				
Impotence				
Vaginal dryness				
BONES AND TEETH				
Mid-back pain				
"Bad" teeth				
Frequent fractures				
Bleeding gums when brushing teeth				
Bad breath				
SKIN				
Acne				
Rashes				
Dry skin				
Oily skin				
EYES				
Dry eyes				
Eyestrain				
Red eyes				
Decreased central vision				
Difficulty adapting to light changes				
Difficulty reading				
Shade/color contrasts are fuzzy				
FEELINGS/THINKING				
Sense of well-being (good or bad)				
Depression				
Anxiety				
Memory				
Concentration (good or bad)				
Mood swings				

How You Can Expect to Feel After a Natural Health Makeover

What can you expect after completing this makeover plan? It all depends on you, your current health, your age and sex, and how diligently you stuck with this layout. I find that patients who take my advice to heart invariably feel better. Here's some of what I hear:

- More energy
- Constipation improves or resolves
- Digestion is better
- Sleep is more sound
- Headaches decrease or leave
- Thinking clears
- Skin clears
- Get sick less often
- Sex drive increases
- Pain diminishes
- Hope returns

There are occasionally instances when health doesn't improve—usually for a reason. Look at the end of each chapter where I summarize the steps you've just taken. Also listed here are references to conditions related to the body system you just made over. If following these two steps doesn't set you right, seek the counsel of a natural health practitioner or your physician. A list of laboratory tests conclude each chapter for your benefit and that of your doctor.

Chapter 3

Defend Your Body for Total Revitalization

Your Multi-Talented Liver

The liver is one of the largest and busiest organs in your body. Tucked under the right-hand side of your ribcage, it makes bile for fat digestion, stores blood, iron, and vitamins like A, B_{12}, D, and K (that's why your mother tried to get you to eat liver), and is involved in most of the body's metabolic functions. This versatile structure is also a respected member of the digestive system. Did you know that the liver helps stabilize your blood sugar levels? Were you aware that the liver breaks protein down into its most basic building blocks— amino acids? Has anyone ever told you that fat metabolism, including cholesterol production, happens in your liver? Arthur Guyton, M.D., author of *Textbook of Medical Physiology*, states that "the liver has so many and such varied function that it is impossible to separate its actions from those of other organ systems."[1]

Natural health practitioners are enthralled by the liver's part in digestion, and its dual role as body defender and blood cleanser. A direct blood line runs from the gastrointestinal (GI) tract to the liver; another feeds this industrious organ with blood from the general circulation. This means the amazing liver must filter and clean a total of one and a half quarts of blood every minute. While blood from the digestive tract is full of nutrients needed by the liver (and rest of the body), it also carries with it bacteria and other undesirables like drugs you've taken and chemicals you've been exposed to. All of these need to be pulled from the blood to keep your body safe. Kupffer cells, the liver's resident immunity guards, are extremely efficient at grabbing bacteria, and handling bothersome substances trying to sneak into the body via the GI tract. Special chemicals in the liver detoxify drugs like penicillin, erythromycin, and ampicillin and toss them into bile which is then carried away. Similarly, several hormones like estrogen, cortisol, and thyroxine are inactivated by the liver so as not to poison the body.[1] Premenstrual syndrome and other conditions aggravated by elevated estrogen are often solved by treating an overburdened liver so it becomes more efficient at breaking down estrogen, which in turn lowers estrogen blood levels.

Bile, which is made by the liver but stored in the gallbladder, is another important piece of the liver story. Besides helping you digest fat, the four cups of bile your liver produces each day also carts toxins away into the feces. This is one reason why a well-functioning colon and regular bowel movements are vital, in addition to a picture-perfect liver. If you're constipated, stool remains in the colon longer than it should—along with toxic bile—and some of those toxins are reabsorbed into the bloodstream.

A Regular Liver Makeover Is a Must

Some of the poisons deactivated by the liver come from your body. But living in today's world has made health problems much more complicated than they were even 20 years ago, partly due to all the chemicals we're currently exposed to. Pollution, medications (over-the-counter and prescription), alcohol, tobacco, drugs, pesticides, food additives, junk food, plastics, solvents, and other factors have placed an additional burden on the modern liver. Some people work in professions where chemical exposure is an everyday occurrence, like factory employees or dry cleaners. When you consider that blood cleansing is only one of the many tasks your liver must perform, you begin to understand why a regular Liver Makeover is a good idea.

Naturopathic physicians talk about a "sluggish," "toxic," or "congested" liver. This doesn't refer to overt liver disease like hepatitis or cirrhosis, but a condition where the liver isn't functioning up to par. Besides asking about possible toxic exposure, naturopathic doctors look at a person's medical history for signs that the liver needs help. One hint is when someone has used or is using therapeutic hormones, like levothyroxine (Synthroid®), estrogen (birth control pills, hormone replacement), or anabolic steroids. Even pregnancy—

when estrogen levels soar—may be reason enough for a liver cleanse. Note: Never embark on a Liver Makeover when you're pregnant or nursing a baby.

A poor diet can add to the liver's burden. The busy liver, and every other bodily organ, needs nutrients to operate efficiently. The liver is no different.

So what are the signs that your body and liver might be toxic? They include unexplained itching, bad breath, headaches, sensitivity to many things—including chemicals and foods, constant fatigue, increased susceptibility to infection, acne, foul-smelling stools and a general "toxic" feeling as if you have a hangover.

Super Healing Foods

The place to start with a Liver Makeover is to screen all the foods you eat. I'll be harping on the need for sound nutrition again and again—that is, after all, the foundation of good health—but for now, let's begin with how foods affect the liver.

As a general rule, the more whole, unprocessed foods you eat—fresh fruits and vegetables; raw, unsalted nuts and seeds; dried beans and legumes; fresh poultry, fish and lean meats; whole grains—the better. While processing supplies us with food when fresh is unavailable, eating products with synthetic preservatives, colorings, flavorings, and other additives is hard on the liver. Study content using the labels on all packaged foods you buy; if you can't pronounce it, you may not want to eat it. Some additives are fine. For example, annatto added for color, or extra vitamins aren't going to hurt you.

When foods have been processed so much that they barely resemble true food, beware. Potato chips, for instance, look like nothing from nature and are worthless when it comes to nutrition. That goes for most of the creatively colored, sugared, and shaped food-like items you find in the grocery store.

As you begin to make the switch from food-like edibles to true foods, find out if your grocer carries organic produce. A recent study published in *Plant and Soil* (Volume 167, 1994) showed that barley fertilized with manure—in other words, organic barley—contained three times as much vitamin B_{12} as the commercial variety fed with synthetic fertilizers; spinach treated the same way had almost twice as much B_{12}.[2] Since only vitamin B_{12} was measured in this experiment, we don't know if amounts of other vitamins and minerals are also higher, but we can assume that some, if not most, probably are. Past experiments have shown us that animals fed organic grains grow much better than those feasting on foods treated with inorganic fertilizers. This has led scientists to believe that good old-fashioned manure, compost, and other natural fertilizers enhance at least the B vitamins in foods. Thus eating organic foods not only allows you to avoid liver-damaging pesticides, but also gives your liver more of the nutrients it needs.

Check for Food Intolerances

Sometimes avoiding pesticides, food additives, and processed foods isn't enough. For reasons we're not entirely sure of, allergies or just plain food sensitivities seem to be on the rise. These intolerances may be due to our modern lifestyle fraught with pesticides, irradiated foods, processed and refined foods, hybridized foods, genetically manipulated foods, stress, poor digestion due to faulty eating habits and general liver overload. Whatever the reason, food intolerance is more common than we think and a party-crasher when it comes to health.

Food allergy symptoms are varied and unpredictable. When I mention to patients that food allergies could be behind their health troubles, they often say, "But my stomach doesn't hurt! How can that be?" Food allergies don't just affect the digestive tract. According to scientific research, they've also been linked to rheumatoid arthritis,[3] migraine headaches,[4] eczema,[5] asthma,[6] irritable bowel syndrome,[7] and several other conditions. Many times when a patient comes to me with a chronic complaint and displays a personal or family history of allergies—not necessarily to food—I suggest testing for foods. Invariably, after avoiding those allergic foods for two to four weeks, they feel better. You'll notice in Part Two that I frequently suggest checking for food allergies when simple measures don't work.

If you suspect you're intolerant to one or more foods, consider food allergy testing. This can be done with a blood test; I recommend the test which measures both IgE and IgG antibodies, and picks up both immediate and delayed food reactions. Or you can test for intolerances on your own using the Elimination and

Challenge diet. If you know or suspect you have severe reactions to certain foods, do not use this method.

- Begin by making a list of foods you eat every day. These are the foods you're going to eliminate for four days.
- Add to this list (if not already included) the foods that most commonly cause reactions in people. These foods will also be eliminated for four days:

> alcohol (wine, beer, and hard liquor)
> chocolate
> citrus fruits (grapefruit, oranges, lemons, limes, tangerines)
> coconut
> coffee and black tea
> corn (often in the form of corn syrup)
> dairy products (milk, butter, cheese, ice cream, yogurt, cottage cheese)
> eggs
> fish
> nuts (including nut oils and butters)
> peanuts and peanut butter—peanuts are a legume, not a nut
> pineapple
> soy (a common additive)
> strawberries
> sugar, and products containing it
> tomatoes
> vinegar
> wheat (bread, pasta, cookies, cereals etc.)
> yeast

- For four days, eat a diet of foods that rarely cause allergies (unless they're on your list of frequently eaten foods). These include:

> apricots
> artichokes
> asparagus

barley

broccoli

carrots (organic only)

grapes (organic only)

honey

lamb and mutton

lettuce

oats

peaches

pears

raisins (organic)

rice

rye

sweet potatoes

- On the fifth day, eat one of the suspected intolerant foods on your list. This is called a Challenge. It helps you determine, after clearing your body of all suspected allergenic foods, which ones are causing you troubles. Keep a detailed journal of what you eat and any reactions you have to any food. If you react (watch for symptoms for two days), remove that food from your diet. If you have no reactions, feel free to keep it in your diet.
- Continue introducing a new food every other day until you've finished the entire list.

This is a very time-consuming process that takes patience, observation, and perseverance. The advantage of the Elimination and Challenge technique is that it gives you immediate, firsthand knowledge of which foods are troubling you. Once you've experienced the stomach upset, headache, or foggy thinking caused by an allergenic egg, you're less likely to eat it again. The downside to this method is the willpower and time involved. Also, this test is not very adept at picking up delayed reactions that last longer than two days, or reactions caused from eating a combination of foods. Most of my patients prefer the simplicity of having blood drawn for the IgE/IgG test, and like the clear black-and-white information it provides. Either way, investigating for food intolerances can make you and your liver happier.

Don's Sensitive Stomach

Don, a 67-year-old retired farmer, came to see me for high cholesterol; the usual dietary changes hadn't helped. However, after visiting with him for awhile it was apparent that a more annoying problem for Don was his sensitive stomach. He had a difficult time taking most medicines or supplements, and eating a variety of foods, because they hurt his gut. This roadblock made it difficult for me to suggest nutrients or herbs for Don, so before beginning any treatment plan, I recommended he be tested for food allergies.

When the test results came back, many foods showed up as highly allergic, including all milk products, eggs, and most grains. Don agreed to avoid these foods for one month to see if that would help his constantly sore stomach. Thirty days later Don came to see me and happily reported that his once delicate abdomen was ever so much better. All gas was gone and he no longer needed antacids. The pleasing side effects of this temporarily restrictive diet were a 75-percent drop in fatigue, clear sinuses, less joint pain, and an end to his once ongoing leg pain. He now found dinner-time enjoyable, and he could take most pills with ease. This first step now allowed me to direct Don to nutrients that would help with his cholesterol problem.

Wash Away the Poisons

The next step to reviving a sluggish liver is to remove all the poisons you can from your life. These include toxins at home, work, and play. Once you have identified these potential poisons, look for safer alternatives.

One of the most common household toxins is cleaners—the window sprays; tub scrubbers; cleaning fluids for the floors, walls, and counters; carpet spot removers; and sink decloggers. Wherever possible, replace these smelly poisons with non-toxic cleaning products either purchased from a natural foods store or homemade. If you're a gardener, consider replacing synthetic fertilizers with more natural alternatives like compost and manure. Call your local gardening shop for options to garden pesticides; there are also many mail order companies specializing in these products. For you interior decorators, be cautious when working with paint, paint thinners, paint strippers, and other harmful solvents. Again, search for safer options. If you can't locate substitutes, be sure to ventilate well while working with these products. Everyone should be cautious around gasoline and similar fuels.

Some people are faced with toxins every day in their work. Anyone who works in a dental office, farms, cleans offices or homes for a living, paints houses or does other building repair or remodeling that involves solvents or chemicals is in danger of hurting the liver. Again, where possible, use safer chemical alternatives. Otherwise, practice safety techniques when handling these chemicals such as ventilation, wearing protective clothing, gloves and masks, and taking breaks from exposure. Discuss using less toxic substances with your employer.

Last, take a close look at any medications you're currently taking. The liver must break down most of these drugs when your body's done with them. One way to protect your liver is by minimizing the number of synthetic medicines you take. You should have less need for some medicines after completing your Natural Health Makeover. In the meantime, consider using natural treatments instead when you're sick (see Part Two). For help with serious health conditions, consult with a practitioner knowledgeable in natural therapies.

■ *Makeover Hint # 3—Less Is More*

Many times we use poisons unnecessarily. You don't have to use a spray cleaner every time you wash the kitchen counter. You don't have to spray insecticide around your house every month to prevent ants from creeping in. You don't have to bleach your clothes every time you wash them. Adopt the motto: Less is more, especially when it comes to chemicals and your liver's health.

Your Liver's Favorite Foods

Your liver has many favorite foods that nourish it and help it work better. Brussels sprouts, cauliflower, cabbage, and other members of the brassica family boost its detoxifying abilities.[7] Beets, both the greens and red-staining root, are famous as liver foods due in part to their nutritious state.

If you're looking to spice up a bland meal and heal your liver at the same time, lace your food with onions and garlic. These smelly bulbs are loaded with sulfur that help restore the liver's sulfate reservoir, necessary for detoxification. Turmeric, that yellowish-orange spice that gives prepared mustard and curry their festive colors, contains curcumin. This bright pigment works by enhancing the liver's bile flow.[8]

A favorite liver beverage is green tea. Japanese research tells us that the more cups you drink each day, the more your liver is protected. When subjects drank very high amounts of this tea daily (10 cups and more), laboratory tests showed that serum markers like aspartate aminotransferase were favorably influenced.[9]

■ Makeover Hint #4—Make Ruby Beet Soup

For those cold winter nights, prepare a steamy pot of ruby beet soup. You'll please both your tummy and liver with these ingredients.

Add the following items to one quart of stock (chicken, beef, or vegetable). Add more liquid as needed. Let simmer for two hours (or six hours in a crock pot), and serve with a crusty loaf of bread. Add a dollop of sour cream to your soup bowl if you like.

2 cups of beets, cubed

1 cup of red and/or green cabbage, shredded

3 cloves of garlic, diced

1 onion, diced

1/2 cup carrots, diced

Season to taste with sea salt, fresh ground pepper, and other favorite spices.

Fill Up on Fiber

Your liver, your digestive system, in fact your entire body adores fiber. Fiber, also known as roughage, is the indigestible stuff found in whole grains, beans, legumes, and fresh vegetables and fruits. Unfortunately, the more we tamper with these virgin foods, the more likely they are to lose both fiber and other nutrients. The vitamins and minerals you lose when you eat fiber-less, processed foods is reason enough to become a roughage enthusiast. However, there are other reasons as well.

More fiber means less chance of constipation. Efficient digestion decreases both your body's and liver's exposure to toxins either created by the bacteria in your colon or those consumed. A healthy serving of fiber several times daily also helps sweep away bile, which carries with it more toxins for disposal outside. The water-soluble fibers in particular, found in vegetables and fruits, increase bile secretion. Finally, too little roughage creates an upset in the bug population in your intestine. There are over 400 good bugs residing in your GI tract keeping the bad bugs at bay. When delinquent germs increase in number and take over, they make poisons like endotoxins—one more thing for your liver to deal with. Yeast overgrowth and infections from pathogenic bacteria are also more likely.

Here are 10 easy ways to increase your fiber intake:

- Munch on carrot and celery sticks before each meal (when you're hungry).
- Eat brown rice instead of white; or mix it half and half with the white.
- Have a piece of fresh fruit instead of juice for breakfast.
- Add beans or barley to your homemade soups.
- Eat hot oat bran cereal for breakfast (or as a snack).
- Eat whole-grain bread, not white.
- Top your yogurt with fresh banana slices or other fresh fruit.
- Crumble shredded wheat on top of casseroles.
- Eat the skin on your baked potato (this is safest if the potato is organic).
- Add a tomato slice, lettuce, cucumber slices and/or bean sprouts to your sandwich.

Super Nutrients for Your Liver

The next step in revitalizing your liver is to ensure that you're giving this hardworking organ all the vitamins and minerals it needs.

Antioxidants top the list—those that fight organ-damaging, make-you-look-older-than-you-really-are free radical molecules. These super nutrients are found far and wide in nature, both in foods and herbs. The most brightly colored fruits and vegetables contain the most antioxidant carotenoids (the autumn-colored pigments) and flavonoids (red, blue, and purple colorings). Be sure to feast on these brilliant foods. For added protection look to the antioxidant nutrients selenium, vitamins E and C, and glutathione. Your whole foods diet should keep you well stocked. Look to a well-balanced multiple vitamin pill as additional insurance. The more diverse the antioxidants you consume, the better they work.

There's also a class of liver nutrients called lipotropics which guard the liver from fatty buildup. Exposure to toxic substances like pesticides or birth control pills increases fat infiltration in your liver and drags down function. Lipotropic compounds include choline, folic acid, vitamin B_{12}, methionine, betaine, and carnitine; lipotropic formulas often include other liver-friendly herbs and nutrients as well. If you feel a need to use such a formula, start by taking one pill a day and gradually increase dosage by one pill daily until you reach the recommended amount. Unless you are under the guidance of a health practitioner, take lipotropics for no more than two months. If you experience any adverse effects while taking these pills, like nausea, decrease your dose. If this doesn't help, discontinue taking them.

Four Helpful Liver Herbs

Some plants serve as both food and herbs; we find several among the liver herbs. You can use some of these in everyday cooking like turmeric, known in professional circles as *Curcuma longa*. Or, if you prefer, take the active pigment found in turmeric, curcumin, as a pill. You can eat artichokes, *Cynara scolymus*, or take its leaves in medicinal form—pills, tea, or tincture. Researchers suspect that cynarin, one of artichoke's active ingredients, is what boosts bile secretion.[10]

One of the most fascinating liver herbs is milk thistle, or *Silybum marianum*. Researchers have discovered that milk thistle actually protects the liver from poisonous substances by offsetting free radical damage, and through regeneration of new liver cells.[11] You can see that milk thistle is a most valuable plant to have around for both liver damage due to diseases like hepatitis and cirrhosis, or exposure to toxins ranging from alcohol to drugs to chemicals. I have a very low tolerance to anesthetics, and typically feel spacey and ill afterward. A few years ago I needed a sebaceous cyst removed from my scalp, and was dreading the operation only because I knew I'd be injected with a local anesthetic. As an experiment I took milk thistle several days before and directly after the procedure. That day and the few following, when I usually took to my bed, I felt fine. Milk thistle had done its job.

A simple way to start using this herb is to include milk thistle seeds (available at many fine natural foods markets) as part of your daily meals. Merely grind up a week's worth in your coffee blender or food processor. Sprinkle one tablespoon of this seed meal on your food each day. Store unused portions in the refrigerator.

Dandelion (*Taraxacum officinale*) is famous as a liver herb. The root of this "weed" works in three-step fashion: by promoting bile production in the liver, its flow to the gallbladder (where it's stored) and finally release from the gallbladder into the digestive tract.[12] Remember that without proper bile flow, toxic substances can't be adequately flushed from your body. Drink dandelion root tea made from the unsprayed weeds in your backyard, one to three cups a day. If you're unfortunate enough to have a dandelion-free lawn or are worried about what the neighbors will think, look to your local herb or health food store. You can also spruce up salads with a few dandelion leaves thrown in.

■ Makeover Hint #5—Live on the Wild Side

The first place to look for liver herbs is your backyard. Those #$%@ dandelions, specifically the long tap root clogging up your lawn, are some of the best medicines for your liver. During the summer collect your dandelions, cut off the root and cut it into small pieces or chop up in a blender. For a fresh cup of liver tea, boil a pot of water, add a handful of root, and simmer for 30 minutes. Drink three cups of tea daily for one to two weeks. If you'd like to dry the root for later use, split it longitudinally first.

Practice Regular Inner Cleansing

Like regular exercise, routinely cleansing your body by eating simple foods is a healthy idea. By doing this you decrease the toxic burden on your liver and ease up on digestion. Think of this as a liver vacation. In fact, I suggest you follow a cleansing diet for a day or two each month instead of attempting an annual week-long cleanse.

There are several types of cleansing routines. Fasting with water only is the most traditional way to cleanse. It's simple and requires minimal preparation. The disadvantage is that some people find the idea of going without food both difficult (due to hunger and social pressures to eat) and frightening. Some find drinking only water boring. I don't recommend you embark on a water fast without professional supervision.

Another choice is to follow a liquid-only diet where fresh vegetable and fruit juices, vegetable broth, herbal teas, and water are on the menu. This requires slightly more preparation, but it also gives you some nutrients and a variety of tastes. Again, be cautious before starting this sort of cleanse. Only do it if you're experienced; alternately try this plan for one to two days.

A third option is to follow a simple cleansing diet. While not as effective as a fast, this menu is less apt to induce hunger because it includes food. Also these cleansing foods are highly nutritious and can actually help your liver (and other organs) function more efficiently. But most important, a cleansing diet such as this retrains your taste buds to appreciate the whole foods we should all eat most of the time. After a few months of regular cleansing "vacations" you may find that your everyday menus don't vary appreciably from your monthly cleansing weekends. Those of you unaccustomed to a high-fiber diet may find this cleansing regimen causes bloating and gas. Drink plenty of water, chew your food well and drink gas-relieving teas like peppermint and ginger.

Here is a list of foods you can consume during a cleanse. Eat mostly vegetables, with small portions of other foods. Drink one to two quarts of fluid daily. Eat organic foods where possible:

- Amaranth
- Brown rice
- Dried beans and legumes (soaked, then cooked)

- Fresh raw fruits
- Fresh vegetables (raw or lightly steamed)
- Fresh vegetable juices; can include small amount of fruit in these juices to taste
- Herbal teas
- Homemade vegetarian soup or broth
- Kamut
- Millet
- Oils such as canola, flax seed, and olive—cold pressed (use sparingly as seasoning or dressing). Don't heat flax seed oil.
- Nuts (raw and unsalted; not peanuts)
- Quinoa
- Seeds (raw and unsalted)
- Water (pure—either distilled or filtered)

■ **Makeover Hint #6—The Mini-Cleanse**

Can't stand the idea of a two-day cleanse? Then start out small, very small. Begin with a one-meal cleanse, say breakfast. The following week or month, follow your cleansing routine for two meals—breakfast and lunch. The third month, cleanse for an entire day. Continue at this snail's pace until you're cleansing for a whole two days.

How to Calm an Angry Liver

Natural and conventional medicine both recognize that emotions affect overall health. According to Chinese medical philosophy, the liver is the governor of emotions, and when feelings are excessive or insufficient, they generate illness. Or conversely, when the body is unwell, the emotional state is affected.

Traditional Chinese Medicine has developed an even more specific guide to emotions and various body organs. Seven different emotions—fear, fright, grief, joy, sadness, pensiveness, and anger—are thought to be tied to five different organs. The liver is said to be the seat of anger, and is considered, along with the heart, to be the most susceptible to emotional disruption. An angry outlook, according to Chinese Medicine, is thus responsible for liver problems. Or if the liver is "congested," you may experience frustration, anger or extreme mood swings.[13]

Use Edgar Cayce's Castor Oil Treatment

The castor oil treatment is an old-time treatment for the liver, though it can be used on other body parts and does affect other systems. I include this historical, and somewhat mystical, treatment because: (1) it works, and (2) it's tied to such an interesting story.

Edgar Cayce, born in 1877 in Hopkinsville, Kentucky, was a lay healer. The difference between him and others was that he could only offer therapeutic suggestions under a self-induced trance. With the help of his wife, Gertrude, and secretary, Gladys Davis Turner, Cayce performed almost 9,000 readings over a 40-year period for the sick that visited him. According to historical records he helped an enormous number of people, so much so that the Association for Research and Enlightenment, or ARE, Clinic in Arizona, was specifically set up to offer Cayce's health principles and remedies to patients. This clinic still thrives today.

Although used for thousands of years, the castor oil treatment was one remedy frequently suggested by Cayce. A recent study published in *The Journal of Naturopathic Medicine* proved that castor oil packs increase the number of white blood cells called lymphocytes in the body—one part of immunity.[14] This treatment is also thought to work as an antitoxin.

■ *Makeover Hint #7—How to Make a Castor Oil Pack*

To make your own castor oil pack, begin by collecting:

- Cloth—36" × 12" inch piece of plain wool or cotton flannel
- Bottle of castor oil
- Plastic sheet (Saran Wrap™ or plastic bag opened up)
- Towel
- Two safety pins.

Fold the cloth so you end up with a pack of three thicknesses that measure one foot by one foot. Pour the castor oil into a bowl, and dip the pack into it until it is saturated, but not dripping, with oil. Next, find a comfortable and quiet place where you can lie down for 30 minutes to an hour, and apply the castor oil pack over the right upper area of your abdomen. This would include the bottom portion of your right rib cage where your liver is housed, overlapping slightly to the area just above and to the right of your belly button. Place a piece of plastic sheet over the pack. Wrap the towel around your torso and fasten with a couple of safety pins.

For a suspected toxic liver, practice this therapy daily for a week to a month. Save your pack in a plastic bag between treatments. Oily skin can be washed with a baking soda wash, two teaspoons of soda added to a quart of warm water.

Lois Halts Hair Loss With Amazing Liver Treatment

After quitting a 10-year stint on birth control pills, 27-year-old Lois noticed she was losing her hair, so she decided to consult a naturopathic physician. Upon learning of her history, the naturopath immediately recognized that Lois's liver needed help. A decade of synthetic hormones had compromised her liver function. First the doctor prescribed a lipotropic supplement. Next she advised that Lois use a castor oil pack over her liver region. Lois followed the doctor's directions exactly. When she returned to the doctor's office two months later, she reported that her hair felt thicker and wasn't falling out at the same rate as before.

Liver Makeover Checkup

How did you do? These are the steps you've just taken to invigorate your liver:

- Began eating more whole foods, and fewer processed foods, and fewer additives.
- Checked for food intolerances.
- Checked home and work for poisons.

- Started eating liver-friendly foods like Brussels sprouts, beets, onions, and garlic.
- Ate more fiber.
- Added more antioxidant foods and nutrients to regimen.
- Took a lipotropic supplement.
- Tried some liver herbs like turmeric, dandelion, and milk thistle.
- Vowed to eat a cleansing diet for one to two days each month.
- Learned about the relationship between anger and the liver.
- Tried a castor oil pack.

For Related Problems, See

- Acne
- Constipation
- Eczema
- Headaches

Laboratory Tests Your Doctor Can Order

- Liver Detoxification Profile
- Food Allergy Panel
- Liver Enzyme Levels

Chapter 4

Revitalize Your Digestive System

Your Intestinal Lifeline

Did you know there's an 18-foot tube filled with a jungle of wildlife—at least 400 species at last count—inside of you? This is your digestive tract. The digestive system goes by many names: the gastrointestinal tract, GI tract, the alimentary tract. This remarkable body system is responsible for converting all that you eat and drink into tiny units that can be utilized for fuel, to repair broken bones and other injured tissues, make sex hormones, create the cells that defend you from germs, grow hair, and perform a staggering number of other everyday functions. When the digestive tract doesn't do its job, not only do you feel it in your gut, but in the rest of your body as well.

The Healing Power of Your Kitchen

There's a joke about a gentleman who visits his doctor. He informs the physician that he hasn't felt well for the last month and can't figure out why. After asking numerous questions, the doctor finds nothing unusual in his patient's medical history. Laboratory tests are all perfectly normal. Finally the doctor conducts a physical exam. Blood pressure is normal, temperature is fine, as are heart rate and respiration. However, when the doctor peeks into the gentleman's ears, he's surprised to see carrots lodged inside. A glance up his nose reveals bits of parsley. And when the doctor asks his patient to lift his arms, a piece of watermelon falls out.

"I know why you don't feel well," the physician announces.

"Why?" asks the desperate patient.

"You're not eating right!"

This punch line applies to many people: They feel bad because they're not eating right. The Standard American Diet—the SAD American diet—and that of most other industrialized nations is quite different from more traditional menus. In his superb work, *Traditional Foods Are Your Best Medicine* (Ballantine Books), Dr. Ronald Schmid talks about the benefits of ancestral diets—be they vegetable-based or more meat-laden. When compared to modern ways of eating, these traditional foods contained more fiber, and less fat overall. "Whether one ate more in the manner of hunter-fisher-gatherer, or more in that of the agriculturist," says Schmid, the result was people who "were healthy and largely resistant to diseases prevalent today."

The difference between eating healthy and not isn't determined by whether you're a vegetarian or one who loves meat. For each of us has our own nutritional requirements based on cultural and ethnic roots, individual physiology, and current health needs. Some people do fine eating red meat, while others thrive on strictly plant foods. It's how food is grown, handled, and processed that impacts health the most.

Before the turn of the century, most people ate foods that were whole and mostly unprocessed. This meant fresh, home-grown vegetables and fruits, wild or free-range meats, raw dairy, whole grains. Milling wheat to produce white flour wasn't available on a large scale until 1910; this process strips the wheat berry of its bran and germ, as well as of nutrients like vitamin E, B-vitamins, and minerals. Consumption of refined sugars, vegetable oils, hydroxygenated oils and margarine, additives, irradiated foods, and quick-to-fix foods in general has soared in the last 100 years.

During the last century, many indigenous peoples have moved to the city and adopted modern menus. One result has been a dramatic rise in diabetes.[1] The landmark work of Weston Price, D.D.S. revealed similar disturbing news. This Canadian dentist discovered that swapping "primitive" foods for modern, refined ones not only adversely affected people's teeth, but contributed to the swell of rheumatoid arthritis, heart disease, cancer, and other modern diseases we see today.[2] More recently Professor Sylvia Guendelman from the University of California at Berkeley reports that Mexican women who emigrate to the United States are much healthier than their American counterparts, with their low-fat, high-protein diets brimming with zinc, calcium, and folic acid. However, as these new residents become more Americanized, their diets and health deteriorate.[3]

In response to increasing ill health and the realization that food is one cause, there has been heightened interest in nutrition by both the public and researchers. Scores of articles fill the pages of both alternative and conventional medical journals; scientists probe and prod our food trying to learn which nutrients keep health humming. Magazines scramble for the newest information on nutritional advances, and how the latest vitamin, mineral, or food can cure this or that sickness. Caught in the middle of this is you—the consumer—confused and feeling guilty about not eating as well as you could.

Do you feel like giving up? Many people do. During a nutritional lecture I gave, several audience members expressed their frustration at maintaining a healthful diet amidst a culture that entices its members with commercials, restaurants, and billboards to consume more sugar, more pop, more fast food, more candy, more beer—all those things you're told to avoid. This is in addition to the bewilderment over "What foods should we eat anyway?"

Eating doesn't have to be complicated or mysterious. Or guilt-provoking. This is not an issue of morality, it's one of health. As you launch into your Digestive Makeover, keep these simple thoughts in mind:

- Choose whole foods, as close to their original state as possible, for more nutrients and fewer additives. For example, pick a baked potato over potato chips, a steak over a hot dog, an apple over a candy bar.
- Pick fresh foods. Nutrient levels fall with processing and storage.
- Include raw foods in your meals (vegetables, fruits, nuts, seeds); when you must cook, don't overdo it. Nutritional value is lost with the heat of cooking. (There are exceptions to this minimal cooking rule: poultry and eggs, for instance.)
- Select regional and seasonal foods, that is, items grown in your area and in season. Out-of-season foods and ones that must be shipped long distances are often treated with unwanted chemicals to prevent spoilage, and are less nutritious due to storage.

- Eat organic foods. This is the best way to avoid harmful pesticide and chemical exposure; there's also evidence that organic produce is more nutritious than commercially grown foods.

Remember: As you improve the quality of your food using the above suggestions, you may find the quantity of what you eat declines. Try that piece of whole grain bread; it's much more filling than white.

Signs That Your Digestion Needs a Face-lift

Most patients in my general practice complain of digestive troubles—regardless of their main complaint. Come to think of it, most don't even complain. Among the people I care for, digestive problems are so common as to be considered normal. But they're not. Does dinner give you gas and bloating? Just plop-plop-fizz-fizz your way back to comfort. Suffering from occasional irregularity? That overnight laxative will do the trick. Got a little heartburn? Pop an antacid. Some of the most important information I collect about a person's health, regardless of why they came to visit, centers around digestive function. For how and what you eat not only affects the GI tract, but the body at large. I look for clues that their digestion needs a makeover: indigestion, gas, bloating, constipation, diarrhea, nausea, cramping, or other abdominal-centered complaints.

Besides examining what people eat, I try to figure out if they're digesting, absorbing, and utilizing their food. You can eat the best diet in the world, but if your body can't use the food it does you no good. Read on for steps to improve your diet, and clues that you need help digesting and absorbing your food.

Record Everything You Eat for One Week

Before you can make dietary changes, you must know what you eat now. You can do this two different ways: Record everything you ate during the past week based on recall, or fill out a Diet Diary as you go. Both scientists and doctors recognize that retrospective data (remembering what you did) is much less reliable than prospective information (recording as you go).

Most people don't realize what or how much they eat until they actually write it down. I use Diet Diaries not only to learn what a patient is consuming, but to educate him as well. When a patient is slightly embarrassed about her Diet Diary, and tries to explain away the results with "I really don't eat like this . . . there was Aunt Martha's birthday on Friday and I had two pieces of cake. We ordered a pizza on Wednesday—we hardly ever do that. And, well, Joan brought in these fantastic chocolate chip cookies on Friday—I couldn't resist and had four," I know I'm getting the truth.

Use the Diet Diary on the following page as your guide. You must record everything that goes into your mouth including food, all beverages (water, alcohol, coffee), medicine, and vitamins. Amounts are important, too. It also helps to mark down how you felt after eating—either digestive or other symptoms, bowel movements, and emotions. After a week of using your Diet Diary, you may discover how certain foods are affecting you both physically and emotionally. You'll also see how much you eat and what foods you eat on a regular basis. You may be surprised to learn that you're drinking 10 cups of coffee daily and eating sweets every three hours. It may shock you to discover that you're low on protein. Or you might be pleased that you are actually eating five servings of vegetables and three of fruit each day.

Hang on to this record, along with your Before-and-After Chart. Use it as a blueprint during your Digestive Makeover. Begin by circling one item you'd like to change—for instance, fewer sweets. Then get to work. If it helps, use the Diet Diary throughout your Digestive Makeover as a testimony to the changes you're making.

Getting Ready with a Grocery List Makeover

You know what you eat. The next step in your Digestive Makeover is altering your shopping habits. I decided to put this step here so you'll be prepared to buy new foods as I discuss them later. Before I do that, let's stop for a moment and establish a few ground rules.

You may be feeling slightly overwhelmed, maybe even depressed at this point. Your Diet Diary isn't as sparkling as you'd hoped, and forgoing your favorite foods isn't particularly appealing.

Table 4.1
DIET DIARY

Date	Time	Item	Amount	Feeling
EXAMPLE				
Nov 11	8am	coffee, white toast, jam	2 cups, 1 slice, 1 tbsp	Jittery

You don't relish the idea of sprouts and tofu for the rest of your life; you don't want to be deprived of delicious dishes forever.

- Rule number one—Eating should be enjoyable. I don't know about you, but I love food. And I do my utmost to prepare and select delectable dishes. The trick, of course, is finding healthful foods that are fun.
- Rule number two—Shopping should be an adventure. I love to grocery shop. I find beauty in fresh vegetables and fruits, and love discovering new and interesting foods. Try new stores (specialty, gourmet, bakeries, health food); add one new food a week to your list.
- Rule number three—Cooking should be simple. I hate to cook, as much as I love to shop. Perhaps it's the everyday drudgery of it. Whatever the reason, I promise to show you easy, convenient ways to prepare nutritious Digestive Makeover foods.

To begin your Grocery Shopping Makeover, change nothing. That's right, just shop as usual—but make sure you make a list of what you plan to buy. (You do make lists, don't you? Like a good shopper?) The only difference with this list is that I want you to put your foods into categories: produce (mark fresh, frozen, canned, or other—sorry, ketchup and potato chips don't count), protein foods (meats, poultry, fish, beans, legumes, nuts, and seeds), dairy, grains (bread, rice, cereals, pastas), beverages (coffee, tea, water, juice, pop, alcohol) and miscellaneous. This will help you see how much of each you're buying, and where you'll want to make changes in the future. For instance, the bulk of your foods should be in the produce sections, with a good portion under grains and protein; if you're buying mainly miscellaneous items like chips, we need to talk.

Week number two, start making menus for the week and incorporate some of the Digestive Makeover ideas that follow. Rather than white bread, buy whole wheat. Add a crisp green salad to dinnertime. Stock up on fresh fruit and dish it out for between-meal snacks. Based on these dietary changes and your seven-day menu, write up your grocery list. I do this myself, and find it saves me time, money, and frustration over what to cook that night. In addition to my seven selected dinners for that week, I add a couple of easy back-up meals in case I'm too busy to make a complex meal or we feel like eating something different. Purchase ingredients for these meals, too.

Many of the items I use in everyday cooking I order in bulk or have on hand. I'm also a very lazy cook, and so in the name of convenience, supplement my nutritious cooking with some healthy convenience foods like spaghetti sauce, fixings for burritos, items to make a panful of vegetable stir-fry. Besides enjoying sandwiches and soups for lunch, I double my dinner meals for either lunch-time leftovers or freeze for future use.

Continue to make gradual changes to your shopping list as you take steps to make over your digestion and eating habits. Think of each shopping trip as a safari, with you as the hunter out to bag the wild tofu or exotic quinoa. Try foods on for size, check out their flavor and texture, and see if they fit your tastes. When you do this, keep these thoughts in mind: Number one—just because a food tastes *different* doesn't mean it tastes *bad*. Many foods are an acquired taste. (Remember the first time you tried shrimp or spinach or some other non-kid food you love now?) Number two—you don't have to enjoy every food. Some people love tofu, others don't. Bean sprouts aren't for everyone, and barley may not be your cup of tea. But there are plenty of healthful, delicious foods out there, enough for everyone's liking.

■ *Makeover Hint #8—Buy Organic*

An easy first step when making over your groceries is to shop organic. Organic foods are grown—by and large—without synthetic fertilizers, pesticides, livestock feed additives and/or growth regulators. The idea is to produce safer foods while preserving our environment and agricultural lands. Organic produce and meats may be slightly more expensive than commercial items, though not always. You can find these foods in health or natural foods stores, farmers' markets, and some grocery stores. Also ask your neighbors and friends who raise organic gardens if you can buy their leftovers; or grow your own.

Seven Ways to Make Cooking Easy

Do you remember Peggy Bracken's *I Hate to Cook Book*? She wrote a humorous cookbook thirty years ago, generously seasoned with complaints about cooking. One of her chief beefs was recipe books with beautiful pictures of perfect, impossible-to-prepare food; her answer was dozens of simple meals in place of those too-hard-to-cook recipes. Her easy tips hit a chord with American women, and we haven't looked back since. I've gone one step beyond Peggy's advice, and developed these seven ways to keep meals healthy, yet simple to prepare.

- Always serve raw vegetables. They're easy to make—just cut them up, no cooking involved. They're nutritious, and after they get used to them, kids and spouses love them. Try green salad, carrot and celery sticks, hunks of jicama, or tomatoes and cucumbers in an olive oil and balsamic vinegar mix. Throw together vegetables that don't belong for a new dish—for example, carrots, red peppers, and cucumbers.

- Prepare whole grains ahead of time. Brown rice, millet, and other whole grains take more than one minute to cook. I don't want to miss out on their goodness, so I make a large pot early in the day and feast on it during the week.

- Cut your meat down to size. Small pieces of chicken, ground turkey, or dabs of beef or lamb cook much faster than larger chunks.

- Crock-pot magic. I love my slow cooker—especially on cold winter days. I can throw a bunch of vegetables, stock, beans, and meat into it in the morning for soup or stew, and let its savory aroma embrace me all day long. The best part is I don't have to cook another thing.

- Undercook your vegetables. A quick steaming for broccoli (three minutes over boiling water), seven minutes for corn on the cob, keeps veggies crisp, nutritious, and saves you time in the kitchen.

- Serve fresh fruit. Dish up a platter of fresh fruit instead of vegetables during dinner or lunch. In-season melons, grapes, slices of apple, cherries, kiwi are all delicious and require little prep.

- The less the better. You don't need to serve four different platters of food at each meal. Soup and bread; stew and salad; rice and stir-fried vegetables are plenty, and easier on your digestive system (and budget).

■ *Makeover Hint #9—Prepare a Basic Snack*

There is such a thing as fast healthy foods. Instead of potato chips and candy bars, turn to these simple snacks, or make up your own:

- Fresh fruit
- Raw vegetables
- Nuts and dried fruit
- Rice cake with peanut or nut butter, sprinkled with raisins
- Celery sticks filled with soy cheese or brie
- Whole wheat toast with sugar-free jam
- Plain yogurt mixed with pineapple and sunflower seeds

A Makeover for Every Favorite Recipe

Simple cooking is important to stay motivated during your Digestive Makeover. However, there are probably several old recipes you'd like to hang on to. Making dietary changes doesn't mean giving up on old favorites; merely make over your recipes to fit with your new way of eating.

As with meal alterations, slow and steady is the key to changing any recipe. If you make too many changes at once, results can be disastrous. Instead, modify one ingredient or measurement each time you cook a dish. In pencil, record on the recipe sheet what you've altered—amount and ingredients. Jot down comments about how successful (or not) you were. For example, your great banana bread may taste wonderful with 3/4 of the flour as whole wheat and 1/4 white; any more and it's too heavy. For new, untried recipes, cook exactly as directed the first time. Then make modifications. Here are some ideas on how to convert old standbys into digestively-pleasing dishes. Natural health cookbooks offer many suggestions also.

- Substitute whole grain flours for white. Start by replacing half the white flour only, then work your way up.

- Substitute canola oil for shortening or lard.
- Use butter instead of lard.
- Substitute apple sauce or a smashed banana for one egg or fats (oil, lard, butter).
- Replace cream with low-fat milk or soy milk.
- In place of one egg, add two egg whites.

■ *Makeover Hint #10—Sneaky Vegetables*

There are hundreds of ways to sneak vegetables into your meals. (See importance of vegetables discussed later.) You can feed them to hungry kids pestering you for dinner. You can slip garlic, onions, celery, peppers, and mushrooms into spaghetti sauce. When no one's looking, throw extra potatoes, yams, carrots, peas, onions, into the stew. Serve vegetable soup. Make healthy zucchini bread or carrot cake. Chop up red cabbage, fresh tomatoes, yellow peppers, leaf lettuce, alfalfa sprouts for tacos or burritos. Carry fresh fruit and bunny carrots with you while traveling; offer them to starving passengers before you hit the ice cream shop.

Seven is a Lucky Number for Fruits and Vegetables

Adam, my older son, and his young friend, Josh, were watching me make dinner one day. Josh watched with particular interest as I put together my famous vegetarian lasagna. The next day, Josh's mother reported her son's reaction. "He came home with a puzzled look on his face," she said. "Then he looked up to me and replied, 'Mom, Lauri puts *green* stuff in her lasagna!'" When I heard that, I knew I was on the right nutritional track trying to feed my family seven servings of produce a day.

The Food Guide Pyramid says we should each eat two to four servings of fruits and three to five servings of vegetables for a total of five to nine servings of produce daily. Only 10 percent of us manage to consume five servings each day, much less seven or nine.[4] Since World War II, Americans on average eat 40 percent fewer vegetables and 45 percent less fruit. Whole grain consumption has also declined dramatically. The average American has filled this void with pastries, soft drinks, potato chips, as well as more fat, salt, and sugar.[5]

As nutritional research expands and matures, it is becoming increasingly evident that those vegetables and fruits your mother coaxed you into eating held more than a parent's guilt. Vegetables and fruits possess a host of vitamins, minerals and, of course, fiber. They retain enzymes that aid digestion. The *Journal of the American Medical Association* published a study in 1996 that found persons whose blood was highest in beta-carotene—the pigment found in vegetables like carrots and yams—were less likely to die young when compared with individuals with the very lowest beta-carotene blood levels.[6] People who eat produce rich in vitamin C, like alfalfa sprouts, citrus fruits, and broccoli, are significantly protected against cancers of the esophagus, larynx, mouth, pancreas, stomach, rectum, breast and cervix, according to the National Cancer Institute.[7] And just when you feel grown-up enough to say "no" to a helping of spinach, a dozen scientists prove that the more you munch on this dark leafy green (and its relations), the less chance you have of developing macular degeneration—a very serious and blinding condition.[8]

These and other studies that hammer home the phrase "Eat all your vegetables" are wonderful and welcoming. But I like what Kristen McNutt, Ph.D., J.D. has to say on the subject. She explains that it isn't enough that we tease apart foods—like fruits and vegetables—looking for which nutrients do what in the body. It may be that various food components are interactive, meaning that they don't act alone. Also, there are likely many nutrients and other substances in foods, herbs, and spices "for which functions have not yet been recognized".[9] It's not enough to pop vitamin pills. You need to keep eating your fruits and vegetables, and one day we'll figure out all the reasons why they're good for you—though we already have some pretty good ones.

Look to Makeover Hint #11 to learn what a serving is. And use Table 4.2 to play Vegetable One-Upmanship—a fun and easy way to increase the amount of vegetables you eat each week.

■ *Makeover Hint # 11—What's a Serving?*

Part of your Digestive Makeover is finding ways to eat seven servings of vegetables and fruits every day. If you're a light eater, five is fine. For those with a big appetite, aim for nine.

So what's a serving? Depends on what you eat. A serving can be:

- One medium piece of fresh fruit
- One cup of lettuce, spinach, kale or other fresh, raw leafy vegetable
- 1/2 cup of cooked beans, split peas, lentils, or other legumes
- 1/2 cup of cut-up fruit
- 1/2 cup of cooked corn, carrots, or other dense vegetables
- 3/4 cup of pure, fresh vegetable or fruit juice

How to Play Vegetable One-Upmanship

Rule #1—Pull out your Diet Diary and count how many vegetables and fruits you eat on average each day. Write it down on your Weekly Produce Chart on the following page under Week One.

Rule #2—Pick a time during the day to eat one more serving of vegetables. Remember: Carrot sticks and salads count.

Rule #3—Eat that extra vegetable serving all week long. Write it down on Your Weekly Produce Chart.

Rule #4—Pat yourself on the back, or reward yourself in some non-food way. (A movie, new shirt, calling your best friend long-distance count; a chocolate sundae does not.)

Rule #5—Continue to add one more fresh produce to your menu each week, and record and reward appropriately. Stop when you reach seven. If you wish to continue, that's OK too.

Table 4.2
YOUR WEEKLY PRODUCE CHART

Week #	Veg 1	Veg 2	Veg 3	Veg 4	Veg 5	Fruit 1	Fruit 2
1							
2							
3							
4							
5							
6							
7							
8							
9							
10							
11							
12							
13							
14							
15							
16							
17							

Switch to Well-Dressed Grains

Grains fulfill us in so many ways: a bowl of steaming rice, home-made bread, savory pasta, sweet banana bread. These are all fine complex carbohydrate foods—if eaten as their unrefined selves. Grain-containing foods that have been processed to achieve a whiter product, say white bread or white rice, lack the fiber, vitamins, and minerals of whole, untouched grains. To make up for this loss, many manufacturers "enrich" their breads or noodles with a smattering of thiamin, riboflavin, and other nutrients. This nutritional improvement, however, is a poor substitute for the real thing. Enriching processed grains is like mugging people, taking their clothes and money, then giving them back their raincoats and saying "You're enriched."

The next step to better digestion is to switch to well-dressed, whole grains.

Of the more than one dozen grains available to us, most people only take advantage of a very few, mainly wheat, rice, oats, and corn. Get out of your grain rut and explore some of those exotic grains and grain-like foods found in your grocery store or natural foods markets. These grains can be enjoyed in their whole state—solo or mixed together—or in related products like breads and pastas; you can also use the flour to make your own creations.

- Amaranth—actually a cereal-like herb, this teeny beige seed tastes woodsy. Cook one cup of dry amaranth in three cups of water for 1/2 hour to partake of its high protein, calcium, iron, and fiber.

- Barley—a great addition to soup; aim for whole barley rather than pearl for its higher nutrient content. In a one-to-three ratio of whole barley to water cooked for an hour, you can fix yourself a wholesome bowl of barley mush.

- Buckwheat—famous as a pancake ingredient, this seed is related to rhubarb. For buckwheat porridge, cook as you would for amaranth.

- Cornmeal—lots of colors available in the corn family: yellow, white, and blue for starters. Eat corn as is, as popcorn, or make into a porridge.

- Kamut—this ancient high-protein cousin to wheat looks like a large version of rice. It tastes chewy and rich.

- Kasha—this is a hulled, toasted version of buckwheat. Its reddish-brown color provides lots of high-quality protein, iron, calcium, as well as vitamins B and E.

- Millet—another high-protein grain, it is a yellow, small, bead-like, nutty grain loaded with potassium, B-vitamins, magnesium and phosphorus. Cook for one hour, with one cup of dry millet added to five cups of water.

- Oats—oatmeal and oat bran are already breakfast favorites among Americans. Look for whole, versus rolled, oats for your morning mush.

- Quinoa (pronounced "keen-wa")—like amaranth, this is really an herb. Varieties range from the black type to one that's more creamy in color. This delicate tasting food sports more protein than other grains, as well as greater quantities of iron, B-vitamins, calcium and phosphorus.

- Rice—besides brown and white rice, there are many colorful and fragrant varieties to choose from. Try jasmine, basmati, jasponica, and wehani. Wild rice, by the way, is really an aquatic grass seed but valuable as a nutritious food. Cooking times and amounts vary; start with one cup of rice to two of water and simmer for 30 to 60 minutes.

- Spelt—another cousin to wheat, but higher in nutrients. This whole grain is like rice but nuttier.

- Teff—this Ethiopian grain comes in white, red, or brown. All taste somewhat nutty; loaded with iron and calcium and high in protein. Cook for 30 minutes to make porridge.

- Wheat—a very familiar grain to Americans. But did you know it also comes as couscous, cracked wheat, and bulgur? Try one and see what you think.

If you're used to eating white bread, white pasta, and white rice, this step may be difficult for you. Whole-grain foods are much heavier, more robust, and taste fuller than their paler cousins. Go slowly as you make the crossover to more complete grains. Mix your white rice half and half with brown. Buy a whole wheat bread that's only 60 percent whole wheat. (Beware of the label "brown" for bread; it may only be white bread with coloring added.) Add a handful of barley to your soups and stews. And use some of the Flour Power hints listed below.

■ *Makeover Hint #12—Flour Power*

The whole grain is more nutritious than the ground flour. But if you like to bake, play around with flours made from the above grains as well as those made from arrowroot, chestnut, chickpea, fava bean, and soy bean. Each flour has its own particular taste and texture. Keep an open mind, have fun, and stay healthy with these tips:

- Buy fresh, or grind your own. Flour can turn rancid with time.
- Keep flour refrigerated or store in a cool, dark place.
- Toss unused flour after three months.
- Avoid flour-based products if ill with a cold or hay fever as they tend to promote mucus production.

Try Some Magical Beans and Other Plant Proteins

Next in your Digestive Makeover is adding the mysterious bean to your diet. Vegetarians, and natural health writers and practitioners love beans. Pound for pound they're higher in protein than eggs and most meats—17 to 25 percent—without the saturated fat. They have plenty of calcium, iron, and B-vitamins. They're a valuable fiber source. And they help keep unsteady blood sugar levels even— something meat can't do quickly.

Patients are often incredulous when I suggest beans as one solution to their gastric distress. "Beans?" they sputter. "The gas! The pain! . . . I'll have no friends left."

Not necessarily so. It's all in how you cook them. Let's take a look at these 10 helpful hints:

1. Choose fresh beans. If more than 12 months passes between harvest time and dinner-time, gas will also pass.

2. Store beans in a cool area in a sealed container. Pretty jars are fine; I use my mother-in-law's old Mason jars and display them on my counter top.

3. Wash beans before cooking. Remove any floating beans. Wash again if water is particularly grubby.

4. Soak beans several hours or overnight before cooking (four cups of water to one cup of beans).

5. Drain soaking liquid. Rinse beans again.

6. Add fresh water or other liquid (same proportions as for soaking).

7. Bring beans to a boil and skim off all foam. Turn down heat and simmer. Add water as needed to keep beans covered.

8. Add kombu, a sea vegetable, for flavor, minerals, and less gas.

9. Add 1/4 to 1/2 tsp of sea salt to last five minutes of cooking beans; works like kombu. If you add salt too soon, it'll make the beans hard. This isn't a seasoning, it's to improve your social life.

10. Serve beans first as a side dish or ingredient in an entree. Start with a small amount, and work your way up so your body acclimatizes to the beans.

Look to the many wonderful cookbooks available for specific bean recipes. Or use your imagination, and season at will.

■ *Makeover Hint #13—An Easy Dinner*

This idea comes from Dr. Amrit Devgun of Minneapolis. As a busy doctor, she doesn't have time to cook dinner at night for her husband and herself. So many mornings she prepares this easy meal in her slow cooker. From her many jars of beans and grains, she tosses in a handful of a mixture of dried beans (rinsed); the same for longer-cooking whole grains, such as wild rice, millet, and barley. Depending on her mood and cupboards, diced vegetables, crumbled seaweeds like kelp or wakame, and herbs are also part of the mix. You may chop the veggies by throwing them in a food processor and giving it a few spins. She fills her crock pot half way with water to cover the ingredients. During the week when she's gone all day seeing patients, she turns her slow cooker on low for seven to eight hours. For those lazy weekends, medium heat is fine for three to four hours. This potluck supper contains all the makings of a well-rounded vegetarian meal—and it's never the same twice. Or in Dr. Devgun's words: "Voila, you have a lovely hot soup, ready to serve when you get home!"

Remember to Chew

A major reason for indigestion is eating too fast. In order for food to digest, you must chew it properly. Incorporating more chewy, fibrous foods into your meals will help you do this. Chewing is so important because the mouth is where you begin to break down food. In fact, your mouth prepares for whatever succulent morsel you feed it before the food even touches your lips.

Has your mouth ever watered from the smell of dinner? This is saliva spurting forth from the parotid gland in your cheek and sublingual and submandibular glands hidden under your tongue, and jaw. Bite into a juicy apple, and your teeth tear it into tiny pieces for easier digestion, and along with your cheeks, lips, tongue and jaws mix it up with saliva into a soft, wet ball for easy swallowing. Before that happens, however, amylase, an enzyme in saliva, starts to chemically break the apple down—as well as any other sugars or starches that come its way. Salivary lipase, the fat enzyme, is also released, ready to disintegrate fats. (Apples, unless dipped in caramel, are fat-free.) Chewing also signals other digestive enzymes and organs to prepare. Thus the more thoroughly you chew, the better digestion will be further down the GI tract.

■ *Makeover Hint #14—Avoid the No-Time-to-Taste Syndrome*

In this day and age of fast food and faster eating, we often lose the pleasure of tasting our food. Here's a flavorful tip to slip into your Digestive Makeover: Sit down and enjoy the taste of your food. Savor each delicious mouthful, and pay attention to the subtle tastes and textures of every bite. There are four types of taste buds on your tongue: sweet, sour, salty, and bitter. Take advantage of these. Slow and lazy eating also gives your gastrointestinal tract a chance to ready itself for digestion.

Sprinkle Your Food with Laughter

Once you find the time to chew your food, you might extend your meal breaks and invite a friend or guest to join you. Congenial companionship is another way to improve digestion. The American Association of Therapeutic Laughter says humor and laughter improve digestion. Eating in the company of people you enjoy, laughter, and even prayer beforehand relaxes your stomach. Investigators at Queen's Hospital in Belfast would agree. They found that patients who complained of heartburn of unknown cause had poor social support compared to individuals whose heartburn was brought on by acid reflux.[10] More of a heartache, than a heartburn, you might say. Avoid stress and you also decrease your chance of developing constipation, irritable bowel syndrome, inflammatory bowel disease, ulcers, and indigestion.

Use Natural Digestive Aids

Laughter is wonderful. But sometimes you may need additional help digesting. Throw out your antacids. Once again, Mother Nature has blessed us with an array of foods that promote digestion and enhance enzyme release, all very naturally. To begin your meal, sip on a glass of water spiked with a squeezed wedge of lemon. Serve a heaping plate of salad before the main course (see Makeover Hint #15). Munch on pineapple and papaya as an appetizer 10 to 15 minutes before a meal for their natural fruit enzymes bromelain and papain. Include plenty of raw vegetables as part of your meal—salads before, carrot sticks, jicama, cucumber, radishes—for their enzyme content. Sip on some digestive teas like ginger, chamomile, and peppermint either before a meal, or at its conclusion. Herbal bitters include gentian, barberry, and golden seal. A small glass of wine prior to eating is also a digestive aid.

   If these steps don't help with that full or bloated feeling, consider combining your foods differently. Eat simpler combinations, refrain from refined carbohydrates and fatty foods, and try this food-combining approach.

Eat vegetables and starchy foods together

Eat vegetables and protein foods together

Eat vegetables with grains and legumes

Eat fruits alone

Avoid combining starches with protein foods

Also try drinking liquids before meals, but not during. Wait one to two hours before drinking fluids again.

As a last resort, try supplemental digestive enzymes and/or hydrochloric acid. Some products contain both. Take between two and five capsules, depending on the size of your meal. Swallow the pills, one by one, throughout the meal. If you're still experiencing gastric distress, increase this amount slowly to a maximum of seven. If this still doesn't work, try a different brand. Note: If you have an ulcer or experience increased gastric distress after doing this, avoid hydrochloric acid supplements.

■ **Makeover Hint #15—The Advantage of the Raw Deal**

Make it a habit to eat a salad before every meal. It's elegant, fashionable, and so very, very healthy. A raw vegetable salad gives you fiber to stay regular and enzymes to aid digestion. Most green leafy vegetables, including lettuces, encourage enzyme release from your digestive tract due to their slightly bitter quality and taste. The more biting the leaf, the better it works. Try endive, radicchio, escarole, watercress, and dandelion greens.

Custom-Tailor Your Food

While certain basic rules on eating can apply to everyone, not everyone should necessarily eat the same foods, or the same amounts. As a finishing touch to your Digestive Makeover, take into consideration these idiosyncrasies and how they apply to you. Make adjustments as needed.

1. Ethnic and cultural background. What did your ancestors eat? If you come from a tradition of feasting on fish, perhaps you should eat more.

2. Blood type. Dr. Peter D'Adamo writes about how blood type can affect food choices in his book *Eat Right for Your Type* (G.P. Putnam's Sons, 1996). This is based on ancestral heritage, and one more way you can determine what's best for you. Briefly, Dr. D'Adamo says that people with type O blood are like the hunter-gatherers of long ago and do well eating meat. This is the majority of the population. Blood type A does better on a vegetarian diet; type B thrives on dairy products. And the most modern and least prevalent blood type—AB—can consume a variety of foods comfortably.

3. Individual physiology. If you find you don't feel well eating bread, but do fine with beef, that may be your body talking. People with unstable blood sugar often need more protein spread throughout the day than the average person. Take into account all digestive symptoms; be sure to listen to the rest of your body, too.

4. Personal health. The healthier your digestive (and overall) health, the more foods you will tolerate. Some people are intolerant or allergic to certain foods, and do better when those are avoided or eaten only occasionally.

■ Makeover Hint #16—Start Your Own Nutritional Support Group

Making food changes is lonely. Gather together your like-minded compatriots and form a nutritional support/educational group. Meet weekly and exchange recipes, spots to shop, how to prepare tofu—any helpful tip to make your Digestive Makeover easier. Choose a theme for each meeting—grains, vegetables, food allergies—and ask members to take turns leading the group in discussion. If you like, use this book as a guide. Or begin a weekly Natural Health Makeover party.

Cold or Hay Fever
  Avoid flour based products,
     they promote mucus production

Cooking Beans
  Add Kombu a sea vegetable
   for flavor, minerals + less gas
  Add 1/4 - 1/2 tsp sea salt for soft beans
   to last 5 minutes of cooking
     Works like Kombu
Serve beans first as a side dish

The Highlander Band

West Milford Township High School
West Milford, New Jersey

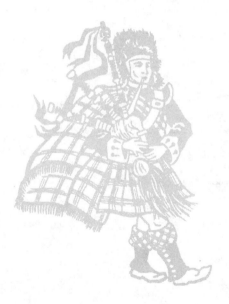

The Highlander Band Thanks You
For Your Continued Support!

Digestion Makeover Checkup

You're on a roll. So far, you've wiped away the poisons and found new ways to soothe digestion. These are the steps you've taken in your Digestive Makeover:

- Filled out a diet diary.
- Made over your grocery list.
- Cooked simple, nutritious meals and snacks.
- Converted some favorite recipes.
- Began increasing the vegetables and fruits you eat each day.
- Discovered a world of grains—and enjoyed them!
- Found more protein foods. Made beans without the gas.
- Chewed each bite 10, 20, 30 times.
- Shared a meal with a friend.
- Tried some natural digestive aids.
- Customized your eating style and needs.
- Gathered together friends for nutritional support.

For Related Problems, See

- Constipation
- Diarrhea
- Food Poisoning
- Heartburn
- Hemorrhoids
- Indigestion
- Ulcers

Laboratory Tests Your Doctor Can Order

- Complete Digestive Stool Analysis
- Intestinal Permeability Test

- Lactose Intolerance Breath Test
- Bacterial Overgrowth of the Small Intestine
- Breath Hydrogen/Methane Test
- Helicobacter Pylori (for ulcers)
- Comprehensive Parasitology

Chapter 5

Better Inner Cleansing

Scouring the Body with the Kidneys

The underrated kidneys are remarkable organs. Not only do they help the body toss out garbage, in the form of metabolic waste products and other foreign substances, via urine, but they also have a hand in maintaining proper body fluid balance—including volume, pressure, and composition. The kidneys also help change vitamin D to its active form, assist with red blood cell production, aid with insulin breakdown, and influence blood pressure.

Normally, the kidneys are very good at what they do, no matter how much or what you eat or drink. For instance, when you drink more water than usual, you expel excess fluid with additional trips to the bathroom. Thirst is your cue to drink more water when fluid levels drop. The anti-diuretic hormone (ADH) is a very descriptive term for the pituitary chemical that puts the brakes on when enough water (that's urine) has been released. The adrenal hormone, aldosterone, helps kidneys out by monitoring sodium and potassium excretion.

To do all this, the kidneys must filter and monitor approximately two gallons of fluid each day. Most is reabsorbed into the body, while a quart or so is discarded as urine. Besides hanging on to most of your body's water, the kidneys also reabsorb most of the nutritionally important substances like protein and sugar. Toxins and artificial substances, many of which are made water-soluble by the liver, are released into the urine for disposal.

Cleansing the body and blood so thoroughly is a daunting task—and one the kidneys do well. Most of the blood that enters the kidneys is reabsorbed. Excess water, waste products, and toxins are sent through a tube called the ureter into the bladder, a hollow muscular balloon, for storage. This happens all day and all night, drip by drip. When the bladder is full (just over a cup), the sensation of "having to go" begins and urine is released through the urinary tract, or urethra, and out.

You Need an Elimination Makeover When This Happens

There are several serious kidney diseases that require you visit your doctor immediately, such as:

1. Acute kidney failure, when the kidneys stop working

2 Chronic kidney failure, when the kidneys stop working gradually

3. Hypertensive kidney disease, when kidney disease causes high blood pressure but not kidney failure

4. Nephrotic syndrome, when the glomeruli are so porous that large amounts of protein are lost in the urine

5. Specific tubular abnormalities, when reabsorption of certain substances by the kidney is abnormal

You certainly can't diagnose these problems on your own. Some people with kidney problems have no symptoms. But you can still be aware of what to watch for, particularly if members of your family have kidney disease. Patrol your body for these symptoms: dull mid-backache or side ache, fever, malaise, changes in urination amount. Changes in urine color should also be checked out with your physician, though be aware that color is also influenced by food and drugs. Other signs to be alert for include general body swelling, sudden or unexplained weight loss, weakness, fatigue, shortness of breath, loss of appetite, nausea, vomiting, itching, or convulsions.

Other more subtle signs to watch for that may indicate you need a Kidney Makeover are: frequent urination (normal is four to six times daily), getting up during the night to void, urgency, urinary dribbling, difficulty starting urination, weak urinary stream, pain or itching upon urination, a "full" feeling in the bladder, a sensation that not all urine has been expelled. Some of these symptoms can indicate a urinary tract, bladder, or kidney infection. When men reach middle age (50 and above), a weak urinary stream, difficulty starting and stopping urine, and inability to completely empty the bladder, can point to an enlarged prostate which subsequently presses down on the urinary tract. Again, visit your doctor for a proper diagnosis in these cases.

Also, if you have a history of exposure to toxic materials, chemicals, drugs, or medications—substances that your kidneys must expel—a Kidney Makeover is warranted.

Don't Hold It

The first step toward healthier kidneys is common sense. When you have to urinate, do so, don't hold it! This may sound like ridiculous advice, but I've met plenty of people who've admitted to resisting the urge to void because of time, work, inconvenience or other annoyances. Part of maintaining good health means listening to bodily urges (be it urination, defecation, thirst, or hunger) and carrying through. This is particularly important with urination as the urine holds waste products, substances you don't want to voluntarily hold onto.

Water—Nature's Own Cleanser

The next phase in maintaining healthy, body-cleaning kidneys is learning how to drink water. Don't laugh. In this country, soft drink consumption exceeds water intake1 and from what I've seen in clinical practice, many people forgo water in favor of other beverages. Water should always be your first, thirst-quenching choice—not pop, not juice, not milk, not coffee, not beer. Besides their stimulating and sedating effects, respectively, coffee and alcohol are diuretics causing fluid loss, not gain. Soda, with its sugar and artificial additives, is another diuretic and impairs health in other ways. While milk provides protein and calcium, it's best served as a food, not as a primary beverage. Fruit juice is fine occasionally, but eating fresh fruit is preferable to gain fiber.

Here are eight more reasons why water is a superior fluid for your kidneys and body:

1. Water (not soda or juice) makes up 70 percent of the adult body.

2. Water helps clear the body of waste material.

3. Water helps fight constipation and aids digestion.

4. Water helps lubricate joints.

5. Water aids cell function and is an important solvent in the body.

6. Water vapor in the lungs helps control oxygen concentration there.

7. Water helps control body temperature.

8. Inadequate water intake may result in fatigue and general body aches.

Working toward the recommended six to eight 8-ounce glasses of water each day seems impossible to many people. This may be partly habit, i.e. they are used to drinking other beverages; perhaps they've been downing tap water and the taste is disagreeable; maybe they mistake thirst for hunger. It could be that their sense of thirst has diminished and they truly don't yearn to drink. Whatever the reason, you can begin to teach your body to enjoy and even desire water again.

Start by choosing only clean, pure water. If you know of a reputable bottled or mineral water to buy, that'll do. Otherwise, rely on filtered or distilled water cleaned in your home. (See Chapter 12, Makeover Hint #65—How to Ensure You Have Clean Water.) Next, make sure you have water available to you at all times. Third, reintroduce water to your life slowly. If you're currently drinking one or two glasses a day, begin by drinking three cups for awhile. Then up it to four. Continue this trend until you're drinking six to eight glasses each day. Also, make note of thirst. And, like urination, don't ignore it.

■ **Makeover Hint # 17—The Sip Tip**

To ensure you drink enough water during the day, carry a special bottle filled with delicious, clean water, and sip liberally. If the idea of carting water around is embarrassing, maybe this story will help. During a getaway to Minneapolis, my husband and I decided to treat ourselves and checked into the downtown Hilton. Being thirsty folks, each of us, in addition to our luggage, toted a hefty jug of water. We did our best to blend in as we casually walked through the lobby of this posh hotel, where well-dressed ladies and gentlemen strolled and limousines were the preferred mode of transportation. No one gave us a second glance. Who says class and good health don't mix?

Cindy's Restaurant Trick

Cindy doesn't make a habit of bringing her own water to hotels, but she has discovered a way of getting her family to drink more water and save money at the same time. As a working mother, Cindy and her husband take their three children out to dinner about once a week. Instead of allowing her sons and daughter to order pop, it has been a long-time tradition that each family member asks for water. Her children, says Cindy, don't even think twice about asking for soft drinks and are very content with water as their quencher. (If you're concerned about the quality of a restaurant's water, ask if it serves tap, filtered, or bottled water. For spots where only tap is available, pull out your own or wait until you leave to drink.)

Prestigious Protein

Protein is certainly a vital nutrient; its name—literally "of first importance"—tells us so. It is the raw material used to build and repair muscle, bones, teeth, blood, and bodily fluids. It form enzymes and hormones. When sick or injured or stressed-out, our body cries out for more protein so it may regain health. Kidneys, particularly when under-the-weather, do better when fed the right protein. Consider this.

British scientist Dr. W.G. Robertson surveyed over 2500 vegetarians about their eating habits and whether or not they'd had kidney stones. Judging from the answers received, Dr. Robertson discovered that vegetarians (this group included pure vegetarians—vegans—as well as those who ate eggs and/or dairy) were about half as likely to get kidney stones as their meat-eating counterparts.[2] As part of your Kidney Makeover, incorporate more plant proteins into your daily fare: beans, legumes, nuts, seeds, soy products like tofu, tempeh, soy cheeses and soy milk, nut milks, and whole grains.

■ **Makeover Hint # 18—Eat a Handful of Nuts**

Raw, unsalted (preferably organic) nuts like walnuts, almonds, Brazil nuts, and hazel nuts are an admirable choice for a snack high in protein and healthy essential fatty acids, vitamins and minerals. You can even mix them with a sprinkling of dried fruit like raisins or figs. Use your cupped hand as a measuring device to approximate how much to eat each day.

The Cranberry-Kidney Connection

If you're prone to any type of urinary system infection, you'll want to read this. Cranberry juice is a well-known anecdotal cure for urinary tract, bladder, and possibly kidney infections. The question remains, however, does it really work? According to doctors at Harvard Medical School and Brigham and Women's Hospital in Boston, 10 ounces of *Vaccinum macrocarpon* (cranberry) juice every day did the trick for 60 women with chronic urinary tract infections (UTIs). After six months, these cranberry-drinking individuals had significantly fewer bacteria in their urine than a matched group that sipped on fake juice, and their antibiotic use for urinary tract infection was half.[3]

Ocean Spray™ products, which contain one-third pure cranberry juice, are typically used in these studies. Unlike what's available in grocery stores, these juices were sweetened with saccharin, not sugar. Sugar is known to depress immunity[4,5] and saccharin has the potential to promote cancer. Your best bet is to purchase cranberry juice that has been sweetened with other juices, rather than sugar or artificial sweeteners. You can eat fresh cranberries too.

If 10 ounces of cranberry juice every day is too much for you to stomach, take heart. Another study found that four to six ounces of cranberry juice was enough to prevent future UTIs and bladder infections.[6] If blueberry juice or blueberries are more to your liking, try them instead. They have also been found to deter these infections.[7]

How Cathy Fought Back

Cathy was always getting urinary tract infections. They would begin with a tingling sensation when she urinated, followed by burning, and the urge to run to the bathroom constantly. Every month or two, it seemed, she was also running to the doctor's office for a new antibiotic prescription. After a year of this, Cathy decided to pursue other options. Not only were these treatments getting expensive, but she was concerned about the long-term use of antibiotics. In her reading, Cathy learned about the cranberry-kidney (and urinary tract) connection. She made a habit of drinking one or two glasses of cranberry juice each day, as well as switching from soft drinks to a couple of quarts of water. To her pleasant surprise, Cathy's troubles diminished to the point where such infections bothered her only once or twice a year—a vast improvement from earlier.

Foods That Help the Kidneys Cleanse

One way the kidneys cleanse the body is through diuresis, the act of urination. You can urge urination on by drinking lots of pure water. Alcohol and caffeine are also diuretic substances, but their less-than-desirable health effects and the fact that they don't hydrate the body like water does make them beverages to avoid.

Physicians often use diuretic medications to enhance urination and help patients eliminate surplus fluid for conditions such as hypertension and congestive heart failure.[8] Many herbs and foods also have this ability—albeit much gentler. As we scrutinize fruits, vegetables, grains, and beans, it's becoming increasingly apparent that edibles also possess physiological effects. Consuming foods with a mild diuretic action helps the kidneys flush your body of poisons; drinking water has a similar effect.

Maybe you're eating some of these foods already? Celery sticks are naturally diuretic, as are parsley and asparagus. Note that parsley can promote kidney stones in some people; yet asparagus is a natural kidney stone therapy. Artichokes encourage urine flow, and folklore says corn does the same thing. Not too many people toss fresh dandelion leaves into their salads, but if you do, you'll enjoy their diuretic properties too.

Parsley is often set on dinner plates as a garnish—and left untouched. It is, however, a flavorful ingredient you can add to many dishes including salads. Here's one of my favorites.

1 cup red leaf lettuce, torn

1 cup fresh spinach, torn

1/2 cup radicchio, torn

1/2 cup fresh parsley, chopped

1 medium tomato, cubed

1/2 cucumber, diced

Mix the above ingredients and toss in a large salad bowl. Serve as a side dish with an olive oil and balsamic vinegar dressing, or enjoy as a snack or main entree.

Gorge on Garlic for Greater Kidney Gusto

Eating a couple of cloves of germ-stopping garlic each day adds cleansing power to your kidneys. Bugs that succumb to garlic include bacteria,[9] yeast,[10] and other fungi,[11] protozoa like *Entamoeba histolytica*[12] as well as flu viruses and the herpes bug.[13] In addition, garlic promotes cleansing through its diuretic effects.[14] Raw garlic is always best; cooking steals away some of its medicinal attributes. The fresh-extract garlic pills are another option, though certainly not nearly as tasty. (And a true makeover, I believe, should incorporate as many dietary and lifestyle alterations as possible, and rely less on pill popping.)

Garlic is a tasty and outlandish topping you can add to your homemade pizza. Simply dice the garlic finely and sprinkle it on your pizza creation while you add other healthful and tasty ingredients, such as pineapple, green peppers, fresh tomatoes, shiitake or portabello mushrooms, onions, red cabbage, crumbled tofu, artichokes, and parsley. With a pizza like that, who needs pepperoni? For more kick and therapeutic effect, add garlic after the pizza has been cooked or five minutes before it's done. Serve with Parsley Paisley Salad (see Makeover Hint #19).

Watch for Kidney Poisons

Because the kidneys are elimination organs, they're particularly susceptible to poisoning. For example, uranium (used in industry), aluminum (in cookware, aluminum cans, foil, baking powder, and deodorant), mercury (in alloy plants and some batteries) and other heavy metals poison the kidneys.[15] Cadmium, found in glass factories, metal alloys, electrical equipment, and cigarette smoke, can concentrate in the kidneys and cause problems like kidney stones.[16] Other kidney toxins to watch for include lead, arsenic, thallium, copper, nickel, antimony, and silver. Be careful of lubricants and solvents, paints and petroleum-based mineral oils.[15] A colleague of mine was a landscaper years before she entered naturopathic medical school. The pesticides she was exposed to during her gardening days caused her kidneys to fail years later.

The kidneys are also the route of excretion for many medications. Unfortunately, during the cleansing process, the kidneys not only excrete but must consolidate medicinal leftovers. This is a dangerous job because the kidneys are then swimming in toxic concentrations of these substances. When medication doses are high or use is prolonged, the kidneys are harmed, a condition called toxic nephropathy. *Brenner & Rector's: The Kidney* (5th edition), a respected textbook on the subject, offers an entire chapter on the subject. Here is some of what this authoritative tome has to say.

Immunosuppressive drugs used during kidney (ironically) and heart transplants, like FK-506, can damage kidneys. Cisplatin, cyclophosphamide, streptozocin, and other chemotherapeutic agents are also guilty. Those using gold, penicillamine, methotrexate, and high doses of pain-killers like aspirin and acetaminophen for rheumatoid arthritis need to be cautious. Even antibiotics, like neomycin, cephalosporin, and amphotericin, need to be prescribed with care. When antibiotics from the gentamicin and tobramycin family were first introduced in 1969, kidney injury among patients was 2 to 3 percent. Almost 25 years later, this number rose to 20 percent. Even acyclovir, used to treat herpes, is risky. While we all must be wary and work with our doctors to avoid such problems, those at greatest risk are the elderly, people with existing kidney troubles, diabetics, patients with cancer or congestive heart failure, and anyone who's dehydrated.[15]

Nature's Own Pantry

What's more delicious than a big, juicy T-bone steak served with mashed potatoes swimming in gravy, white dinner rolls dripping with melted butter, followed by a big hunk of apple pie a la mode, all washed down with a brew? In my younger days, I too enjoyed such a feast and my South Dakotan husband regularly points out the steakhouses he and his father used to frequent 20 years ago. Unfortunately, if this is your normal supper, your kidneys are probably in need of a face-lift. (By the way, I'm not adverse to T-bones, just a daily diet or them.)

Adhering to a simple, whole-foods eating plan full of fresh fruits and vegetables keeps the most common type of kidney stones—90 percent are composed of calcium—to a minimum.[17] It has been demonstrated by noted scientists that some of our favorite foods—white buns,low in fiber;[18] gravy, butter and T-bone steak—high in fat;[19] apple pie,refined carbohydrates;[20] sugar[21]— increase calcium in the urine and thus calcium stones. Alcohol is another culprit.[22] Calcium supplementation and vitamin-D enriched foods seem to aggravate this problem in susceptible individuals.

Read Chapter 11, and you'll see that some of the same foods that cause calcium stones rob the bones of calcium. In other words, the calcium is being pulled from the skeleton into the urine for excretion, where it runs the risk of concentrating in the kidneys and forming a stone.

■ *Makeover Hint # 21—Follow This Menu for a Day*

You've already been introduced to the idea of cleansing diets in Chapter 3 (see Makeover Hint #6—The Mini-Cleanse). At the risk of repeating myself, I offer you a slightly different version here and a few more reasons why both are a good idea. When implemented in a non-threatening, sensible manner, they also help you readjust your eating patterns (get you used to all those fruits, vegetables, and whole grains) and give your kidneys a rest. Follow this menu for 24 hours, with plans to do the same every month or two.

Begin the morning with a glass of water flavored with a slice of fresh lemon. Enjoy a piece of fresh fruit.

Breakfast is a large bowl of oatmeal or other whole grain cereal, topped with fresh fruit and soy milk.

Morning snack consists of one piece of fruit or raw vegetable sticks.

Lunch is a raw vegetable salad. Use your imagination.

Afternoon snack is one cup of steamed or raw vegetables.

Dinner can be vegetable soup or steamed vegetables and a large bowl of brown rice or millet.

During this cleansing time, drink fluids liberally: pure water, vegetable broth, and vegetable juice. Fruit juice is all right, if diluted half and half with water. Avoid taking nutritional supplements and unnecessary medications. When I have patients dependent on strong medication—prednisone, for example—I modify this plan for them. If that describes you, work with a skilled natural health physician.

Kidney Stones and Calcium

High-calcium foods and supplements have the reputation of adding to kidney stone problems—particularly since 90 percent of stones contain calcium. So what should you do if you're, on the one hand, concerned about maintaining strong bones (see Chapter 11 for other skeletal strengthening tips), yet don't want to harm your kidneys? One way is to carefully choose your calcium source. On the food side, select dark leafy greens like kale and collard greens, and serve them with your favorite tofu dish. (The body absorbs calcium from kale better than from milk.) As far as calcium pills go, calcium citrate stands head and shoulders above other calcium forms. For one, citrate limits calcium stone formation,[23] even though calcium citrate is better absorbed than calcium carbonate, found in most calcium-containing antacids.[24] Another way to keep your kidneys safe is to take supplemental calcium with meals.[25]

With the increasing threat of osteoporosis—especially for aging baby boomers—doctors are recommending that their patients drink more milk and take antacids for extra calcium. Yet taking these supposedly bone-building steps may increase your chance of developing kidney stones through a condition called milk-alkali syndrome.

Kidney Makeover Checkup

Do you feel cleaner after your Kidney Makeover? These are the steps you took to get there:

- Urinating as soon as the need hits.
- Drinking at least one quart of pure water daily.
- Eating more of those darn'd beans and tofu.
- Sipping on cranberry or blueberry juice as needed.
- Turning to celery, asparagus, and other cleansing foods.
- Gorging on garlic.
- Watching for kidney poisons.
- Taking one more step toward whole foods.
- Taking calcium supplements with meals.

For Related Problems, See

- Backaches
- Fever
- Gout
- Urinary Tract Infections

Chapter 6

Maximize Your Immunity

Fight Off Sickness Naturally

Have you ever noticed that not everyone gets sick during cold season? Why is that? Is it the luck of the draw, or is this something you have control over? Your body, when in tip-top shape, has the ability to fight off most bugs and noxious substances. Individuals who are most susceptible to sickness need an Immune System Makeover.

When natural doctors talk about "the body healing itself," in effect they're praising immunity. To be "immune" means you're protected. In the case of the body, the immune system guards you from germs like bacteria, viruses, fungi, and parasites, and diseases like cancer. It does this through a complex collection of organs, cells, lymphatic vessels, and other factors that work together with help from non-immune body parts, such as searing stomach acid and skin.

Don't Let Your Immunity Down

One of the first signs that you need an Immunity Makeover is when you seem to catch everything that's going around: a cold, the flu. People with poor immunity also have a difficult time shaking illness—the cold that never goes away. Or you might just be tired all the time. If it takes a long time for a cut to heal up, it could be your immunity is dragging. Chronic infections, too, can be a signal that either your defenses are low or the infection itself could be causing depressed immunity. Watch for recurring warts, cold sores, genital herpes, athlete's foot, fungal infection of the nails, or yeast infections (anywhere—vaginal, intestinal, skin or mouth). If you've had mononucleosis in the past, and have never felt well since, think Immune Makeover. Those with AIDS or infected with HIV should also groom their immunity.

If you have multiple sensitivities either to food, chemicals, inhalant substances, or all of the above, consider the following. Some white blood cells—members of your immune system—can create an allergic reaction. This is an overreaction by your immune system to harmless matter. Also remember, for reasons we don't quite understand, the immune system sometimes turns against its host—you. These are called autoimmune diseases and can include rheumatoid arthritis, multiple sclerosis, diabetes, lupus, Hashimoto's thyroiditis, pernicious anemia, Goodpasture's syndrome, and others. Caring for your immune system, and removing other suspected allergens from your life—be they foods, chemicals, or inhalants—often help these conditions.

Kick the Sugar Habit

The simplest way to bolster sagging immunity is by avoiding or minimizing the sugar you eat. This includes white, yellow, and brown sugar, corn syrup, fructose, honey, maple syrup, dried fruit, and fruit juice. Also look for sugar aliases, especially in packaged foods, such as dextrose, sucrose, maltose, turbinado sugar, raw sugar, glucose and cane juice. In some cases, side-stepping sugar, particularly at the first inkling of illness, is enough to turn a slumped immune system around. Try it and see.

More than 20 years ago a group of dentists showed us that sugar doesn't just cause cavities. Using dental students as their subjects, they discovered that drinking a 24-ounce container of soda depressed the germ-eating activity of some white blood cells called neutrophils by 50 percent. This occurred 45 minutes after downing the pop[1]. That's a substantial kick-in-the-pants to your immune system. It's especially rattling when you consider that not only does the average American consume 120 pounds of sugar yearly, but that pop outdistances water as the beverage of choice.[2]

Further research by Loma Linda University in California revealed that sugar's effect on immunity lasts for at least five hours, possibly longer. This pattern occurs not only with white table sugar, but fructose, glucose, and honey as well.[3] Again, the implications of a sweet tooth are great when you consider that a dose of sweetness every three to four hours dampens your defenses all day long. Last but not least, sugar is the preferred food of bacteria[4] and yeast.[5] Eating sugar is like stoking the infectious fire.

■ *Makeover Hint # 22—KO the OJ*

At the first sign of a cold you should start drinking lots of orange juice. That's the conventional wisdom. But according to the Loma Linda study, orange juice is just as damaging to immunity as other sugars. And the vitamin C you gain from this beverage is minimal. So skip the OJ, and drink plenty of water with a frequent dose of vitamin C—in pill form—when you start feeling sick.

Watch the Fats

Too much fat in your diet or on your body appears to hamper the immune system. Not only does your susceptibility to infection increase, but various immune cells and tissues are depressed. Obviously the fats we usually associate with illness—dietary cholesterol and saturated fats—can interfere with immunity. Even polyunsaturated fats, the healthful lipids found in vegetable oils, may impair immunity when eaten in excess. However, don't cut these fats out of your diet entirely. Eating foods and oils that supply you with a balance of omega-6 and omega-3 essential fatty acids, like fish, flax seeds, flax seed oil, walnuts, and other nuts and seeds, should be a regular but moderate part of everyday eating. These essential fats, when deficient, interfere with some aspects of immune operations.[6]

How about when you're ill? Researchers from the University of Texas Medical School in Houston demonstrated that a low-fat diet was best for immediate healing.[7] Why is this? First, stress caused by disease or surgery lowers your body's fat metabolism. Also, scientists have shown the liver's energy reserves, in the form of glycogen, are lower when a lot of fat is consumed. This means an ailing body has less energy to draw from. Carbohydrates, not fats, spare protein. The body has more raw materials for rebuilding wounded or diseased parts when glycogen levels are up. Finally, some experts theorize that high-fat diets may increase free radical levels, those internally produced molecules blamed for accelerated aging, cancer, and impaired healing.

■ *Makeover Hint #23—How to Keep Your Oils Healthy*

Have you ever sniffed a bottle of vegetable oil that smells funny? This is a sign that your otherwise healthy oil is rancid and full of free radicals, those harmful molecules that contribute to degenerative disease and aging. To get the most out of healthful oils, be sure to follow these steps:

- Buy only cold-pressed, when possible, organic oils.
- Store your oil in a cool, dark place such as the refrigerator.
- Use only fresh oil. Toss unused portions two to three months after purchase or if the oil smells "off."
- Take two vitamin E capsules, cut them open and empty the contents into your bottle of oil. This antioxidant quenches free radical molecules and is good for your heart.

Rest and Resist Disease

Rest. Sleep. Laze around. This is the next stage in making over your immunity. Sound hard? It shouldn't be, yet most adults find it difficult to fit rest, relaxing breaks during the day, and eight hours of nighttime sleep into their busy lives. Whenever I'm tempted to skimp on my shut-eye, I need only turn to my three-year-old son for guidance. Willie is a remarkable toddler with an uncanny knack for sleeping. (Actually, this trait runs in the family.) If Will starts coughing or his nose begins to run, he promptly takes a nap. And I don't mean a cat-nap; William is a super napper, dozing for three to five hours at a stretch. When he awakes, he's perky and he's usually symptom-free.

Studies show that Willie is on the right track. Animal research has provided considerable evidence that sleep and immunity are inseparable. It's been just recently that scientists have explored the same connection in humans. Nevertheless, exciting studies are confirming that not only does sleep support immunity and help you fend off illness, but that parts of your immune system may regulate sleep.[8] Just as the field of psychoneuroimmunology (see Battle Stress for Better Defense following) has demonstrated the scientific link between emotions and the immune system, investigators are now drawing similar conclusions about sleep and immunity.[9]

■ *Makeover Hint #24—Nip Sickness With a Nap*

The signs are there. A tickle in your throat. A wave of fatigue. Loose stools. You're getting that cold that's going around the office. There's no stopping it, right?

Wrong! Taking heed of those very warning signals and stopping it in its tracks are a vital part of being a health makeover artist. The best thing to do is listen to your tired body and take a nap. A snooze today could prevent a sick day or more tomorrow.

Don't Starve Your Immune Soldiers

The many cells, glands, and vessels that comprise your immune system are a hungry bunch. That's why it's important to eat nutritious foods, and when necessary, take a general vitamin/mineral supplement. The immune system requires a wide range of vitamins, minerals, and other nutrients to keep it operating in ideal fashion.

One of the most dramatic illustrations of this was a 1992 study done at Johns Hopkins University by Professor Ranjit Kujmar Chandra. He gathered together 96 healthy and independent people 65 and older. To half he gave a multiple vitamin and mineral pill every day for a year; the other 48 received a sugar pill. This minor lifestyle adjustment produced major results. The women and men who took a moderate helping of extra nutrients each day for 12 months were sick half as many days as their placebo counterparts. Also, they used antibiotics less frequently and blood tests showed a significant reduction in nutrient deficiencies, especially vitamins A, B_6 and C, iron, zinc and beta-carotene.[10]

Lest you think nutrients only help the immunity of the elderly, know that your immune soldiers can starve at any age. Young medical students, between 18 and 21, who took 1000 mg of vitamin C everyday for one and a half months enjoyed a substantial immunity boost.[11] Young children who are deficient in vitamin A (a problem that can be solved with minimal supplementation) are more susceptible to illness.[12] The best way to ensure that your immunity is well fed is first, to eat a varied and wholesome diet; second, to add a comprehensive multiple vitamin and mineral supplement as an insurance policy.

■ *Makeover Hint #25—If a Little Is Good, Is More Even Better?*

There are still gaps in our knowledge of immunity and nutrition. However, we do know that single nutrient deficiencies, excessive amounts of certain vitamins and minerals, and a general imbalance among the range of nutrients can upset your defense system.[13] Don't take too many extra vitamins or minerals unless you know what you're doing. Too much of a single nutrient can be as detrimental to your immunity as too little.

Nancy's Swiss Chard Account

Nancy discovered an easy and secret way to keep her family— husband, two daughters and son—healthy all winter long using Swiss chard. During the summer months, Nancy planted a mound of this zesty beet-like vegetable. Throughout July and August she watched the deep green leaves grow, and picked the young shoots often to add to salads and the older ones for other dishes. One year, after a successful vegetable garden, she was saddened to think that all the leftover chard was going to go to waste. Suddenly she had a thought. She'd recently purchased a food dehydrator, so she decided to dry the extra chard she had in the garden. She carefully stored her dried treasure in airtight containers.

That winter, Nancy pulled out her Swiss chard jar whenever she made any dishes that required seasoning, be it stew or soup, and sprinkled the highly nutritious spice-looking substance on it. To Nancy's delight, her family never once complained about the unusual addition to their meals. In fact they seemed to like it because the chard made her dishes taste slightly salty. So without their knowing it, Nancy was able to boost her family's defenses against winter-time germs.

Protein is a Positive Step

A forgotten nutrient when making over immunity is protein, found in beans, legumes, nuts and seeds, eggs, milk and dairy foods, meats, poultry, fish, and whole grains. So many of the cells, tissues, and other parts of your defense system rely on protein for their structure and function. Illness, hemorrhaging, surgery, broken bones, infection, and severe burns accelerate protein breakdown[14] and increase your body's need for good-quality protein. Indeed, being sick tends to depress appetite and thus protein consumption, when protein is most needed. Diarrhea contributes to this problem as well.

During immune-demanding times, look for these signs that you need a protein boost. Enhance your protein intake through either meals, or a protein drink if appetite is down.

- Weight loss
- Skin changes (moist, or dry and scaly)
- Increased susceptibility to infection

I'm sure you're somewhat confused reading this information, only because our culture has been shooed away from protein (and fat). I've had patients, who feast mainly on vegetables, breads, and fruits, look at me as if I'm crazy when I suggest they increase their protein intake. The trick, of course, is finding suitable protein sources and amount that are healthy not only for your immunity but for the rest of your body.

Begin by following my basic rule of eating: stick to whole foods. When you apply this to meats, it means avoiding processed meat products like hot dogs, bologna, and luncheon meats. Many of these contain undesirable additives. Eating rule number two: choose fresh, organic sources. This applies to meats, dairy, and eggs as well as fruits and vegetables.

You can even combine your protein foods. There's no rule saying that tofu can't join chicken or hamburger in an entree. As part of your Recipe Makeover, replace half the meat in all hamburger recipes with crumbled up tofu or tempeh. If you don't say anything, I'll bet your family won't be able to tell the difference.

Also, load your plate up with salads and other vegetables as well as a good portion of lean steak, broiled salmon, skinned chicken, or braised tofu. Continue to snack on fruit as well. Scatter your protein throughout all meals so you're consuming some at each meal and snack; this means breakfast too. This will avoid that draggy feeling between meals. In order to fit all this good-quality protein and vegetation into your menus, you'll have to toss more and more refined foods out.

■ *Makeover Hint # 26—How Much Protein is Enough?*

There's no easy answer to the "how much protein is enough?" question. Each of you has individual requirements; it'll take a little experimentation to determine your optimum amount. If a high carbohydrate diet with 12 percent or so protein is what you've been eating—this is what most Americans do—and you don't feel so great, try boosting that to meals with one-third protein calories, 40 to 50 percent carbohydrates, and 20 to 30 percent fats. If you're overweight, have heart problems, are diabetic, have blood sugar problems or feel sickly, you may need more protein. Also take into account individual differences, activity levels, health or other needs. See Table 6.1 for how much protein is found in common protein foods.

Table 6.1
PROTEIN SOURCES

- 1 cup of soy milk is almost 8 grams
- 1 cup of whole cow's milk is 8 grams
- 1 cup of cottage cheese is 25 grams
- 1 cup of cooked lentils is 15 grams
- 1 cup of cooked beans (e.g., kidney, navy) is 14 grams
- 8 ounces of chicken (light meat) is 12 grams
- 8 ounces of turkey (light meat) is 20 grams

Table 6.1, cont'd.

- 8 ounces of sirloin steak is 41 grams
- 8 ounces of venison is 47 grams
- 1/2 cup of almonds is 13 grams
- 1/2 cup of walnuts is 7 grams
- 1/2 cup of pumpkin seeds is 20 grams
- 1 egg is 6 grams

Vegans can also look to vegetable protein powders, tofu, tempeh, and other soybean-based products for additional protein.

Battle Stress for Better Defense

It's a well-documented fact that stress is an enemy of your immune system. In fact, there's a field of study solely dedicated to the relationship between psychological stress, the nervous system, and the immune system called psychoneuroimmunology (PNI). During the past twenty years, PNI scientists have connected the dots between tension and cancer,[15] upper respiratory infections,[16] periodontal disease,[17] psoriasis[18] and slow wound healing[19]—to mention a few.

Hans Selye, M.D., Ph.D. changed our lives forever when he published his 1956 work *The Stress of Life* (McGraw-Hill), and planted the word "stress" in our minds. Stress is many things, said Selye. It can be emotional turmoil, mental anguish, pain, surgery, a car accident, arthritis, a bad cold, starvation, overeating, or just overdoing it. It's also a poor diet, a couch potato existence, not enough sleep, or any of those other lifestyle no-nos. Stress is anything that fits a very broad category of factors that upset your body's natural balance.

Forty years later, we're confirming Selye's original contention that not only can stress be caused by many things, but it also has widespread effects in the body. Besides rattling the adrenals (see Chapter 7) and other hormone-producing glands, stress stomps on the thymus gland, lymph nodes, white blood cells, and other members of the immune system. So many ways to get sick, so little time.

You'll never remove stress from your life, and you wouldn't want to. A little bit of tension is good; it's what keeps you primed for life. It adds spice to everyday living. You wouldn't want to avoid that thrilling Caribbean cruise just because thinking about it makes your heart race a little bit faster, would you? The trick is to keep your stress load to a level where it doesn't impede immunity and health.

The "Cold" War Experiment

In 1991 a group of American and British scientists proved what most of us already know—stress can make you sick.

They began by choosing almost 400 people and asking them how stressed-out they felt, either from past major events or current demands. Then these perfectly healthy individuals were purposely inoculated with cold viruses. Isolated from the everyday world, this group of human guinea pigs was observed to see if any sneezed, coughed, or showed any other signs of a cold. The scientists even counted how many tissues their subjects used to blow their noses. After one week, it was discovered that those who felt the most stressed-out were most likely to get a cold.[20] In other words, stay calm and you remain well.

■ *Makeover Hint #27—The Stress-O-Meter*

To keep stress—be it physical, mental, or emotional—at arm's length, keep an eye on your stress-o-meter. These are some signs that the stress in your life is passing into the danger zone:

- Exhaustion
- Tension headaches
- Insomnia
- Lack of concentration, forgetfulness
- Mood swings, and erratic emotional behavior
- Nightmares
- Recurrent infections, like colds
- Tearfulness
- Tight muscles
- Muscle spasms
- Vague pain

Minimize the Negative;
Accentuate the Positive

The next phase in your Immunity Makeover is to minimize those substances that put a strain on your defense system (and other body parts, like the liver). These range from tobacco to recreational drugs to unnecessary medications. I realize that abandoning an addictive habit, like smoking, is easier said than done. And offering a comprehensive plan for battling addictions is beyond the scope of this book. However, a short treatise on why taking such a step is best for you and your immune system is outlined below.

Tobacco

Cigarette smoking is the main avoidable cause of death in the United States[21], and possibly an immunity depressor.[22] Nicotine is most often blamed for tobacco's deleterious effects. However, carbon monoxide, tar and an array of other toxic materials support nicotine's role in inviting a variety of cancers, heart disease, atherosclerosis, cataracts (see Chapter 13), chronic lung disease, and increased susceptibility to illness in general.[23] In addition, cigarette smoking steals from you immune-hungry nutrients, such as folic acid and vitamin B_{12}.[24]

This advice isn't just for smokers, but also for those who live with second-hand smoke—so called passive smokers. No longer is it cool to sit among your smoking friends; for doing so also tramples on your immunity. Passive tobacco smoke may increase your risk of lung cancer.[25] Children who live in smoking homes are more prone to ear infections, inflamed tonsils (which are often removed as a result), respiratory infections, Sudden Infant Death Syndrome, as well as asthma in susceptible youngsters.[26] Stop smoking tip: Sip on dandelion tea to help remove tobacco toxins.

Recreational Drugs

Marijuana, heroin, cocaine, and other fun-drugs can make your immune system miserable. It's the opinion of some experts that these recreational substances may be what makes an individual vulnerable to AIDS and other viruses.[27] Intravenous cocaine, for instance, decreases the white blood cells called lymphocytes in rats; the more they're given, the greater the fall.[28] Other immune-devastating drugs include the opiates (morphine, opium), marijuana, and nitrite inhalants ("poppers").[29] Besides their direct bombardment on body defenses, these drugs rob immune vitality by pilfering away vitamins and minerals[30]—the very same nutrients used to uplift your germ guard.

Alcohol

Alcohol often goes hand in hand with smoking and drug use; well over 80 percent of alcoholics also smoke.[23] So, what's that got to do with an Immunity Makeover? Plenty. Besides depleting nutrients used to fuel your defenses, alcohol has been shown to slow down white blood cells in nutritionally intact people.[31] So much for that hot brandy cold cure.

Medications

An Immunity Makeover accomplishes many things, one of which is better health so you have less need for strong medication. Unfortunately, there's a Catch-22 when you're ill. Often the very medicines you rely on for relief come with a laundry list of side effects, including immune suppression. Our most common painkillers—aspirin, acetaminophen (Tylenol®) and ibuprofen (Advil®, Motrin®)—also stomp on body defenses. Australian researchers discovered that taking aspirin and acetaminophen for achiness during a cold not only crushed subjects' defenses, but *increased* nasal stuffiness.[32] While antibiotics are a welcome treatment for serious bacterial infections, their overuse has created "super-bugs" resistant to this medicine. In addition, chronic[33] and frequent[34] antibiotic use diminishes the body's ability to resist such bugs—super or otherwise.

Then there are medications prescribed purposely to impair immunity. I see many patients using these drugs, like gold and methotrexate for rheumatoid arthritis; prednisone used to curtail inflammation, or steroid nasal sprays for chronic sinus infections also harm immunity.

While I make it a policy never to suggest that a patient or reader discontinue medication prescribed by their other physician, I do encourage everyone to learn about the adverse effects of these substances and help each find safer, immune-friendly options. These may include lifestyle changes (as discussed in this chapter), herbs, and nutrients. Part Two offers many ideas for a variety of conditions. However, anyone who is afflicted with a serious condition or who has been taking a prescription medication for months or more should work with the prescribing doctor and a practitioner experienced in natural therapies before making changes. We want to make over your immunity, but not at the expense of your safety.

■ Makeover Hint #28—Fewer Chemicals, More Immunity

Get rid of the superfluous chemicals in your life, and you'll enliven your immunity. California researcher Aristo Vojdani, Ph.D., found that individuals chronically exposed to industrial chemicals— trimellitic anhydride, formaldehyde, aromatic hydrocarbons—from working in computer manufacturing plants for a decade or more suffered from significant immune system malfunction.[35] For hints on how to rid your life of poisons, see Chapter 3.

Boost Your Immunity with Plants

One final step to defending your immune system is through the use of herbs. Mother Nature has covered our world with immune-strengthening plants to keep us healthy and cure us when sick. Barrie learned the value of one such herb when she and her one-and-a-half-year-old son were both sick with pneumonia. Barrie knew a little bit about medicinal herbs but hadn't used them much. Her young son wasn't getting better from the penicillin the doctor prescribed, so she began giving him capsules of garlic and Echinacea, a wildflower native to the state where she lived, South Dakota. Within three days, Barrie saw an improvement in her son; a couple of weeks later he was completely well. And he's been pneumonia-free ever since. Now Barrie always relies on this formula to treat her family when they come down with winter illness. "It takes a little longer before their symptoms turn around," she admits, "four days, compared to the 48-hour improvement you see with antibiotics. But their sickness doesn't recur, something I never saw with penicillin."

The purple coneflower (Echinacea) works by not only killing bacteria and viruses (antibiotics only attack the former), but also by kickstarting your immune system into action—something most medications can't do. You can also turn to goldenseal (*Hydrastis canadensis*), licorice (*Glycyrrhiza glabra*), *Astragalus membranaceous* and *Ligustrum lucidum* to stimulate your defenses. Unless you are skilled in herbal medicine, reserve these herbs for acute infections, taking them for a maximum of 10 straight days. If you want to repeat this cycle, take a four-day rest first.

Many foods are natural immune beautifiers and can be a regular part of meals. Garlic takes first place as an immune-enhancing bug fighter, in addition to its role in warding off cancer and protecting your heart from disease. Take heed: don't cook the medicine out of your garlic. That pungent, garlicky smell comes from volatile oils like allicin and is responsible for most of garlic's good deeds. The more you cook it, the less healing it is. Also, crush it prior to eating for the most benefit.

Campbell's (of soup fame) is now distributing fresh shiitake mushrooms (*Lentinus edodes*), found in many grocery stores. While rather expensive, these succulent, meaty fungi contain a polysaccharide called lentinan that supports immune function.[36] If you can't find shiitakes in your local market, try a natural foods store or Asian shop where the dried versions are often sold. Revitalize these dried mushrooms by submerging them in water for three hours or overnight; add both the fleshy mushroom and soaking water to your cooking.

Inflammation, be it from a nasty cut or arthritis, is part of immunity and can be tempered with ingredients in your spice cupboard. Ginger, as a powder, root, or tea, has been shown to decrease joint and muscular swelling when eaten daily for several months.[37] Turmeric also works this way.[37]

■ *Makeover Hint #29—Brew a "Cuppa" Purple Coneflower Tea*

To keep your immune system humming, drink purple coneflower tea on a regular basis. This majestic daisy-like wild flower is an attractive addition to any garden, for those who enjoy growing their own herbs. Or you can purchase the dried plant loose or in tea bags from most health food stores and some grocery stores. For prevention drink a cup every other day; as a treatment drink three cups a day while sick or during stressful and susceptible times like winter. Here's how you make it:

- Add one tea bag or one tablespoon of dried herb to a mug.
- Fill your cup with boiling water.
- Cover, and let steep for 10 minutes.
- Relax and enjoy.

This tea recipe works for most teas containing the leaf, flower, or other soft parts of a plant. If your dried herb is made of the hard woody portions, boil and then simmer it in a covered pot for 30 minutes. Strain before drinking.

Sunbathe Sensibly

Contrary to what you've read about avoiding sun exposure, sunlight is essential to our well-being. For example, 15 to 20 minutes of the sun's warm rays help our bodies convert vitamin D to its active form. However, too much of this good thing may harm immunity. Studies suggest that long-term exposure to the sun's ultraviolet-B (UV-B) rays not only increases risk for sunburn, skin cancer, and eye damage, but dampens immunity as well.

People with a history of basal or squamous cell skin cancer are most susceptible. Skin pigmentation is not protective. Ironically, UV radiation (both therapeutically and with sunlight) is used medically to treat skin conditions like acne and psoriasis. However, research now suggests that over-indulgence lowers resistance especially to infections like herpes, and may in fact increase how often, how long, or how severe each outbreak is.[38] So what should you do? Practice moderation with daily, short periods in the sun.

Immunity Makeover Checkup

You should be feeling sick-free and alive. These are the steps you've just taken to get there:

- Kicked the sugar habit.
- Watched your fats.

- Took naps, breaks, and slept eight hours each night.
- Kept working on your diet. (I told you I'd harp on nutrition.) You added a general vitamin/mineral multiple to your day.
- Made sure protein levels were adequate.
- Took a look at the nicotine, alcohol, and drugs in your life; assessed medications and consulted with your doctor if needed.
- Tried some immune-boosting herbs.

For Related Problems, See

- Bronchitis
- Canker Sores
- Colds & Flu
- Coughing
- Ear Infection
- Fever
- Hay Fever
- Sore Throat
- Urinary Tract Infection
- Yeast Infections

Laboratory Tests Your Doctor Can Order

- Complete Blood Count
- Food Allergy Panel (combined IgG4 and IgE)—ELISA
- Adrenal Test: Comprehensive Hormone Profile

Chapter 7

Lasting Stress Relief

Your Body's Stress Alarms

Perched on top of each kidney is an adrenal gland. While they perform many functions, their role as "stress alarms" is particularly pertinent to modern-day life. The middle portion of the adrenals, called the medulla, produces the hormones epinephrine (adrenaline) and norepinephrine during fear or stress. Your body reacts to these hormones with a "flight or fight" response—pounding heart, faster breathing—all indications that your body is preparing to either go into battle or run from it. A pounding heart means your muscles are getting more nutrient and oxygen-rich blood; increased breathing pulls more oxygen into your lungs.

As stress alarms, adrenal glands are lifesavers during real crises—like a bear attack. But in our world, danger is less tangible. Things like a demanding boss, traffic jams, and money troubles can't be beaten off with a stick (I suppose you could, but this creates a whole new set of crises) or fled from easily. And because of that, the adrenal alarm system seems primitive. For one, all that heart-pounding adrenaline just sits there while your blood pressure soars during rush hour. During a bear attack, running or fighting wears it off. Secondly, today we are faced with many more intangible hazards than the average bear fighter of long ago.

But the adrenals are more than stress alarms. They're responsible for producing steroid hormones such as aldosterone, which maintains normal blood pressure by balancing sodium, potassium, and fluid levels. Glucocorticoids, namely the hormones cortisol and corticosterone, regulate blood pressure, support normal muscle function, promote protein breakdown, distribute body fat, and increase blood sugar as needed. This hormone class is most noted for its anti-inflammatory properties, hence the popularity of artificial cortisone as a medication. Adrenal glands also make sex hormones, namely testosterone and estrogen, and dehydroepiandrosterone (DHEA), which is currently gaining fame as an anti-aging supplement.

Signs Your Adrenal Glands Need a Makeover

Speeding through life, while at times exhilarating, is also tiring. Yet rather than learn how to relax and take time to sleep, we cover the dark circles of fatigue with make-up and rely on caffeinated energy. Minor aches and pains are ignored—after all, we're not getting any younger—or temporarily treated with a pain pill. Then we wonder why this swift and surface-like way we care for our bodies results in bigger problems down the road.

Relentless stress without outlet also tires out your adrenal glands and causes them to atrophy or shrink. A little stress is OK, and in fact saves us from danger. But when these alarms are rung continuously without a bear in sight—kind of like the little boy who cried wolf—then the adrenals get tuckered out. What you feel is exhaustion, stomach upset, insomnia or sleepiness, irritability, headaches, and that all too familiar stressed-out feeling. Some women may develop premenstrual syndrome as elevated cortisol levels leave the body progesterone-poor. Others develop allergies easily or are open to every cold, flu, and other infection floating by (see Chapter 6). Look at making over your adrenals, as well, if you've taken prednisone or other cortisone medications for a long time.

Secrets of Stress Reduction

What is stress? That's easy, you might say. It's the boss yelling at me, the kids yelling at me, my spouse yelling at me—any situation that makes me uptight. True, but stress is not strictly mental or emotional. It's anything, physical, mental, emotional, environmental, social, that attempts to push your body out of balance. This means illness is a stress. Injury, be it a cut or broken leg, is a stress. Surgery, traveling, Christmas (whether you like it or not), getting married, having a baby, winning the lottery, drinking alcohol, smoking cigarettes, eating a bag of chips and a 24-ounce cola are all stresses. Why? Because they challenge your body. Fatty foods, in fact, have been shown to hurt your ability to deal with stress.

Beth Tannenbaum, a neuroscientist from McGill University's Douglas Hospital Research Center in Montreal fed 60 rats a high-fat diet; another 60 were served low-fat fare. She placed some of her subjects in tense situations and found that the fat eaters recovered more slowly from stress than those rats that watched what they ate.[1]

So does this mean all this stuff is bad for you? Not necessarily. Certainly you want to keep junk food down, and stick as much as you can to a wholesome diet. But when it comes to mental/emotional stress, it can be a good thing. It's what keeps us animated and alive. It's the reason for living. I, for one, wouldn't mind winning the lottery at all, and would welcome the stress it brings. For I know that our adrenal glands and body are equipped to handle a certain amount of pressure, and when healthy, bounce back rather nicely. The trick is for you to recognize the stresses in your life, and to keep them in line so they don't overtax your adrenal glands. This is the first step in your Adrenal Makeover. (For more hints on dealing with stress, see Battle Stress for Better Defense and Makeover Hint #27 in Chapter 6.)

■ Makeover Hint #30—List Your Stress Excesses

Take 15 minutes, and write down everything that you feel creates tension in your life and on your adrenals (besides making lists). Include pressures at work and home, dietary indulgences, too much or too little exercise or sleep, illness, surgeries, drugs (prescription, over-the-counter, or otherwise). You get the idea.

When you're done, star everything you have some control over. Then start making changes that will turn your stress excesses into vitalizing tension.

Six Adrenal Super Nutrients

In order to carry out all their duties, the adrenal glands rely on you to feed them well. Specific to their diet are vitamins B_6 and C, magnesium, and zinc. If you feast on alfalfa sprouts, citrus fruits, and broccoli, there'll be lots of vitamin C in your meals. Whole grains and green leafy vegetables give you B_6 and magnesium. Zinc is found in abundance in soybeans, pumpkin, sunflower seeds, and eggs. Lean meats gives you additional B_6 and zinc.

Potassium, plentiful in most produce, particularly bananas, as well as in whole grains, dried fruits, legumes and sunflower seeds, is another plus for hard working adrenals. In tandem with this, it's important to limit salt and salt-laden foods like pickles, processed cheeses and most canned foods. So eating canned (high salt) vegetables (high potassium) is rather pointless.

But the vitamin that appears most vital for proper adrenal operation is pantothenic acid, or vitamin B_5. When this nutrient is low— for those of you who avoid whole grains, legumes, salmon, eggs, tomatoes, and sweet potatoes—the adrenals shrink and tell-tales signs of adrenal exhaustion appear. Of course, as you slowly improve your eating habits and include whole foods, not only will your adrenals make a recovery, but your entire health will transform during the makeover process. For times when stress is particularly cruel to your adrenals, load up on these nutrients by using a high-potency vitamin and mineral multiple supplement.

■ *Makeover Hint #31—Whip Up This Adrenal Appetizer*

For some zing when you're zapped, create this flavorful snack full of adrenal-pleasing nutrients. Mix together:

1 banana, sliced up (rich in potassium)

1 cup strawberries, diced (lots of vitamin C here)

Top with a mixture of:

1 Tbsp Brewer's yeast (vitamin B_6 and zinc)

1 Tbsp of wheat germ (vitamin B_5 and more zinc)

1/4 cup of ground-up nuts, especially almonds (for magnesium)

Don't Burst your Balloon

I want you to think of yourself as a balloon, and stress as air. The more stress you add to your life, the fuller you get until one day the pressures of life are so numerous you feel like you're going to burst—not unlike an overblown balloon. The trick to managing stress, then, is to constantly gauge how full your balloon is and not let it get so full that it'll pop. How do you do that?

There are a couple of ways. One is to keep an eye on the number of stressors in your life, and to keep these to a manageable amount. (See Makeover Hint #30). The other is to make sure you have enough reserves to handle these demands. Remember, one sign of a healthy person is someone who is resilient enough to handle unexpected physical and emotional demands, like the flu, a sick child that's awake all night, bad news, a long car ride, a piece of birthday cake. You can take care of this by following all the Adrenal Makeover suggestions in this chapter; the other way is to implement some of these ideas:

- Get eight hours of sleep each night as often as possible.
- Make a wholesome diet the rule, not the exception.
- Schedule in restful breaks throughout the day.
- Pretend exercise is as important as brushing your teeth—then do it as often.
- Don't sweat the small stuff.

■ *Makeover Hint #32—Play Bullseye Bingo*

Part of stress control comes from deciding which demands in life need attention, and which do not. One way to help you prioritize, and thus lower tension levels, is to play Bullseye Bingo. My husband, Chris, a business trainer, taught me this method and uses it all the time during his Stress for Success seminars. You can use this game to gain perspective with the people in your life, work, household chores, and other time-eating, stress-inducing factors.

Grab a blank piece of paper and pen. Draw a bullseye like the one on the following page.

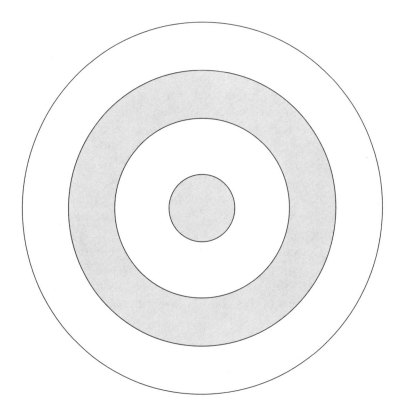

Then select a category of stress, say, the people in your life. Write your name at the center of your bullseye. Next, jot down the people most important to you in the next circle. Continue to do this with all the individuals you deal with regularly or are emotionally tied to. The farther away they are in the bullseye from you, the less important they are to you. For example, your children and spouse may be in the circle directly next to you. When there's discord between them and you, it's worth the energy and time it takes to iron out differences. On the other hand, the mailman has no VIP status in your life and sits on the most outer ring of your bullseye. It's not worth your emotional energy to ensure that you and your mailman have a smooth relationship.

This kind of diagram allows you to gain perspective on what's really significant in your daily life, and what's worth your time and energy. You have only so much time; using it indiscriminately creates stress and a drain on your adrenals.

Give Coffee a Break

"A cup of coffee is a miracle," say Heinrich Edward Jacob in *Coffee, the Epic of a Commodity*. Unfortunately this miraculous beverage and its caffeinated cousins do a number on adrenal glands. Save your adrenals, and cut coffee, black tea, colas, chocolate, and cocoa down or out of your routine. Here's why.

Sanford Bolton, Ph.D., and his colleagues from St. John's University in New York were curious about how exactly caffeine affects our stress alarms, so they enlisted the help of 11 volunteers. After serving them the equivalent of one cup of coffee a day for a week, the researchers found that adrenal function declined in subjects who were not regular caffeine users. Subjects who labeled themselves as moderate to high users (two to six cups daily for two or more years) were unaffected, probably because their adrenal function was already diminished—by chronic caffeine consumption—before the experiment began.

One of the researchers, Dr. Martin Feldman, reported that 65 percent of his new patients who complained of fatigue drank three or more cups of coffee or black tea each day. As these patients' fatigue worsened, they increased caffeine to boost their energy. Caffeine bolsters adrenal function by increasing epinephrine and norepinephrine release.[2] Not the thing for stressed-out, adrenally-sapped individuals.

■ *Makeover Hint #33—Drink a Soothing Cup of Tea*

Instead of sipping on coffee during breaks, look to herbal teas as a non-stimulating, adrenal-friendly way of relaxing. Teas with a calming influence include peppermint, chamomile, valerian, passion flower, or skullcap. Drinking these teas also helps you avoid the over-stimulating effects of caffeine.

Curing the Blood Sugar Blues

If missing a meal makes you grouchy; if you shake, rattle, and roll between meals; if your eyes glaze over, your mind shuts down, and you collapse within an hour of your coffee and Danish breakfast;

you may well be part of the "dysglycemic club." Dysglycemia (literally "bad blood sugar") is one of the new labels being used in place of hypoglycemia, a state where blood sugar must be boosted every couple of hours with food. You may have heard the terms Syndrome X, carbohydrate intolerance, hyperinsulinemia, or insulin resistance describing this condition too. (These latter two descriptors technically apply to a state where the hormone insulin—which lowers blood sugar—is ineffectual.) I bring this subject up here, because there is a link to your adrenal glands.

Those same stimulating hormones—epinephrine and norepinephrine—that get you hot and bothered during stress, also raise your blood sugar. The idea is that you need plenty of available food to keep you going as you run from (or fight) that bear. So if you're under a load of stress, for whatever reason, your poor adrenals are going to be pumping out higher-than-usual amounts of adrenaline. Eventually your adrenals are going to get tired; less adrenaline means less blood-sugar-raising back-up.

Adding to this is a diet heavy in sugars and refined carbohydrates (that's white bread, pastas made with white flour, white rice). Eating these foods causes blood sugar to shoot up; the pancreas counters with a burst of insulin and blood sugar drops. Next the adrenals step in with their stimulating hormones to bring plummeting blood sugar to a halt and try to hoist it back up. And so begins the vicious bad blood sugar cycle. The liver, thyroid, and pituitary glands are also affected. All of this sounds like a play-by-play description of a sporting event. Candy Bar 1. Adrenals 0.

Besides keeping that stress in check, see Low Blood Sugar in Part Two for practical suggestions on how to solve this problem.

Soothing Herbal Help

Besides drinking relaxing herbal teas, like chamomile and valerian, you can turn to other plants for adrenal help. Borage boasts a pretty little purple flower, but it's the leaves that hold promise for your adrenal cortex. This herb is used to renew worn-out adrenal glands, whether due to unyielding stress or extensive cortisone use; it's also a good convalescent remedy. Licorice is the other adrenal-helper that comes to mind. Some of the compounds in the licorice plant, called glycosides, are very similar in structure to steroid hormones in the body. Like borage, licorice helps make over adrenal health after steroid medication or merely a trying time. Note: Don't use licorice for more than six weeks without a one- to two-week break as it can cause water retention, sodium retention and elevated blood pressure in some people. Eating plenty of high-potassium foods— most vegetables and fruits—helps offset this potential effect. Anyone who currently or previously had kidney problems or hypertension, or is now taking digitalis, should likely avoid licorice.

Wild yam provides the raw materials for drug manufacturers to make birth control pills, steroids, progesterone, and other medicinal hormones in the laboratory. Some herbal companies sell wild yam claiming the untouched version possesses these hormonal properties. There's no firm evidence that this is so. However, many herbalists add wild yam to their adrenal restorative formulas.

Ginseng is the other well-known herb used for Adrenal Makeovers. Actually ginseng refers to a group of plants, the most common of which are *Panax ginseng* (Asian ginseng) and *Eleutherococcus senticosus* (Siberian ginseng). These tonic herbs—also referred to as adaptogens because they help you *adapt* to stressful situations—are useful for those physically and emotionally draining times. And unlike stimulants like caffeine, ginseng energizes you only during time of stress, not when you take it.

■ Makeover Hint #34—How to Use Ginseng

There are many ginseng products on the market with varying prices to match. Since ginseng only works well if you purchase a good-quality product, follow these tips to get the most out of what you buy:

- Make sure you're getting the right species. See Appendix A for how to assess herbal quality.
- Use only as directed to avoid over-stimulation. Albeit rarely, some users may experience insomnia, irritability, morning diarrhea, skin rashes, or anxiety. If you do, stop using the ginseng for two weeks, then try it again at a lower dose.
- If you plan to use it over a long time, take it for two to three weeks, with a one- to two-week rest in between.
- Women should use eleutherococcus rather than Asian ginseng, as the latter may cause abnormal periods and cyclical breast pain.[3]

Revitalize With Hormonal Extracts

In addition to or in place of herbal help for your adrenals, you can try using adrenal glandular supplements. These products are derived from cattle, so may not be preferred by anyone eating a vegetarian diet. Nevertheless, using endocrine glands (adrenals, thymus, thyroid, pancreas, ovaries, testes) or their hormones is common practice in both natural and conventional medicine, though orthodox medicine favors the latter.

Adrenal (and other) glandulars provide your body with hormones, enzymes, building blocks for hormones, and nutrients required by that particular endocrine organ. For maximum effectiveness, you need to choose a product that has been prepared in such a way that these vital components have not been destroyed. According to Dr. Michael Murray in his excellent work, *Encyclopedia of Nutritional Supplements* (Prima Publishing, 1996), the "predigested soluble concentrates" are the most effective. For a more in-depth discussion on this topic, refer to his book.

I can personally attest to the benefits of using adrenal glandulars. Immediately following graduation from naturopathic medical school, I was a wreck. Although I attempted to stick to a healthful existence during my training (after all, that is what I was taught everyday), the stress of study, a new marriage, the death of my husband's mother, and a long list of other pressures finally wore me down. I was exhausted and my adrenals were shot. On the advice of a colleague, I began taking an adrenal glandular supplement. Within one month I felt considerably better. After three months, I was well on the road to recovery. Of course, putting my natural health ideas into practice—like managing stress, breathing, eating right, exercising, sleeping—was mandatory; yet, I believe the glandular supplement was a helpful boost.

■ *Makeover Hint #35—What about DHEA?*

You may have heard about dehydroepiandrosterone (DHEA), an adrenal hormone that is the precursor for other hormones, and in some cases mimics other hormones (see Chapter 10 for more info). Because of its central role in hormonal biochemistry, supplemental DHEA has many effects on people, most reported of which is a sense of well-being. It's also tempting to use DHEA as an adrenal rejuvenator. DHEA is sold in most health food stores and drugstores. But before you run out and stock up, read this:

- DHEA is a hormone, not an herb or vitamin.
- We don't know the long-term effects of indiscriminate supplementation.
- It is most effective in people who are deficient. You can be tested for this by your doctor.
- DHEA is helpful as a treatment. Sometimes dosages are very high; you should not take more than 10 mg of DHEA a day without professional supervision.
- Women have more side effects from DHEA than men. (DHEA is an androgen or male hormone.)
- It's better to first try boosting your DHEA levels naturally by reducing stress and following the other suggestions in the Adrenal Makeover.

The Laughter Remedy

Laughter truly is the best medicine. Norman Cousins, author of *Anatomy of an Illness*, helped popularize the notion that laughing and humor were crucial to healing. Diagnosed with the crippling disease of ankylosing spondylitis, Cousins was informed by his physician that he had one chance in 500 of recovering completely. Interestingly, Cousins was familiar with Hans Selye's work and knew of the connection between stress and adrenal function, and Selye's contention that negative emotions adversely affected the body. So Cousins' solution to his incurable condition was to chuckle his way to wellness, together with other immune-enhancing, adrenal-replenishing steps.[4] As an epilogue to his recuperation, Cousins spent the last dozen years of his life exploring the science behind laughter at the UCLA Medical School in the Department of Behavioral Medicine with his Humor Research Task Force.[5]

The American Association for Therapeutic Humor (AATH) has taken Cousins' work a step further with its membership of 600 physicians and health care practitioners who'd like to see laughter become part of every treatment plan. A good belly laugh not only relaxes you, but helps immunity (and adrenal function) by lowering cortisol levels.[6, 7] Many nurses and others in the medical field are taking therapeutic humor very seriously. Besides incorporating buffoonery into their protocols, practitioners can attend Clown Camp at the University of Wisconsin in La Crosse, subscribe to several newsletters and books on the subject, listen to tapes of funny songs by and about their peers (there's Nursing Notes and the Chordiac Arrest), and attend conferences. See Appendix C for more information on the AATH and humor-related newsletters, and visit the AATH website at http://www.callamer.com/itc/aath for a great collection of jokes.

■ *Makeover Hint #36—Jump Start Snickers*

Mirth doesn't always appear at the drop of a hat. If you're having difficulty getting into the mood, try this to jump-start your laughter.

- Stand up.
- Put your hands on your belly.
- Say "Ha" several times slowly until you can feel your belly move under your fingers.
- Now increase the speed and volume of your "Ha's" until they jump-start into continuous laughter.

Warning, this technique works best in a crowd.

Still Not Laughing?

Need a few more tips on how to handle stress? Try these on for size:

- Make a list of things you've already done.
- Bill your doctor for the time you spent in his waiting room.
- Use your Visa to pay your Mastercard.
- When someone says "Have a Nice Day!" respond that you have other plans.

Adrenal Makeover Checkup

Once you've stopped laughing, scan this list to make sure you've done all you can for your adrenals.

- Taken control of stress.
- Added adrenal nutrients and foods to your life.
- Put people and situations in perspective with Bullseye Bingo.
- Given caffeine a break.
- Tried a few adrenal-pleasing herbs.
- Considered adrenal glandulars.
- Learned how to laugh.

For Related Problems, See

- Anxiety
- Fatigue
- Headaches
- Insomnia
- Low Blood Sugar

Laboratory Tests Your Doctor Can Order

- Adrenal Test: Comprehensive Hormone Profile
- DHEA Levels or DHEA-Sulfate Levels

Chapter 8

Improve Circulation and Live Longer

Understanding Your Heart and Circulation

Heart disease is the number one killer in the United States. For that reason alone, you should pay close attention to this chapter. The heart is a muscular pump that drives blood through an intricate highway of vessels in your body, what we call circulation. If blood vessels are the body's highways, then blood is the truck that carries food particles, gases, garbage, hormones, and other chemicals from place to place as needed to keep your body going.

Arteries form the first section of circulatory highway, running from the heart to the rest of the body carrying oxygen-rich blood. Capillaries are the bridges between arteries and veins, and are the place where the body pulls oxygen and nutrients out of the blood in exchange for waste and carbon dioxide. Veins then cart the body's debris back up to the heart (and liver) for disposal.

There are four chambers in the heart: two atria and two ventricles. The right atrium, a kind of primer pump, is the first to receive "used" blood from the body. Its job is to push blood into the heart's power pump, or right ventricle. From here blood is sent up to the lungs where carbon dioxide is exchanged for oxygen. The body uses oxygen as fuel for various metabolic functions; carbon dioxide is what's left over. Once blood is recharged with oxygen, it travels down to the second primer pump, the left atrium, where it's given a boost to the left ventricle. Then this most powerful heart pump forces the blood through the rest of the body.

The Plus Side of a Good-Hearted Makeover

Once you understand what your heart and circulation do, you can see how important it is to maintain optimum cardiac function. When the highways of your body are clogged or your pump is too weak or diseased to work well, then the body can't get enough oxygen or nutrients, or dispose of its refuse.

One of the most common circulatory conditions is atherosclerosis, where blood vessels become thick and hard. Unfortunately, symptoms are often silent until heart or blood vessel disease is advanced. Most Americans can assume they have some degree of atherosclerosis; studies have shown that this insidious disease is even apparent in some children.[1] Your chance of developing this and other heart-related conditions increases when you have high blood pressure, high total cholesterol, LDL (bad) cholesterol (the kind that sticks to artery walls) and triglycerides, and low HDL (good) cholesterol (which travels to the liver for disposal). However, according to research that began appearing over a decade ago, our current method of testing blood fats is incomplete. We also need to measure something called "apolipoproteins." These molecules may actually be better markers for detecting coronary artery disease than cholesterol and triglycerides, according to the research team at the Mayo Medical School in Rochester, Minnesota.[2]

If you smoke, have diabetes, or are overweight, then your risk of heart troubles goes up. We mustn't forget that genetics play a part in heart disease; not everything's your fault. On the other hand, a sedentary lifestyle and eating a high-saturated fat, low-fiber, nutrient-void diet do make matters worse.

Now let's talk about some not so well-known risk factors for heart disease. Did you know that higher-than-average levels of insulin in the blood, called hyperinsulinemia, disturb your heart and vessels? In addition, insulin resistance—that is, insulin that doesn't do its job very well—is a problem.[3] Insulin is the hormone produced by the pancreas that helps cells grasp glucose (from broken-down food) and ultimately lowers blood sugar. When insulin is high, hypoglycemic symptoms are common. (See Chapter 7.)

Protecting you against oxidative damage (that's where antioxidants come in) helps keep your blood vessels clear and healthy.

Artery disease and high blood pressure are often attributed to blood vessel damage caused by everyday wear-and-tear and an inadequate repair system. Smoking, alcohol, rancid fats, and poor nutrition contribute to this.

If you have a personal or family history of chest pain due to angina, heart disease, or heart attack, then a Cardiovascular Makeover is for you. Fortunately, your heart and circulation are greatly influenced by lifestyle. The authors of the scientific paper, "Can lifestyle changes reverse coronary heart disease?" answer this question with a resounding probably—if you adhere to a healthful diet, regular exercise, and stress control, instead of letting stress control you.[4] So whether you have high cholesterol, high triglycerides, high blood pressure, or actually feel fine, take the Heart Makeover plunge for a longer and stronger life.

Good Fats, Bad Fats—Which Ones to Eat

Eat a low-fat diet! That's the standard recommendation of most heart specialists. And while I agree somewhat with this statement, you must also realize that there's more to the fat scenario than eradicating it from your meals. Fats are vital nutrients in every diet. The trick, especially if you're prone to heart problems or have a family history, is how to eat enough of the good fats and stay healthy. Let's start with a lesson in fats.

Fats are divided into two main categories: saturated and unsaturated. The saturated fats are solid at room temperature, and primarily of animal origin; tropical oils like palm, palm kernel, and coconut are exceptions. Plant and animal fats contain *both* saturated and unsaturated portions; some also possess naturally occurring trans fatty acids. The difference is that more animal foods like egg yolks, shellfish, whole dairy products, lard, red meats, and poultry skin are top-heavy in saturated fats, while plants favor unsaturated oils. Unsaturated fats are typically liquid at room temperature and mainly of vegetable origin. There are polyunsaturated fats like the oils from safflower, soybean, sunflower, sesame, and corn. Macadamia oil, canola oil, and olive oil are considered monounsaturated fats—liquid at room temperature, but solid in the fridge.

Piling on the vegetables and whole grains will naturally shove aside many fatty foods. But don't eliminate fats entirely. Dine cautiously on the saturated fatty foods mentioned above. And when you do, remove excess fat. Skin your chickens and turkeys. Trim that marble of fat off your steak and lamb chops. Drink non-fat milk. Fill in the fat gaps with the essential fats that your body can't make but needs. Select raw, unsalted nuts and seeds. Use olive and canola oils in your cooking and salad dressings; they don't harm arteries or raise blood fat levels. Instead they help create the HDL cholesterol that protects your blood vessels. And eat all the fish you like (see Makeover Hint #41.)

There has been some research indicating that eating too much polyunsaturated oil (safflower, sunflower, soybean) may lower helpful HDL-cholesterol. This may be because these oils tend to turn rancid faster than monounsaturated oils, and rancid fats produce free radical molecules—not good for your heart or circulation.[5] Consuming rancid oils, fried foods, and high amounts of saturated fats adds to damaging oxidation, specifically of no-good LDL cholesterol, and ultimately atherosclerosis.[6] Also, be cautious when cooking with oils, since heating them increases oxidative damage.

I should mention a third category of fats, the trans fatty acids or hydrogenated vegetable oils (they also come in the partially-hydrogenated style). These fats are vegetable oils that have been altered so that they are hard at room temperature, just like saturated fats. Hence you have margarine, and the hydrogenated fats added to many processed foods like breads, salad oils, mayonnaise, and snack foods. It's been a century since the invention of hydrogenation—the method that performs this trans fatty magic—but only 20 years of a rocket-like increase in consumption. As we search for heart-friendly foods, we've been told by margarine manufacturers to use their healthful alternative to butter. In truth, trans fatty acids boost LDL and total blood cholesterol, and drag down the good HDL cholesterol.[7]

Talking about cholesterol, do you remember all the hoopla in 1989 when we were told that avoiding cholesterol-rich foods was really unnecessary? First realize that *your body* makes most of the cholesterol you own. That's right, your liver makes up to 1500 mg of this fat-like substance from saturated fats and simple sugars;

most people don't absorb more than a third of that from foods in a day. Without cholesterol your cells would collapse without their rigid covering; you'd have no sex life because you couldn't make the sex hormones estrogen, progesterone, and testosterone (see Chapter 10); you couldn't handle stress because you'd be void of cortisone (see Chapter 7); your kidneys would be at a loss in handling fluid levels without needed aldosterone (see Chapter 5); your skin would look terrible (see Chapter 12); your bones would crumble and fall (see Chapter 11); your liver couldn't make bile for fat digestion (see Chapters 3 and 4). Without cholesterol, you'd be a mess.

It's not so much eating cholesterol that raises blood cholesterol, it's saturated fats and, possibly, refined sugars (see below, Do You Have Low Blood Sugar or High Blood Pressure?). Many cultures thrive on diets with more meat, whole dairy, and fat than we as Americans (and Canadians) think is healthy, yet don't have our high cholesterol problem. This, I think, goes back to our tendency to eat processed, refined foods rather than vegetables, fruits, meats and grains in their original and organic forms. When you get your cholesterol checked, be sure to have your doctor do a complete lipid panel (see below, Laboratory Tests Your Doctor Can Order); make sure it not only includes a total cholesterol, but HDL, LDL, and apolipoproteins. All of this information together means more than cholesterol level alone.

■ **Makeover Hint #37—Eat Better Butter**

Can't give up butter? You don't have to if you use this recipe to convert your butter into this healthier version—and use it sparingly.

BETTER BUTTER

1/2 lb butter, softened

1/2 cup canola oil (fresh)

Place both ingredients in a blender or food processor. Mix until blended. Store in refrigerator. Use like pure butter. Toss unused portion after two months.

Give Your Heart the Oxygen
It Loves

Get a move on! That's the next step to a healthier heart. A sedentary existence of reading, watching TV, writing (oops), eating, sitting at the computer (me again), sewing, playing cards, or working at a desk is more than your heart and health can handle. Your muscular heart requires a regular workout and aerobic activity, that is, oxygen-filled exercise, to feed it. The Institute for Aerobics Research in Dallas knows this and proved it when it followed more than 10,000 men and 3100 women. After eight years of watching this large group, there was no doubt that the more fit one is, the lower the risk for cardiovascular disease (and cancer). According to this investigation, you can reach top physical conditioning with a mere 30–60 minute brisk walk each day.[8]

■ *Makeover Hint #38—Do the Potato*

The trick to having a healthy heart is to *do* the potato, not *be* a potato. In other words, find ways that keep you physically moving, not sedentary, during the day. For you, the potato might be a funky dance you enjoy practicing to an old Beatles tune while no one is looking. Someone else might find a brisk walk around the block four times a refreshing pick-me-up. Whatever it is, try not to sit still for more than 30 minutes at a time. Other aerobic activities include:

- Running or jogging
- Biking
- Rowing
- Cross-country skiing
- Jumping rope
- Rollerblading (or skating)
- Racing after children (I hope this counts)

Remember, if you haven't exercised on a regular basis for a long time, consult with your doctor first.

Feast on Fiber

I'm going to say it again: eat more fiber. There is no doubt that loading up on roughage each day helps not only your digestive tract and liver, but your heart as well. So if you haven't managed to insert fresh vegetables and fruits, whole wheat bread, brown rice, barley, oat bran, beans, legumes, and other high-fiber foods into your diet, for your heart's sake, now is the time.

Do you remember the oat bran craze of the early 1990s? It began, in part, because of a study done at Rush-Presbyterian-St. Luke's Medical Center in Chicago. Dr. Michael Davidson and his colleagues proved that people who ate just two ounces of oat bran (equivalent to three ounces of oatmeal) each day could lower their LDL-cholesterol by almost 16 percent in only six weeks.[9] Topped with a few walnuts and a sprinkling of raisins, that sounds like a mighty tasty way of staying fit. Beans, psyllium and vegetables have been shown to have similar effects.[10]

Young Andrew Barely Notices Barley in Healthy Cookies

Say the word "fiber," and many people cringe. What they don't know is that this essential heart nutrient can be delicious. One of my favorite ways to slip fiber into my children's diet is by substituting barley flour for white flour in cookies, muffins, waffles, and loaves. A couple of summers ago, I was doling out fresh homemade barley cookies. Adam's friend, Andrew, was visiting and, knowing that we served "healthy food" in our house, was slightly hesitant about sampling my baking. Nevertheless, he took a cookie and began nibbling. A few minutes later I felt a tap on my shoulder. "Mrs. Aesoph," he said, "can I have another cookie?" Of course I agreed. With a large grin on his face, Andrew ran over to the cookie dish, grabbed two, then three, and escaped outside with my son. Barley wins out again.

Eat Heart-Felt Nutrients Everyday

For years, medical experts believed malnutrition posed no threat to the heart. Modern research has proved beyond a doubt, however, that hearty eating is vital if you want your circulation and its pump—

the heart—to serve you well. The first step is to follow those nutritious steps outlined in previous chapters. Next, take a close look at specific vitamins and minerals that affect blood flow and the heart.

Antioxidants, like vitamins A, C, and E, beta carotene, and various flavonoids, are recommended not only to prevent cancer and premature aging, but also heart disease. The reason? Once again, it's because of their free radical scavenging abilities. Those darn free radicals, remember, are highly reactive molecules that damage cells all over the body, including the heart and vessels.

So where do we find free-radical fighters? The best place to start is always food. Colorful vegetables and fruits are among the most flavonoid-rich, antioxidant-full edibles available to us. Dutch researchers gave us hard evidence why eating your greens (and oranges and reds and purples) is heart-friendly. These scientists followed more than 500 men and wrote down what they ate. Five years later, they found that men who ate the most flavonoid-rich foods were half as likely to have a heart attack or die from coronary heart disease as were those eating the least amount. Flavonoids are thought to prevent atherosclerosis and reduce blood clot formation.[11]

Vitamin E, also an antioxidant found in asparagus, avocados, tomatoes, and green leafies, is famous in cardiovascular circles as a heart protector. A Scottish study revealed that men with the lowest amounts of vitamin E in their blood were two and a half times more likely to suffer from angina, or chest pain, than those with high levels.[12] Vitamin C's place in heart health is as an antioxidant, blood pressure reducer, cholesterol shrinker, and a nutrient that helps the body hold on to vitamin E.[13] Oranges, grapefruit, and other citrus fruits are vitamin C warehouses.

Magnesium deficiency has been linked to hypertension, arrhythmias, and congestive heart failure.[14] This mineral is thought to enhance blood flow, relax blood vessel walls, prevent abnormal heart rhythm and even stop blood clots from forming. Some doctors use intravenous magnesium in cases of suspected heart attack to help reduce death rates by one half.[15] Luckily, high fiber foods, like dark green vegetables and whole grains, are also high in magnesium. In addition to these nutrients, chromium, taurine, vitamin B_6, niacin, L-carnitine, pantethine, calcium, copper, and lecithin all play roles in cardiac health. Of course, these nutrients are best taken in food, or a well-balanced nutrient supplement. For specific, individualized recommendations, see a nutrition-wise cardiologist.

When nothing seems to help bring your cholesterol or blood pressure down, ask your doctor to run a homocysteine test. Too much of this, a metabolite of the amino acid methionine, hurts your arteries, and can ultimately lead to atherosclerosis and heart attack. The solution is supplementation, with the right nutrients, based on your laboratory test. Vitamin B$_6$ urges homocysteine to convert to cystathione (that's good), while folic acid pushes homocysteine back to methionine.[16] Vitamin B$_{12}$ may also help.

Treating High Blood Pressure or Low Blood Sugar?

Fats are often the bad guys when it comes to rescuing your poor heart. But several studies point the finger at sugar as well. Next step to your Heart Makeover is to throw out the Valentine chocolates and look to the Low Blood Sugar section in Part Two for advice. Italian scientists examined the sugar-heart connection more closely. Their preliminary evidence showed that in some cases high blood pressure is caused by insulin resistance.[17] This means hypertension is more of a blood sugar problem than one of blood fats. When I spoke with Dr. Jonathan Wright, a well-known nutrition-expert a couple of years ago, he told me that as a matter of course he runs a glucose-insulin tolerance test on all his patients with essential hypertension. This is the most common type of high blood pressure—90 percent of cases—and has no "known" cause. More than half, he says, come back with high insulin levels and/or low blood sugar. When Dr. Wright then treats these patients for these problems, their blood pressures invariably fall.

Another interesting tidbit. Several animal and human studies have implicated sugar as the accessory in salt-related hypertension. There's a strong suggestion that white table sugar especially, in combination with salt, raises blood pressure substantially.[18] So is it the salt or the sugar? Salt-sensitive animals are more susceptible; that may be the case for people too.

■ *Makeover Hint #40—What is a Glucose-Insulin Tolerance Test?*

The standard way to test for low blood sugar is by checking blood glucose levels with the glucose tolerance test (GTT). Most doctors look not only for a glucose level that's fallen to 50 milligrams or less per 100 milliliters of blood, but also for symptoms to occur while the glucose level is at this low point. Some natural health physicians feel this method only looks at half the picture. They also want to see insulin levels, which can rise abnormally (while glucose levels are normal) and cause hypoglycemic-like symptoms. This is the glucose-*insulin* tolerance test.

The QT on Q10

A safe and effective treatment for some types of heart disease, like angina, congestive heart failure, and high blood pressure, is coenzyme Q10. It's also known as ubiquinone because of its ubiquitous nature—it's naturally found in all plant- and animal-based foods. Specifically, it's an essential ingredient of the mitochondria or energy packs that run the cells and body; it's especially high in the heart. Heart disease increases your need for this enzyme.[19] If you decide to try this supplement, give it at least one to two months before you expect results; 50 to 100 mg daily is the usual dose.

Add More Onion, Garlic, and Spice

The heart and blood vessels love well-seasoned cooking; if you do too, you're in luck. My grandfather has been growing garlic for decades; once a week he sups on a goodly amount. It's not just his Ukrainian heritage that drives him to this bulb; he knows garlic's reputation for lowering the fats in blood—cholesterol and triglycerides—more effectively than diet alone. A group of German researchers proved this with 10 of the 20 patients they treated with garlic; all were also treated with diet. Cholesterol levels fell for all 20 patients, though more so in the garlic group. However, only the garlic-eaters saw their triglycerides fall as well. This thrilled the University of Munich scientists, who commented: "Drugs used to do this are almost invariably burdened with side effects—some of them just a nuisance but jeopardizing compliance, some of them serious, possibly out-weighing the therapeutic benefit by increasing the incidence of non-cardiovascular death. In this dilemma a harmless but efficient antilipid medication (*like garlic*) would be appreciated."[20] Onion, a cousin of garlic, offers much the same protection.[21]

For those who enjoy hot and spicy foods, you'll be happy to note that cayenne pepper is a wonderful Heart Makeover condiment. Capsaicin, one of cayenne's many constituents, promotes heart health by decreasing the clumping together of platelets,[22] tiny disk-shaped particles found in blood that assist with blood vessel repair and blood clotting. However, when arteries are damaged and not adequately repaired, for example when nutrient levels are low, platelets congregate in these areas and contribute to clogged arteries. Cayenne decreases this tendency without interfering with platelets' normal duties.

Ginger is another spice to add to your cooking as part of your Heart Makeover. Officially known as *Zingiber officinale*, ginger protects your heart through its antioxidant and tonifying effects[23] as well as its ability to diminish inflammation.[24] Rather than using aspirin as your blood-thinning medicine, rely on ginger. This way you not only avoid gastric bleeding and upset, but actually promote better digestion, help open blocked arteries,[25] and lower cholesterol.

■ *Makeover Hint #41—Spice Up Your Fish*

Eating as little as one or two fish dishes per week may prevent coronary heart disease.[26] For a tasty difference, spice up your broiled fish by flavoring it with a splash of cayenne, a sprinkling of diced garlic (fresh, not powdered) or a few thick slices of heart-loving onion.

How About Hawthorn?

I include a side note about hawthorn here because it once sat in the food category as well, in jam and wine. This plant with the rosehip-like berries is also a traditional cure for many heart ailments. *Crataegus laevigata* (or *oxyacntha*) and *Crataegus monogyna*—all are used—give us their berries, leaves, and blossoms to reduce blood pressure and serum cholesterol, prevent angina, and act as a general heart tonic. You can certainly take it in pill form, but wouldn't a cup of hawthorn berry tea be nice?

Cut Down on Caffeine

Again with the coffee, or should I say caffeine. There's evidence afloat that ingesting the stuff raises blood pressure and the risk of heart disease in people not used to this stimulant. At least that's what Drs. Dan Sharp and Neal Benowitz found in a group of bus drivers. Those who drank caffeinated beverages regularly appeared to have adjusted to this effect.[27] Perhaps it has something to do with adrenal exhaustion (see Chapter 7). I find it interesting that out of the 281 San Francisco bus drivers these doctors selected, only 10 percent used caffeine infrequently, that is, two to four times a week.

Across the Atlantic in the Netherlands, scientists found another reason to be wary of coffee when it comes to matters of the heart. Substances called cafestol and kahweol, that float around in unfiltered coffee as small oily droplets and coffee grounds, raise both cholesterol and triglycerides in the blood. The worst of these coffees are the Middle Eastern coffee brews (Turkish, Greek, and—Israeli mud?) and the boiled Scandinavian type. French press and mocha were next, followed by espresso and percolated. The most sediment-free coffees came from the drip filter; paper filter came out on top with the cleanest coffee and the least grounds.[28]

So there you have it. For a clean bill of health, avoid caffeine and coffee. As a compromise, imbibe occasionally (no more than four times weekly), and use a paper filter. Or try the next Makeover Hint.

■ *Makeover Hint #42—Drink Green Caffeine*

Drinking green tea is another coffee option. Japanese scientists found that the more of this healthful tea their subjects drank, the lower their total cholesterol and triglyceride levels were. More importantly, the good HDL cholesterol went up and bad LDL cholesterol declined.[29] I should note here that green tea does in fact contain caffeine. However, it obviously heralds benefits not found with coffee. If you're concerned about caffeine, try the decaffeinated version of green tea.

Say No to Smoking (and Sitting in a Smoky Room)

Here are two more reasons to give up cigarettes: higher triglyceride levels and less HDL cholesterol—both risk factors for coronary heart disease. Want some more? Years of puffing constricts the blood vessels traveling to your heart, raises your heart rate, and boosts your blood pressure.[30]

For you non-smokers: choose the non-smoking section of the restaurant. Avoid smoky bars and ban smoking in your home and car. If you're worried about being rude, use these facts to fortify your courage. Inhaling second-hand smoke for 20 minutes to eight hours decreases your heart's ability to receive and process oxygen. Do it on a regular basis, and your arteries get plugged, your cholesterol shoots up, blood pressure may climb, and ischemic heart disease is a possible threat.[31]

I know quitting is extremely difficult. But here's what you have to look forward to once you stop:

In 20 minutes—blood pressure drops to normal.

In 8 hours—oxygen levels in blood increase to normal; carbon monoxide drops.

In 24 hours—chance of heart attack decreases.

In 48 hours—nerve endings begin regrowing.

In 2 to 12 weeks—improved circulation.

In 1 to 9 months—energy increases.

In 5 to 10 years—chance of cancer declines.[32]

Advice on Alcohol

This is a confusing topic when it comes to a Heart Makeover. Harvard's Eric Rimm, Sc.D., told us in 1991 that drinking liquor decreases your chance of coronary disease.[33] In France, where wine is consumed like soda is in this country, coronary heart disease is lower than any other developed country. Some have called this the "French Paradox." Why is this? And does this mean that we should be drinking wine or other alcohol every day as part of a Heart Makeover? There is no simple answer.

Certainly wine—even alcohol—has a positive effect on the heart and the good HDL cholesterol in our blood. Red wine, in particular, with its antioxidant flavonoids (from the purple grapes) seems helpful. It could be that in nations where wine is a regular dinner-time beverage, nutrition is better. Maybe drinking wine *with* meals is the trick to lowering blood fats and decreasing alcohol's negative health influences. However, while the French certainly have less heart disease, alcohol abuse is a major problem, as are disease and death from other causes besides heart troubles. Dr. Timothy Regan from the New Jersey Medical School in Newark reminds us that too much booze ups blood pressure and contributes to stroke.[34]

So what should you do?

This is my advice. The occasional glass of wine, especially with dinner, is not harmful for most. Sipping on this or saki (rice wine) before dinner helps digestion, and may improve the health of your heart. The key is moderation. Also take into account your personal health history and risks. Refrain from drinking if you have liver disease or a history of it, a history of alcoholism, or are unable to have "just one." If your immunity is struggling, alcohol could make it worse. Women have special circumstances to consider. Don't drink if you're pregnant or nursing. And the risk for breast cancer does increase substantially for women who drink alcohol.[35]

How to Make Over a Broken Heart

You've heard the story of the elderly woman who dies, and only a couple of months later her husband of many years also passes away, supposedly from a broken heart. Practitioners of Traditional Chinese Medicine believe that the heart not only pumps *blood* throughout the body, but also *emotions* and *thoughts*.

We also read how driving, type A personalities are more prone to heart attacks. Is there any truth to the idea that emotions affect the heart and general health? If you read medical journals, there is.

Harvard researchers discovered that mental stress causes blocked heart arteries to constrict, which in turn reduces blood flow even more. Your heart can't remain well if its life-feeding blood vessels are clogged. Healthy vessels, on the other hand, either open slightly to allow the blood to flow more freely or remain unchanged when things get crazy.[36] High blood pressure jumps even higher in tense situations.[37] And a short fuse more easily triggers the cascade of potentially damaging hormones released when you feel threatened or ready to fight.[38]

Even doctors can get caught in the feelings and heart trap. A Duke University study found that physicians who frequently felt angry, carried cynical mistrust in their hearts, and expressed hostility toward others, had seven times the death rate during a 25-year period than did their calmer colleagues. "Trusting hearts may live longer because for them the biologic cost of situations that anger or irritate is lower," says Redford B. Williams, Jr., M.D., a lead researcher of this study.[39]

What about broken hearts? A research team that fed two bunches of bunnies high-fat, high-cholesterol foods to see how much diet affected atherosclerosis development were shocked to find that one group had 60 percent less damage. It turns out that a graduate student assigned to the less sickly rabbits also fed them large doses of love by regularly taking them out of their cages and tenderly petting them.[41] The moral here is: Keep fat intake low, but if you decide to splurge on ice cream, hug someone first.

Here are some ways to keep your heart from breaking (or to mend it):

- First of all, realize that sadness, anger, and fear are part of the richness of living. Don't avoid them, but rather welcome these emotions, experience them and move on. So-called negative feelings help us grow both personally and within our relationships.

- Second, figure out the best way for you to cope with mental and emotional pressures (see Chapter 7). For some this might mean talking with a friend or writing in a journal. Others might find exercise helpful, or a nap, or deep breathing.

- Third, keep physical stressors low—caffeine, alcohol, junk food, insufficient sleep—when emotional or mental tension increases.

- During times of grief, take a dose of the homeopathic remedy *Ignatia*.

- Last, a healthy heart is more flexible to emotional demands. Follow all the other Cardiac Makeover suggestions above so your heart won't break for other reasons.

Heart Makeover Checkup

Is your heart just bursting with happiness and good health? I knew it would. These are the steps you took to get there:

- Sorted out the good fats and the bad.
- Started exercising.
- Added more fiber to more meals. (I feel like a rabbit!)
- Ate in a healthier manner; still taking a multiple; added a few antioxidant vitamins too.
- Realized that low blood sugar came up again; better read that section.
- Spiced up meals—garlic, onions, ginger, cayenne.
- Got another reminder to give up coffee.
- Decided to avoid cigarette smoke—smokers and nonsmokers alike.
- Cut alcohol down or out.
- Made up my mind to control my anger. . . . grrrrrrr.

For Related Problems, See

- Fatigue
- Heartburn
- Indigestion
- Low Blood Sugar
- Varicose Veins

Laboratory Tests Your Doctor Can Order

- Lipid Profile (total cholesterol, HDL, LDL)
- Apolipoprotein Test
- Homocysteine; Folic Acid/B_{12} Levels
- Glucose-Insulin Tolerance Test
- Other standard cardiac tests as appropriate

Chapter 9

Attain Tiptop Muscle Tone

Staying Active for a Lifetime

You wouldn't go a day without eating, drinking, or sleeping. Yet many ignore the fourth important daily requirement for health—movement. Humans beings are meant to move every day. That can mean walking, laboring, or planned exercise. Movement gives muscles a chance to work. And when we use our muscles, other body systems are indirectly affected. Other makeover musts, like nutrition-rich foods, also help keep our muscles in tiptop shape.

Muscle is a relative term. Your heart has muscle. Then there's the smooth muscle that lines many of your organs—like the digestive tract. But the muscle we'll be speaking of in this chapter is skeletal muscle, the tissue attached to bones that allows you to reach into the cupboard, shake hands, play the piano, use a computer, and move from place to place. Most, though not all, skeletal muscles can be moved at will and are sometimes referred to as voluntary muscles.

Almost half of your body is made up of muscle. Generally speaking, muscles are attached to bone or cartilage via tendons. However, there are exceptions to this rule. The face has muscles that make you smile, chew, and cry; these blend into the skin. The tongue is a muscle too. Within each individual muscle are muscle fibers. The larger the muscle, the more fibers. Smaller muscles, like those in your eye or hand that require precise movement, have fewer fibers.

Your Muscle Makeover

The modern life is typically a sedentary one. This is in large part due to all the conveniences we've adopted: cars, washers and dryers, dishwashers, telephones, vacuums, computers, and take-out food— to name a few. That's not to say we don't all appreciate these time-saving, energy-sparing luxuries. However, because everyday chores don't keep us physically fit anymore, we must schedule "movement time" into each day.

Movement is the foundation of attaining and maintaining muscle tone; food and other things are helpful supporters. But why are toned muscles and exercise so important? Healthy, firm muscles are better able to do their job of getting us from place to place, and protecting joints. You'll also notice, as you work your way through the Natural Health Makeover plan, that movement isn't just tied to musculature. Physical, muscular fitness also revitalizes digestion, maximizes immunity, helps you manage stress and regain sexual vitality, improves circulation, and is one way to live longer. For all you exercise-shy folks who are thinking, "No way. I've never exercised, and I never will. I don't have time. I can't do it!" stop and read on. You don't have to be an athlete to enjoy the benefits of regular movement. When I write of "tiptop muscle tone," I'm not referring to body building. I just want you to squeeze as much physical movement into your daily life as possible; after all, a little bit is better than none at all. Besides wearing off excess calories, the increased oxygen flow will make you look and feel better. Believe me, once you make over your muscles as outlined below, you'll never look back.

There are three main ways to introduce movement into your life: everyday movement—using the stairs instead of the elevator; recreational or play-time movement—golf, gardening, bowling, or biking; and workout time—aerobics class, morning treadmill walk— movement that ensures that you're getting a good, sweaty workout each day.

Foolproof Fitness Test

How do you know you need to move more? Number one, how much do you move now? If you sit most of the day and don't take time for 30 to 60 minutes of planned physical activity (anything from walking to aerobics class) every day or so, then you most certainly have a movement deficiency.

The other way to tell is by listening to your body. Look for these movement deficiency signs:

- Chronic muscle tension or pain (neck, shoulders, back)
- Shortness of breath with minimal movement, for example, climbing a flight of stairs. (This may be a heart problem. Ask your doctor.)
- Insomnia.
- Frequent tension headaches.
- Constipation.
- Weight gain or problems losing weight.
- Fatigue.
- Inability to handle stress.
- Vague body aches and pains.
- Depression.
- Irritability.

Longevity Success Story

Before you take the first step to firmer muscles, I want you to read this story. Mary is a very active, healthy 83-year-old living in Aldergrove, British Columbia. One of the secrets to her longevity and well-being is exercise—not the structured kind, but that old-fashioned hard work that comes from growing up on a prairie farm, living through the Depression, and raising a family. One of Mary's loves, and the source of her daily activity, is her massive vegetable and flower garden.

Mary and her husband Mike live on a four-acre lot, one quarter of which is cultivated. Needless to say, such an ambitious garden needs constant care. Most days throughout the year, Mary dons her wide-brimmed straw hat and heads out to hoe, pull weeds, prune—whatever needs tending. And the way Mary attacks those weeds, gardening becomes a triage of aerobics, stretching, and muscle toning. Because Mary and Mike don't believe in using herbicides, all the food they raise and subsequently eat is organic and deliciously fresh, just the thing for hardworking muscles.

Everyday Energy Boosters

Not everyone can be a Mary. But each of us moves every day—even if it's just to the car and back. The best place to begin your Muscle Makeover is by capitalizing on your current everyday activities. Begin by recording for a couple of days all activity in your life. This could be running down the street to catch a bus, walking up two flights of stairs at work, taking the baby for a walk, or cleaning house. Not only will this tell you how much you move, but it will give you a starting point to make changes. Let's look at the following example.

Joe's Activity Record for April 14, 1997

Walked to the bus from home (two blocks).

Walked from the bus to work (one block).

Got up from desk two times to use copy machine, and one time to use restroom (morning).

Walked to elevator down three flights, and walked from there to cafeteria for lunch. Read the newspaper for half an hour.

Sat in meeting most of the afternoon; got up to use restroom once and to storeroom once.

Walked to bus stop (one block).

Walked home from bus stop (two blocks).

Had dinner, watched TV until bed.

Although Joe is very sedentary, there are several opportunities during his day to sneak in a little extra physical activity. To begin with, his walks to the bus each day. Rather than walking to the closest bus stop near his home, he could walk to the next bus stop a block or two down the road. Similarly, when he exits the bus near work, he could get off a stop earlier. This strategy alone could add a quarter mile of walking to his day. Instead of taking the elevator at work, Joe could take the stairs. Rather than merely eating lunch and reading the newspaper, Joe could begin his lunch hour with a brisk walk followed by lunch. His post-dinner TV watching could be partially replaced by an evening stroll with his wife or a bike ride with the kids.

Other ways you can slip exercise into your day might be shoveling the walk instead of using the snowblower; sweeping the walk with a broom, not the leaf blower—then jumping in the leaves, playing hopscotch with your kids, using your legs, not the channel changer?

■ *Makeover Hint #43—The Underexercising Trick*

Too many people give up on regular exercise before they have a chance to really begin. One reason is they overdo it. The trick to "exercise" longevity is to exercise too little. Let's say you want to jog for your everyday movement. Rather than running one, two, or three miles on your first outing, take an easy quarter-mile jog. If this distance winds you, run or walk even less. Continue running this distance every day until you feel totally comfortable and underexercised. Then very gradually increase your distance a fraction, and run *this* extended distance for a week or more.

I learned to jog this way from my track-and-field-star husband. In high school, he used to push himself so hard that his stomach hurt after a run. Knowing my competitive nature (and complete lack of experience running), he wisely had me follow this baby-step method to running. We began with a quarter of a mile, after which I whined, "Is that all?" (You should too.) But I was so proud that I could run any distance without huffing that I didn't mind too much. We continued with this program for a few months until the day came when I ran a total of three miles without stopping, feeling uncomfortable, or out of breath. What an accomplishment for a person with absolutely no athletic ability at all!

Make Exercise a Daily Occurrence

The next step to tiptop muscles is to add purposeful exercise to your daily routine. This is one of the basic health makeover tips I tell all my patients. For people who complain or give me that "you're-crazy" look, these are the tips I pass on.

- Begin with five minutes of exercise a day.

- If it helps, use a timer to tell you when you're done. When that buzzer goes off, stop regardless of what you're doing.

- Build exercise into your day. Rather than trying to find time to exercise around other commitments, schedule other activities around exercise.

- Don't be rigid. Once you've built your exercise time up, if you only have time for 20 minutes instead of 30, that's fine. A little exercise is better than none.

- Remember, it's more difficult to start something new than continue what you've already established.

While purposeful activity should be a daily habit, it's also reasonable to expect that unavoidable circumstances may prevent you from this goal occasionally. You may find that by planning to exercise every day, you'll actually do it five or six days a week. Better this than planning on exercising three days each week, and only accomplishing it one or two. If you're very disciplined, or after practicing the exercise habit for a month or two, you may decide to schedule one or two days off each week, perhaps the weekend or select weekdays—whatever works for you.

■ *Makeover Hint #44—Timing*

Find the best time of day for you, both schedule-wise ("Mornings are too hectic") and energy-wise ("I can't move after lunch") to exercise. You'll not only enjoy it more, but gain more as well. Also avoid exercising one hour before or two hours after a full meal. A small snack just before exercising is all right if you need an energy boost.

The Exercise Charter

Recording your daily movement for a month or two is a great way to build consistency and develop a good habit. You can either mark your calendar with each event, or use the following Exercise Chart to help introduce daily exercise in a no-sweat way.

Table 9.1
EXERCISE CHART

Activity	Minutes						
	Mon	*Tues*	*Wed*	*Thur*	*Fri*	*Sat*	*Sun*

Vary How You Move

It's no wonder people get bored with exercise. They pick a specific routine and figure they must stick with it for life. This isn't good for your body, and it's certainly not fun. We are naturally drawn to enjoyable activities—at least for the long haul—so a dull physical fitness regimen soon loses its luster and is eventually dropped.

Break the mold and learn to be one of those people who loves to move. Instead of just attending aerobics classes three times a week, mix it up with biking, walking, swimming, and dancing. If you enjoy routine for a short time, then get bored, attend your aerobics class for one or two months and be prepared to jump into a new activity before the excitement wanes. Another way to do this, is change your activities with the seasons. Here in season-rich South Dakota, I love to ride my bike in the summer, go for walks outside in the fall, and when that long, long winter begins, I dust off my treadmill.

Also choose different types of movement to give your Muscle Makeover more power. Besides aerobic activity, incorporate weight training and stretching into your regular routine. This way, not only do you flood your muscles and body with life-giving oxygen and build endurance, but your muscles attain tone and flexibility.

■ *Makeover Hint #45—Rate Your Exercise on the Fun Scale*

Do you exercise because you think you should, or because it's fun? One way to devise an enjoyable activity routine is to make it something you look forward to. Begin by listing all the physical activities you currently do, or could do. These could include walking, running, exercise class, gardening, tennis, dancing, hiking, martial arts, biking, yoga, bowling, making love. Then rate them on the fun scale. Activities you find thrilling rate a 10; activities that bore you to tears get a 1. Assign other pastimes accordingly. Any activity that rates a 5 or less, toss. Concentrate on the most fun activities for you.

Your Super Fitness Plan

Once you've practiced moving more in your everyday routine, and established a time for structured exercise, you need to think about different types of exercises, like aerobics, weight training and stretching, and when it's best to do each. Both stretching and aerobic activity are best done every day, even if it's just a short five- or ten-minute warm-up followed by a 30 minute walk. Weight training, on the other hand, should be done every other day or three days per week (see below for specific suggestions). Lift weights directly after your aerobic exercise. Not only are your muscles already warmed up, but the weight lifting will help prolong your aerobic movement a little bit. If you prefer, alternate stretching and weight lifting days. Your physical fitness schedule might look something like this:

Monday—Stretch 5 minutes; 30-minute walk; 10 minutes weights.

Tuesday—Stretch 5 minutes; 30-minute walk; 10 minutes stretching.

Wednesday—Stretch 5 minutes; 30-minute walk; 10 minutes weights.

Thursday—Stretch 5 minutes; 30-minute walk; 10 minutes stretching.

Friday—Stretch 5 minutes; 30-minute walk; 10 minutes weights.

Saturday—Game of tennis (45 minutes); warm-up included.

Sunday—day off.

Of course, your chosen activities will vary from the above, and can change from day to day, as will the time you allot for each.

Aerobics—Cash in on Oxygen

Other factors to keep in mind when embarking on a structured exercise plan are clothing and breathing. Clothing should be comfortable and loose-fitting, such as jogging pants and T-shirt or leotards. Don't forget shoes that give your feet support. These don't have to be fancy, just functional. Remember to breathe as you work out so your muscles and heart receive the oxygen-rich blood you're working so hard to send their way. Consider too whether you'll get more use from or stay motivated by using a health club, joining forces with a friend or exercising alone with or without exercise equipment. As a busy mother, writer, and physician, I've found a fold-up treadmill the most worthwhile investment for 45 minutes of at-home aerobic activity. I also get bored easily, so I have my machine set up in front of the television where I can catch up on favorite programs I've taped or watch a rented movie. In this same room I perform various yoga positions for stretching, and complete my routine with small dumb-bells and ankle weights. You decide what circumstances will allow you to stick with a daily program.

Last, if you're over 35 or have not exercised on a regular basis, visit your doctor for a checkup and green flag to begin the road to physical fitness.

Stretch It!

Learn how to stretch your body every day, and you'll not only make over your muscles, but release pent-up tension, breathe more easily and gain inner peace. Stretching, whether through simple bends or with yoga, creates more flexible joints and muscles and helps alleviate stiffness that comes with age. Well-positioned stretches are also useful therapeutic tools for bodily aches and pains.

Ideally you want to incorporate a full-body stretch into your everyday routine. It needn't take long—15 to 20 minutes is fine. Here's a routine to get you started.

■ *Makeover Hint #46—The Five Minute Stretch*

For times when you're tense or short on time, use this quickie stretching routine. Find a door and open it. Face the door so that each hand can grasp one side of the door knob. Place your feet on either side of the door. Then very gently lean back so that you're hanging from the door knob. (Don't do this if the knob is insecure—or you are.) Slowly stretch out your back, pelvis, and neck. Hang there for one to two minutes. Pull up slowly.

Now turn around so your back is to the door. Reach behind you and grasp each side of the door knob with each hand. Place your feet on either side of the door, and very gently lean forward with your pelvis. You are now stretching your back and pelvis in the pose opposite to the previous. Hang for as long as you're comfortable. Pull up slowly.

Add a Little Weight to Your Life

It's beyond the scope of this book to instruct you about the ins-and-outs of proper weight training. However, the results are undeniably positive. Whether you're male or female, young or old, weight training can help you build strength, aid in combating chronic back pain and other health problems, give you more stamina, agility, and tiptop muscle tone. This is also an area that you can use as an adjunct to an overall exercise plan, or expand it for a more intense body-building regimen.

For most people, light weights will suffice for general muscle toning. Depending on your strength, choose dumbbells and ankle weights that are one to five pounds each. These are available in most department stores. I'm not an expert in this area, though I do lift weights myself. My advice to you is to incorporate at least 10 minutes of small weight training three times into your week. By lifting weights every other day, you allow stressed muscles to recover and build. Your other option is to lift weights daily, but alternate which body parts you work out. For example, you may want to work on your upper body Monday, Wednesday and Friday, and your lower body on Tuesday, Thursday and Saturday, taking Sunday off.

For specific instructions on weight-lifting procedures seek the guidance of a trained weight lifter or exercise teacher.

■ *Makeover Hint #47—The Soup-Can Lift*

Want to start out slowly? Don't want to invest in a set of dumbbells? Turn to your kitchen cupboard and pull out two cans of soup and use these as light, beginner weights. Just make sure that they're the same size so you're balanced on each side.

Feed Your Muscles

Adhering to a whole-foods, varied diet as described in Chapter 4 is sufficient to feed your muscles. If you suffer from muscle cramps or poor circulation, concentrate on foods high in these nutrients:

1. Magnesium—seafood, whole grains, nuts, dark green vegetables.
2. Calcium—green leafy vegetables, seaweed, nuts, dairy foods.
3. Potassium—vegetables, fruits, whole grains.
4. Vitamin E—fresh vegetable oils, walnuts, hazelnuts, peanuts, eggs.
5. Vitamin C—broccoli, green peppers, tomatoes, strawberries, citrus fruits, alfalfa sprouts.
6. B-Complex Vitamins—whole grains, Brewer's yeast, eggs, organ meats.

Also check your protein intake. Have you been experimenting with this as outlined in Chapter 6: Protein is a Positive Step? If not, now's the time.

How to Prevent Sore Muscles

If you overdo it a bit or are sore after starting your new exercise program, remember this. Be sure you've thoroughly warmed up before and cooled down after each aerobic or weight-lifting session. Also, follow your stretching routine before starting to avoid injuries and soreness.

In addition to these procedural items, there are nutrients and herbs available to prevent these problems from occurring. Katherine Tsoulas, a marathon runner and naturopathic doctor, has found a way to prevent aching muscles. (You don't need to be a star athlete to use these ideas.) She relies on extra vitamin C to strengthen connective tissue and prevent inflammation. Depending on your activity and needs, 1000 to 3000 mg each day in divided amounts should be adequate. Dr. Tsoulas also looks to calcium (1000 mg) and magnesium (500 mg) per day—this is the total amount to take, including what's in your multiple supplement.

Another marathon enthusiast, Dr. Helen Healy from St. Paul, says, "My main advice is to build up slowly and steadily so that a person does not have to deal with a lot of pain in the first place—they just get the enjoyment of the exercise program." She also advises avoiding alcohol and overly salty foods, both of which can cause dehydration. Her favorite drink at marathon time, and one you can use when you're working up a sweat, is the juice of fresh-squeezed oranges and grapefruits. It seems to give her just the right amount of fluid and natural sugars that her body needs, she reports.

If, even after taking the above precautions, you're sore the next day, turn to the homeopathic remedy, Arnica (see Appendix B). You can take this by mouth or apply the cream version directly onto aching muscles. Also helpful are the natural anti-inflammatory and pain-relieving substances curcumin, a derivative of turmeric, and bromelain, found in pineapple; use these instead of muscle relaxants and pain relievers like aspirin. Take both of these between meals. In addition, eat ginger and turmeric, found in curry, as much as you like. My only caution here is that if you're taking strong medications, you may want to avoid bromelain as it can increase absorption of some medicines.

■ Makeover Hint #48—Soak Gingerly

You've had a great workout, but Oh!, do you ache. Relax sore muscles with this simple at-home treatment. Pour yourself a nice hot bath. Make a strong cup of ginger tea, available in tea bags, or use one teaspoon of powdered or diced ginger root in one cup of hot water. Steep for 15 minutes. Pour the tea into your bath and then soak your body.

Follow the Cheap Fuel Rule

Here's an idea for those who not only want to make over their muscles, but delight in saving money and the environment. Instead of driving your car for every errand, follow the six-block rule. If your errand is six blocks or less away, walk (or bike). This is a wonderful way to insert physical activity into your everyday routine. Plus you'll save money on gas and spare the environment some car exhaust. For distances greater than six blocks, you may drive.

Find Ways to Move at Work

One excuse people use to not exercise is work. How about exercising at work? Here are some simple desk-bound movements you can practice each and every day as part of your Muscle Makeover. Remember to breathe during each exercise. Do these at least three times a day, or as needed.

- When no one's looking, stick your hands way up in the air as if signaling a touchdown. Then roll your shoulders back and try to bring your shoulder blades together. Do this slowly five to 10 times. Great for cramped backs caused by too much hunching over important paperwork.

- Neck stretches help unlock tense muscles and remind you to breathe. Pull back from your desk, plant your feet firmly on the ground and sit up straight. Loop your right arm over the top of your head so your right hand covers your left ear. Gently, gently pull your head down so your right ear is moving toward your right shoulder. Stop pulling if painful; this stretch should feel good. Hold for 15 seconds; slowly breathe in and out. Return head to upright position slowly. Do the same on the opposite side.

- For a full neck and back stretch, place laced hands at the back of your head. While sitting tall, slowly and gently pull your head down toward your chest. Feel the stretch, not the pain. Hold for 15 seconds. Return to sitting position slowly.

- For stressed out shoulders that creep higher as the day wears on, try this. Shrug your shoulder and hold for 15 seconds. Release with a big sigh of relief. Do this two more times. If you have a willing co-worker nearby, have her or him push down on your shoulders gently to break up shoulder tension.

Be an Aerobic Tourist

Another excuse for not exercising is travel. Whether you regularly journey for business or are taking a vacation, it's important to bring your exercise attitude along. I've never seen anyone abandon food during a trip; why forgo activity?

Putting aside all the reasons why exercise, or movement, during travel is impossible—time change, no facilities, too busy, too tired, don't want to—let's look at several tricks you can use to keep moving while you're vacationing.

- Pack running shoes and other exercise-type clothing.
- Book your room at a hotel with a gym and/or pool.
- While traveling, try different activities you don't normally do.
- Go swimming, then sit in the hot tub afterward.
- Golf 18 holes—without a golf cart.
- Play tennis or racket ball; if you don't know how, take lessons from a pro.
- Go for long walking tours of the town you're visiting.
- Go for hikes, if in the country.
- Rent a bike.
- If attending a conference or business meetings, go for walks in-between. Take prospective clients for a walk and network.
- Find the exercise channel on your hotel room TV and do floor exercises.
- Go skiing, sledding, or ice skating.

What if You're too Sick to Move?

While it's important to maintain a regular exercise regimen, sometimes you'll want to put your exercise leotards aside for a day or two. If you're experiencing the beginning stages of a cold or other illness, you may find a sweaty workout just the thing to stall it. Couple this with plenty of sleep, and an anti-infection diet (no sugar, caffeine, alcohol, or junk food; take extra vitamin C and drink echinacea tea). For times when illness slams you to the ground (or bed), take care of yourself and give yourself up to bed rest. Sensible exercise habits not only include consistent activity when you're well, but also recognizing when it's OK to sleep and rest so your body can heal. When you're very ill, your body needs all its energy to recover. Part of this mature attitude toward exercise is the ability to re-enter an exercise program once you're well without making excuses. You may need to ease back into your program, depending on how long you've been benched.

These rules also go for when you're severely or acutely injured. Obviously a broken leg is going to stop you from biking or jogging, and immediately following the fracture you won't feel like doing anything. However, there are ways of sneaking some activity into your down-time. Find ways to move the uninjured parts of your body while sitting—including your free leg. Lift small arm weights. Practice stretching your neck, shoulders, and arms. For acute injuries, rest for up to three days depending on how critical the damage; then begin gradually to move again. Ask your doctor or physical therapist for guidance in both of these situations.

Muscle Makeover Checkup

Isn't exercise great? Don't worry, you'll get used to it eventually. In the meantime, continue to practice these Muscle Makeover tips:

- Build on your everyday movement.
- Exercise each day—if only for five minutes.
- Don't overdo it.
- Variety is the spice of exercise.
- Do some aerobics.
- Try stretching.
- Take a shot at weight lifting.
- Are you having fun yet?
- Feed your muscles.
- Take steps to prevent sore muscles.
- Walk, don't drive, when close.
- Move at work.
- Move when you travel.
- Be cautious when sick.

For Related Problems, See

- Backaches
- Gout
- Sprains and strains

Chapter 10

Regain Your Sexual Vitality

Hormone Power

Sex hormones are what make us sexual beings. They help shape our reproductive organs, feed sexual drive, and grace us with those characteristics that make us female—soft skin, breasts, and a menstrual cycle—or male—deep voice and facial hair. Everyone has exactly the same hormones floating around. That's right, men have the female hormones estrogen and progesterone, and women have testosterone and other androgens. The difference between men and women is how much of each they possess.

There are dozens of hormones in the body, chemicals that act as messengers and tell different tissues how to act. Because sexuality is influenced by overall health, an imbalance in any number of hormones can affect your sexual desire. Also consider ways to keep your liver humming (see Chapter 3)—for this is where sex hormones are converted into less powerful forms—and care for your adrenals, another sex hormone factory (see Chapter 7).

What Causes a Lagging Libido

Lack of desire is caused by many things. It may be a sign of discord within a relationship. If so, consider counseling where both partners attend sessions to learn communication skills. Sometimes sex therapy, an adult version of high school sex education, is in order. These classes teach you everything you want to know about sex and desire, including how, why, and when sexual desire waxes and wanes, how

137

an emotional problem, like depression interferes with libido, and how physical illness affects one's love life. A busy routine that barely leaves room for alone time robs many people of not only desire, but the longing to be intimate with a partner.

Low sex drive is also a sign of poor health. People who are healthy tend to have higher sex drives because they feel well. And a well-adjusted sex life is good for your health. If your sexual vitality is lagging, take the following makeover steps.

Know Your Sex Drive Cycle

The first step to achieving sexual vitality is to realize that libido is not a fixed feeling. Sex drive for both men and women waxes and wanes depending on mood, health, and time.

Female libidos are particularly affected by the monthly or menstrual cycle during which sex hormones like estrogen and progesterone peak and then decline. Some women, for instance, find that during ovulation—a couple of weeks after menstruation—arousal increases. This is the most fertile time for women; enhanced libido is Mother Nature's way of ensuring procreation of the species.

A man's sex drive is also affected by changing hormone levels. For example, testosterone in the blood of men peaks between 6 A.M. and 8 A.M., and hits a low 12 hours later.[1] It's also been shown that human sexuality operates on a yearly basis. Sperm count, for one, is highest on average between February and March and lowest during September.[2] These facts explain the appeal of morning sex, and why some couples might find it easier to get pregnant in the springtime.

Since overall health also alters on a daily, monthly, and yearly trend, it makes sense that libido is similarly affected depending on how well you feel. If your mood changes with the seasons, stress, or weather—winter blues being one example—shouldn't your desire for lovemaking also fluctuate?

Sandy and Tom Learn to Give Their Sex Life a Break

Newly married Sandy and Tom didn't know what was wrong. According to surveys they'd read, they should be having sex three times a week. But that wasn't happening, and the young couple was worried that their love and desire for each other was dying a quick death.

Finally, they decided to visit with a marriage counselor who discovered that Sandy and Tom were under a considerable amount of strain. Not only had they both just graduated from college and had no money, but they were brand new parents as well. Sandy was exhausted from waking with the baby at night and Tom was worried about finding a job to support his family. It was a great relief for both Tom and Sandy when the counselor told them a low sex drive, due to fatigue and tension, was perfectly normal. She said that with time their desire for each other would return, and told them to remember there's no such thing as "normal." Each couple has its own unique relationship, and as long as they were happy with each other, nothing else mattered.

Sleep Away the Sexual Blues

The next step to boosting desire is sleep. Without adequate sleep—eight hours nightly for most adults—our bodies are unable to refresh and rejuvenate. Signs of sleep deprivation include declining libido ("not tonight, dear, I'm too tired"), lack of mental concentration, loss of judgment, and decreased resistance to illness.

Spend the next week on sleep therapy. This means establishing a regular bedtime routine. One hour before lights go out, get ready for bed, put on your pajamas, put away work, turn off the TV, and do something relaxing. Try having a hot bath (romantic in itself); sip a cup of soothing herb tea or read a light non-work-related book. Turn the lights out on time, and sleep for at least eight hours.

Laura Finds Sensuality in Rest

Laura, a 26-year-old waitress, was a go-getter. Besides her full-time job, she enjoyed attending aerobics class, biking, reading, and pursuing several hobbies. She also had a tendency to stay up late, either visiting with friends or talking on the phone. The only trouble spot in Laura's life was relations with her husband. George complained that frequently when he asked Laura to make love, she turned him down, saying she was too tired.

Finally, after a couple of months of rejection, George stormed out of the house. Laura was stunned. She hadn't realized how much her busy life and lack of sleep were affecting her relationship with her husband. When George finally returned, Laura vowed to cut down on her activities and concentrate, instead, on catching up on sleep. After four days of eight-hour nights, Laura was pleasantly surprised to discover her flame for George burning brightly. Not only that, but her normally short temper and her body aches disappeared as well.

Alcohol—A Sexual Downer

Thirty years ago, movies treated liquor as sexy. Just think of Dean Martin, Frank Sinatra, and the rest of the Rat Pack, and you'll understand. While alcohol can let down inhibitions, it can also remove some of your sexual edge both directly and indirectly. For starters, alcohol robs you of vital nutrients needed for sexual and other bodily functions by causing inflammation of the stomach, pancreas, and intestines.[3] It also impairs immunity, and contributes to osteoporosis and some cancers.

Closer to reproductive home, excessive or long-term drinking can cripple the liver and its ability to metabolize hormones. Alcohol's tendency to rattle the hormonal cart is described in many studies on women. Judith Gavaler and her research associates from the University of Pittsburgh found that downing less than one drink per week was enough to disturb a postmenopausal woman's normal hormonal levels.[4] Similarly, experts report that many women with PMS have a hard time handling alcohol. They not only seem to become inebriated more easily immediately prior to their periods, but actually crave alcohol.[5]

Men, of course, are not immune to alcohol's effects. In addition to liquor's adverse health influences, men who drink every day or drink more than 20 ounces a week are more likely to experience impotence.[6]

■ *Makeover Hint #49—The Alcohol Substitute*

A glass of wine is very relaxing, and can help you get into the mood. However, it can also break the mood when you drink too much, not to mention its long-term side effects. Try these "mood enhancers" instead:

- Give each other a slow sensuous massage.
- Read love poetry to your loved one.
- Play romantic music and slow dance in your living room.
- Caress your partner's feet with a luxuriously scented oil.
- Sneak a love letter into your loved one's pocket early in the day for love later that night.
- Tell each other secrets.
- Go for a long walk with your arms around one another.

Smoking Isn't Sexy

Lighting up after love-making, according to the movies, seems a natural conclusion to passion. But if you smoke, you could be puffing away your sexuality. Like alcohol, tobacco adds to impotency for men.[6] Smoking also increases your risk for heart and blood vessel disease; this means less circulation to your genitals and everywhere else. Smoking adds to your liver's load, so hormonal metabolism is shaken up. Smoking is neither healthy nor sexy.

The 10 Dietary Commandments for Sexual Vitality

Behind every great sex life is a healthy diet. A deficiency of some nutrients contributes to a lagging sex drive. Wholesome eating also ensures better overall health, which, in turn, boosts sexual function and desire. Follow these 10 dietary commandments to regain sexual vitality.

1. Eat plenty of dark green leafy vegetables and fruits (not citrus) for their boron content. Boron has been found to boost estrogen and testosterone levels in postmenopausal women.[7] Skimping on potassium, abundant in produce, can lead to that dragged-out feeling.[8]

2. Include whole grains, like brown rice, millet, and barley, for B-vitamins to soothe jangled nerves. Whole grains are also high in zinc, a mineral that aids sexual development in both girls and boys.

3. Stay hydrated with at least one quart of pure water daily. This will help drive away fatigue.

4. Get adequate protein. Start with plant sources like beans, legumes, nuts, and seeds. If you enjoy meat, try fish, skinless organic poultry and lean cuts of beef or lamb. Too little protein can decrease testosterone levels in men, thus lowering sex drive.[9]

5. Cut down on caffeine. While a cup of coffee gives you a boost, in the long run it's hard on the adrenal glands—one source of sex hormones. That's not to mention its role in anxiety, headaches, insomnia, and PMS.

6. Try giving flowers instead of candy on Valentine's Day—or any other time. There's scientific evidence that too much sugar harms the liver's ability to deal with estrogen and other sex hormones.[10] In addition, sugar contributes to obesity, PMS, and lower resistance to disease.

7. Go easy on the salt. Water retention caused by excessive salt use is not healthy or attractive.

8. Buy organic foods when possible. Many pesticides act like estrogen, and ultimately upset your endocrine system.

9. Eat the right kinds of fats. Saturated fats (the type that harden at room temperature and are mainly from animal-based foods) are less desirable—stick with lean meats and mix them up with plant proteins. However, essential fatty acids (EFA) found in seeds, nuts, whole grains, and fish, are required for sex hormone production. Male and female infertility is one classic sign of EFA deficiency.[11] Whole grains, seeds, and nuts are also high in vitamin E, necessary for proper sexual function and a useful treatment for menopausal hot flashes and vaginal dryness.

10. Variety feeds vitality. Eat a wide assortment of fresh, whole, organic foods to ensure you're getting all the nutrients you need for reproductive function and overall health.

■ *Makeover Hint #50—A Romantic Meal*

The house is empty and you've both cleared your schedules for a night of love. Begin your night of amore with a romantic meal. Follow these guidelines.

- Prepare a simple meal in advance. Running back and forth from the kitchen disrupts the mood.

- Set a simple and attractive table complete with candlelight. Visual appeal not only heightens your appetite for food, but love as well.

- Choose light foods that won't weigh you down. Raw vegetables with a light dip, skinless chicken strips grilled with a tasty sauce, fancy breads.

- Pick healthy finger foods, like grapes, so you can feed and take care of each other.

- Select foods that will leave you with pleasant breath. This isn't the time for garlic and raw onions. For extra insurance, have a dish of breath-cleansing parsley nearby.

- Avoid foods that cause you or your partner digestive problems. Late-night gas does not add to an evening of love.

Vitamins and Minerals Help Sexuality

Vitamins, minerals, and other nutrients are necessary for hormone production and sexual function. Following the 10 Dietary Commandments outlined earlier as a starting point, the other step is to take a well-balanced, high-potency multiple vitamin and mineral pill. Below are examples of three of the dozens of vitamins and minerals needed for sexual vitality.

At the U.S. Department of Agriculture's research facility in Grand Forks, North Dakota, Forrest Nielsen, Ph.D. conducted studies on a relatively obscure mineral called boron. He found that estrogen levels rose to "levels found in women on estrogen replacement therapy" when postmenopausal women were fed supplemental boron each day.[12] Note: If you have a condition that is aggravated by high estrogen levels, such as estrogen-dependent breast cancer, don't take extra boron.

The antioxidant vitamin E is recognized as a nutrient for sexual ailments. Early studies found that animals couldn't reproduce and males' testicles shrunk without vitamin E in their diet.[11] Vitamin E, both by mouth and applied topically, is useful for menopausal women suffering from vaginal dryness.

The prostate gland contains high amounts of zinc. When zinc levels fall too low, the result is poor sperm production and reduced testosterone levels.[12] Zinc supplementation is also useful in some cases of male infertility.[13] Zinc deficiency can also cause sexual dysfunction in women, a condition that's reversible with supplementation according to Turkish physician Suleyman Dincer, M.D.[14] Ironically, synthetic estrogens used in birth control pills rob the body of zinc.

Exercises for Super Sex

Exercise is a wonderful thing. Not only does it decrease your risk of heart disease, high blood pressure, and osteoporosis, help control weight, and give you strength, but it also makes sex better. This is partly because you feel so good when you're physically fit. People who are physically active on a regular basis also have more life-giving oxygen flowing through their bodies.

See Chapter 9 for how to tone your muscles. In the meantime, take your partner for a romantic walk in the moonlight.

■ _Makeover Hint #51—The Arousal Exercise_

To enhance sexual arousal try Kegels. These exercises train your pubococcygeus or PC muscle, which spans your pubic bone in front to your tail bone. These exercises were originally developed by Dr. Arnold Kegel to help women who had problems controlling urination.

However, some women and men find that following a regular Kegel routine benefits the genital region by increasing circulation there and expanding awareness of feelings in that area. The great thing about Kegels is you can do them anywhere, anytime, and no one can tell. Here's what you do:

1. Identify your PC muscle by stopping the flow of urine next time you urinate. Do this without moving your legs. This is the muscle that shuts urine flow on and off.

2. Practice Slow Kegels by tightening your PC muscle, as if shutting off urine flow. Hold for three seconds and then relax.

3. Practice Fast Kegels by tightening and relaxing your PC muscle as fast as you can.

4. Do five each (one set) of the Slow and Fast Kegels before each meal. You can do more sets each day if you like. Increase the number of Kegels by five each week. So you're doing 10 Slow and 10 Fast Kegels during week two, 15 of each during week three, et cetera.

5. Keep in mind that these exercises may feel awkward or difficult to do at first, and the muscles might feel tired. This is to be expected, as it would be if you started moving any other sedentary muscle in your body. Breathing and patience will help you gain control and more sexual pleasure.

Not Tonight, Dear, I Have a Headache

Feeling bad is a valid, and too common, reason for sitting on the sexual sidelines. If none of the above works for you, ill health or medication could be the cause of decreased desire or pleasure. Any time you're rundown, hurting, or sick, libido is bound to fall.

Prostatitis in young men is a condition where urgent, burning urination invades the groin, scrotum, anus, lower back, abdomen, and legs and is accompanied by painful ejaculation. Such a condition can rob sexual pleasure. Hypothyroidism, an underactive thyroid gland, can drag desire down. Many chronic diseases, such as clogged arteries, affect overall health and slow blood circulation to the genital region.

Medicines can also cut down your sex life. Hypoglycemic agents, vasodilators, cardiovascular drugs, antihistamines, tranquilizers, antidepressants, hormone replacement, and other medications have this effect. Also beware of recreational drugs like cocaine, heroin, and marijuana.

The answer to this dilemma is a complete physical by your doctor, along with appropriate laboratory tests. If you're taking medicines, whether prescription or over-the-counter, find out if they're responsible for cheating you out of romance.

■ *Makeover Hint #52—Practice Safe Sex*

If you're not in a monogamous relationship with a longstanding partner, please, practice safe sex. This means using condoms for men; women, you might consider a diaphragm or cervical cap as added protection. Inquire about your partner's health history before engaging in lovemaking. AIDS, gonorrhea, herpes, genital warts, and a host of other sexually-transmitted diseases are just a few reasons not to make love unsafely.

Should I Take Herbal Aphrodisiacs?

Can herbs electrify your sex life? Probably not—at least not by themselves. Many of the herbs suggested for waning desire work as reproductive tonifiers, calming agents, or as overall health enhancers. What we think of as aphrodisiacs are often urinary tract and genital irritants. *Cantharis*, or Spanish fly, for instance, creates sexual desire in this way but is poisonous in large doses.

An herb that works as an aphrodisiac by promoting general health is Asian ginseng, or *Panax ginseng*. It works by helping the body use oxygen more efficiently, by maintaining blood sugar and cholesterol levels, and by helping manage stress via adrenal gland support. Some people find Asian ginseng overstimulates them to the point of insomnia. If this happens to you, cut down on your dose or stop using it. The safest way to take this herb is two weeks on, one week off. If you have high blood pressure, use ginseng cautiously and have your blood pressure checked regularly.

For impotence due to poor genital blood flow, *Ginkgo biloba* is a logical choice. Its leaves contain compounds so beneficial for circulatory and nervous system problems that it's among the most prescribed and well-researched herbal medicines in the world. Side effects are rare, and when present, mild—upset stomach and headaches.

One of the safest and most effective ways to take this plant is as a 24 percent ginkgo heterosides-standardized formula of ginkgo biloba extract (GBE); this form guarantees a specific amount of potency. Dosage begins at 40 mg three times daily and may take three months for results. Other herbalists prefer using the untouched, whole plant. If you're not certain what's causing your impotence, check with your doctor. If you plan to stay on this herb for a long time, consult an herbalist or other practitioner versed in botanicals.

Yohimbine: What's the Story?

The bark of the yohimbe tree has been hailed as an aphrodisiac for more than a century. Today, doctors prescribe yohimbine, an extract from that tree, to treat impotence. It is thought to energize a man's sexual response by stimulating select portions of his nervous system and increasing blood to erectile tissue. By some estimates, only one-fifth of impotent men completely recover after using yohimbine.[15]

The down side to using this herb-based drug is side effects such as increased blood pressure, racing heart rate, tremors, irritability, headaches, nausea or vomiting, sweating, dizziness, flushed skin and frequent urination. Some medications—like tranquilizers—can interact with yohimbine. Anyone with a heart condition, kidney disease, glaucoma or history of gastric or duodenal ulcers should avoid it because it elevates blood pressure and excites the central nervous system.

If you choose to use this substance, select the herbal form, yohimbe, over the pure extract. Combine it with other herbs like Siberian ginseng or saw palmetto to temper its effects, and to be perfectly safe, use it under the care of an herbal-wise practitioner.

Sexuality Makeover Check-Up

Congratulations! You've just completed another phase of your Natural Health Makeover. Here's a summary:

- Learned about the sex drive cycle.
- Got some more sleep.
- Was careful of alcohol—and tried a few alternates.
- Alerted to watch out for smoking.
- Learned the 10 sexual dietary commandments.
- Made sure your supplement had boron, zinc, and other sexual nutrients.
- Vowed to keep exercising.
- Tried Kegels.
- Had a physical exam and medication screening.
- Looked into herbs like ginkgo and ginseng, if needed.

For Related Problems, See

- Urinary Tract Infections
- Yeast Infection

Laboratory Tests Your Doctor Can Order

- Sex Hormone Profile
- DHEA or DHEA-Sulfate Levels

Chapter 11

Build Stronger Bones
and Teeth

Your Supportive Skeleton

The skeleton is the framework that gives the body support and shape, like the wooden frame of a house. Not only that, but the hundreds of bones in the body are jointed to permit fluid, easy movement. Muscles attached to the end of bone joints are what make movement possible (see Chapter 9).

If you've ever seen one of those dolls on which you pull a cord and the arms and legs flop around, you get an idea of the skeleton's two main parts. The axial skeleton (skull, ribs, backbone, pelvis) is most rigid and provides the main support, in other words the doll's head and body; the appendicular skeleton are the doll's swinging limbs. What you don't see on floppy dolls are the three types of bones. There are flat bones, such as in the skull, breastbone, and pelvis, that protect delicate organs like the brain, lungs, and bladder. Long bones make up your arms and legs, and act as levers allowing you to pick up things and walk. Short small bones comprise the wrist and ankles, and lend strength to these areas. The thirty-three vertebrae stacked up in your backbone not only support most of your body's weight, but allow a wide range of motion from bending back and forward, side to side to twisting. In your mouth are 32 permanent teeth; 28 if wisdom teeth are missing.

But that's not all. Bones are not merely stick-like structures holding up other body parts. They're living, changing tissues that receive and require a wide range of nutrients from the blood vessels that infiltrate them. Most bone is made up of collagen fibers, which give it strength. Ground substance—a collection of chondroitin sulfate and hyaluronic acid—fills in the gaps. Calcium, phosphate and other bone salts like magnesium, sodium, potassium, and carbonate, reinforce this framework.

Teeth are built much like bones, only denser, with a meshwork of collagen fibers and mineral salts. Enamel covers a tooth and protects it against acids (in pop, by the way) and other corrosive substances. Unfortunately, once the very hard enamel is worn away, that's it. It doesn't reform. Nerves, blood vessels, and lymph vessels form the middle pulp of a tooth.

New bone is continually being laid down by special cells called osteoblasts, while osteoclasts—another specialized bone cell—absorb or take bone away. Under healthy circumstances this check and balance of bone give-and-take is equal so that total bone mass stays constant. Unlike bones, only a small portion of teeth contains these special remodeling cells. However, the mineral salts in teeth are constantly being replaced by new ones—though very slowly in the enamel.

Warning Signs of a Crumbling Frame

Several conditions can put your skeleton in jeopardy—rickets, osteomalacia, osteitis fibrosa cystica, hypoparathyroidism, and others. But the most common bone-stealing disease is osteoporosis, a progressive bone loss condition that threatens 24 million Americans[1] and costs them an estimated seven to 10 billion dollars annually in treatment.[2] The irony of osteoporosis is that everyone begins to lose bone at some time in their life. Osteoporosis (literally translated as "porous bone") is merely an exaggerated version of this naturally occurring aging process. Maximum bone density peaks in one's twenties. After that, both sexes begin to lose bone mass at a rate of about one percent per year.[3]

This process, however, is accelerated in women once they reach menopause. Very thin bones caused by menopausal changes, such as drops in estrogen and other hormones, is called postmenopausal osteoporosis. One third to one half of women who've gone through menopause are afflicted.[4] Although twice as many women suffer from fractures due to osteoporosis, this bone disease is an important and growing problem among men as well.[5] Other kinds of osteoporosis, labeled according to what age group they strike, include senile osteoporosis (a condition of the elderly), juvenile osteoporosis (seen in children and adolescents), and idiopathic osteoporosis, a form with unknown cause that strikes people under 40.

The most frightening feature of osteoporosis is its insidious nature. Very often there are no symptoms associated with the disease. It's one of those conditions where you need to do the right thing—lifestyle-wise—just because. Your bones aren't going to give you much feedback. Rather, thinning bones are usually discovered inadvertently on X-rays or as a person gradually shrinks in stature. There are tests available that can tell you current bone density and amount of bone lost over a specific time period. Ask your doctor about these, if you're interested.

Unfortunately, it's only later-stage osteoporosis that creates the most obvious subjective symptoms like mid-back pain or fractures of the hip or wrist. A history of "bad teeth" can be a sign of impending bone loss. There is no one known cause for the most common forms of osteoporosis. Instead this disease develops because of your genetic makeup, age, sex, race, weight, physical strength—and a few factors you can actually control. These are the things we're going to discuss here. If you're concerned about protecting your teeth, beware of bleeding or sore gums, bad breath, and frequent cavities. Below, learn about the steps you can take to make over your bones and teeth.

How to Stop the Calcium Robbers

Calcium is an important bone nutrient, so vital, in fact, that we're constantly reminded to take extra helpings. However, it's equally important to recognize those habits and foods that steal calcium away from bones and teeth. If you can stop calcium robbery, your current calcium supplementation will be more effective.

A good place to start is with caffeine, that stimulating substance found in coffee, black tea, soft drinks (also high in phosphorus, not good for bones), and chocolate. A very large six-year study involving almost 85,000 women discovered that caffeine, particularly coffee, increased the incidence of hip fractures—a sign that bones are weakening. Caffeine does its damage by prompting the body to spill extra calcium into the urine. This occurs on less than one cup of coffee per day.[6] Excessive salt can add to this problem, as can an overabundance of animal-based protein foods like red meat, chicken, eggs and dairy products.[1]

■ Makeover Hint #54—Drink Healthy Orange Soda

Putting aside soft drinks most of the time is a must for women. If you like pop mainly for the carbonation, try this healthy, tasty substitute.

Pour half a glass of orange juice or your favorite fruit juice.

Top off with seltzer (make sure it's sodium free).

Add ice and sip.

I began doing this 20 years ago as an alternate to cocktails and soda. Many of my friends and family members also love this refreshing drink.

Calcium Mysteries of the World

In this country, women are advised to ingest between 1000 and 1200 mg of calcium daily to protect their bones. Yet there are places in the world where calcium intake is much less—and osteoporosis is less frequent. The Bantu women of South Africa, for example, who live on reservations, consume only 220 to 440 mg of calcium per day and are virtually free of osteoporosis. South African women living in cities, on the other hand, have thinner bones and a calcium intake that is two to four times higher.

Why the difference?

Well, the rural-dwelling Bantus are primarily vegetarian, while the South African city women eat meat. Animal protein, say researchers, makes the urine more acidic and thus increases calcium loss from the body.[7] I'd wager that there's more to this puzzle than meat. Citified folk also tend to nibble on more refined foods, sugars, and salts. In *The Paleolithic Prescription*, S. Boyd Eaton, M.D. and his co-authors say osteoporosis was rare among the hunter-gatherers of long ago—these people *did* eat meat. However, they also dined on plenty of wild, calcium-rich vegetation and exercised every day.[8] So if you choose to eat meat, remember the principles of consuming a whole foods diet, and pay attention to the other food on your plate.

Calcium (and Other Mineral Deposits) to the Rescue

Taking calcium for stronger bones is a popular preventive step. Recommended dosage lies between 800 and 1000 mg daily, and increases to 1500 mg per day for high-risk individuals.[9] And for good reason! Calcium is stored mainly in your skeleton, and when your diet falls short of this mineral, it's drawn from bones. Of course the calcium-bone relationship is more complex than popping a pill, as we learned earlier. In addition, the age at which you begin calcium supplementation is also important. As adults, we gain the benefits of a little extra calcium; so do pre-adolescent children,[10] and women well past the age of menopause.[11] Women just entering menopause gain a small, but positive, effect from additional calcium.[12]

Calcium, of course, does not stand alone. Other minerals such as magnesium are required for strong bones. Not only is magnesium an integral part of bone, but it helps form new calcium crystals[13] and the conversion of vitamin D to its active form. Vitamin D aids calcium absorption.[14] Another mineral called boron strengthens bones by decreasing urinary excretion of calcium, magnesium, and phosphorus needed by the skeleton. Boron also keeps bones secure by increasing those hormones—estrogen and testosterone—that enhance bone health.[15]

Also on the bone mineral list are manganese, zinc, strontium, silicon, copper, and vanadium. Paul Saltman, a biologist at the University of California in San Diego, first became interested in manganese when well-known basketball player Bill Walton developed osteoporosis even though he was eating a healthy, macrobiotic diet. Saltman discovered there was no manganese in Walton's blood. After six weeks of changing his eating habits and taking mineral supplements including manganese, Walton was back in playing form although his osteoporosis was not completely corrected. When manganese drops, the cells which lay down new bone—osteoblasts—are less efficient.[16]

Zinc, low in many older folks with osteoporosis, works with vitamin A and D to create normal bone formation.[17] Strontium, not to be confused with the radioactive kind, is abundant in bones and teeth and increases retention of calcium. When osteoporotic patients were fed this mineral in one study, many noticed their bone pain was less.[18] Silicon, a trace element found in such plants as horsetail, seems to disrupt bone growth when too low. (This silicon is different from that used in breast implants.) Too little copper appears to have the same effect. Very low, but definite, amounts of vanadium also appear necessary for stable bones.[19]

Building a mineral-full diet is important. Equally vital is having a digestive system that easily absorbs these nutrients. As we age, stomach acid tends to decline.

■ *Makeover Hint #55—Where to Get Your Fresh Minerals*

The best, most body-friendly sources of minerals are food. Start with a balanced diet packed with these foods for healthy bones.

- Calcium: milk and other dairy foods, sardines, clams, oysters, tofu, canned salmon with bones, dark leafy green vegetables (Swiss chard, mustard greens, kale, collards, beet greens, dandelion greens), broccoli, okra, rhubarb.

- Magnesium: whole grains, nuts, meat, milk, green vegetables, legumes.

- Boron: fruits (not citrus), leafy green vegetables, nuts, legumes.

- Manganese: beet greens, blueberries, whole grains, nuts, legumes, fruit.

- Zinc: oysters, whole grains, meat, lima beans.

- Silicon: high-fiber whole grains, root vegetables.

- Copper: liver, shellfish, whole grains, cherries, legumes, kidney, poultry, oysters, chocolate, nuts.

- Vanadium: shellfish, mushrooms, parsley, dill seed, black pepper.

Vitamins for Healthy Bones and Teeth

We know that minerals, especially calcium, are mandatory for good bone health. What about vitamins? If you remember that bone and teeth are living tissues with nutritional needs similar to those of other organs, then feeding them vitamins only makes sense.

Vitamin D is needed so calcium can be absorbed in the digestive tract. Unfortunately, as we age vitamin D drops as appetites wane. Nutrient malabsorption and problems with vitamin D metabolism are also to blame. Older folks who are house-bound (and us younger stay-at-home ones) spend less time outside than we should; less sun means less fun and vitamin D. Getting enough vitamins, whether through foods or supplements, should begin in childhood. Children who consume adequate vitamin D tend to have harder bones. Still, it's never too late for good bone nutrition. Vitamin D supplementation helps increase calcium levels and reduce bone loss in those with osteoporosis, too.[20]

Another important bone nutrient is vitamin K. A special type of protein found in bone called osteocalcin relies on vitamin K to trap calcium in the skeleton and otherwise function. According to British researchers, people with osteoporosis have one-third the vitamin K they should.[21] When thinking healthy bones, don't forget vitamin B_6, folic acid and vitamin B_{12}. These members of the B-complex family aid in calcium and magnesium metabolism and strengthen connective tissue, a supportive structure for bone.[22] Vitamins C and A are other bone-friendly nutrients that should be included in your regular multiple vitamin/mineral supplement and foods.

■ *Makeover Hint #56—What to Look for in a Bone-Strengthening Pill*

We need many nutrients for strong bones. The place to start is with a wide range of super-nutrient foods. For insurance purposes, you can also take a multiple vitamin and mineral pill. This will not only ensure strong bones, but overall better health. Look for these bone-specific nutrients when you shop. Of course your supplement can contain other nutrients too.

Boron 3 mg

Calcium 1000 mg

Copper 1 mg

Magnesium 500 mg

Manganese 15 mg

Strontium 100 mg

Vanadium 10 mcg

Zinc 15 mg

Vitamin A 5000 IU

Vitamin C 1000 mg

Vitamin D 400 IU

Vitamin B_6 50 mg

Folic Acid 400 mcg

Vitamin B_{12} 400 mcg

Dr. Aesoph's Fabulous Baked Beans

Let me share my famous baked beans recipe with you. It's full of bone-fortifying nutrients. This is an adapted version of my mother's recipe.

Soak 1 1/2 cups dried beans in water overnight (use pinto as the base; feel free to add others: navy, lima, soy).

Next morning, drain soaking water and rinse beans.

Cover beans with fresh water. Bring to a boil, then simmer slowly for 1/2 hour or more, until tender. If you like, add a ham hock.

Drain water, and save. To cooked beans add:

3–5 cloves garlic, diced

1 tbsp. dried mustard

1/4 cup molasses

Enough bean water to mix and keep moist.

Add bean mixture to baking dish with cover.

Bake in low oven (250 degrees) for several hours. I usually make this in the morning, and let it cook until dinner. The longer it cooks, the better it tastes.

Check on beans frequently; add water as needed.

One hour before serving, mix in one can of tomato paste. Serve with corn muffins and a fresh green salad.

Remove Sugar to Save Your Teeth—and Bones

Having a sweet tooth can harm your teeth—no doubt about that. But overindulging in sugar is damaging to bones as well. English researchers at the Royal Naval Hospital in Haslar, Gosport proved that eating white sugar pulls calcium from the body into the urine for excretion.[23] A similar investigation was carried out at the Marquette Medical School and Milwaukee County General Hospital, both in Wisconsin. These researchers fed their subjects 100 grams of sugar—the equivalent of 24 ounces of cola. Not only did the sugar promote calcium loss, but it acted like a diuretic and increased urination. People who had a history of forming calcium-type kidney stones *and their relatives* were affected even more so.[24]

Want to keep your bones strong and hold on to calcium? Simple. Cut sugar, and foods containing sugar, down or out.

■ *Makeover Hint #57—How to Bust a Sweet Tooth*

If you're having troubles breaking the I-have-to-have-sugar cycle, try some of these sweet tooth-busting tips. (See Low Blood Sugar, Part Two, for more ideas.)

- Eat five to six *small* meals every two to three hours throughout the day.
- Include a complex carbohydrate (whole grain, vegetable) and protein food with each meal. For example, a bran muffin and peanut butter. A dish of plain yogurt and fresh fruit. Cheese and crackers.
- Avoid refined sugars (sweets, white flour, white rice), caffeine, and alcohol.
- Carry healthful food with you to avert a sweet tooth attack.
- Eat something sour, like a pickle.

Toss the Tobacco; Pass on the Bottle

Drinking and smoking hurt your bones—one more reason to curtail these habits.

In the past, alcohol abuse was associated with a higher incidence of fractures in drinkers. Lately, moderate alcohol use, less than one ounce daily, has also been a nagging contributor to increased bone breaks and osteoporosis risk. Researchers think this happens because of falls due to inebriation, and liquor reduces bone density over the long haul.[6]

Having a cigarette, with or without a drink, leads to thinner bones in women, likely due to upset estrogen metabolism[25]. This doesn't mean, however, that men are immune. A 16-year study revealed that men who both smoked more than a dozen cigarettes per day and had at least one drink lost bone mass twice as fast as those who smoked or drank less.[5] Both of these habits also deplete your body of folic acid—a bone-loving B-vitamin.[17]

■ *Makeover Hint #58—Acupuncture Helps You Quit Smoking*

Saying you'll quit smoking is one thing; doing it is entirely another. Many people quit cold turkey successfully. If you'd rather engage a little help for the withdrawal cravings from tobacco, consider having needles put in your ears. In other words, use auricular acupuncture.

Auricular acupuncture is a specialized form of acupuncture where several painless needles are placed strategically in your ear and left in for half an hour. Done daily over a 10-day period, this treatment can dampen cravings and smooth out jangled nerves. For information on auricular acupuncture specialists, contact the National Acupuncture Detoxification Association, 3220 N St. NW, Suite 275, Washington, DC 20007; or call (503) 222-1362.

Eat Brightly Colored Fruit to Strengthen Your Skeleton

Make food your medicine. This is particularly true when you feast on delicious cherries, raspberries, blueberries, and blackberries for the sake of your bones. These and other red, blue, and purple fruits contain pigments from the flavonoid family called anthocyanidins and proanthocyanidins. These compounds with the $1000 names brace your skeleton by securing the collagen fibers in bone, those very same strands that give strength to your body's framework.[26]

■ *Makeover Hint #59—Tease Your Palate with a Palette of Fruity Colors*

When berry season hits, feast on the following fruit salad. Also take advantage of fresh fruit in season by freezing as many raspberries, strawberries, blueberries, and blackberries as your freezer can hold.

THE ALL-AMERICAN SALAD

1 cup fresh blueberries

1 cup fresh raspberries

1 cup fresh pitted cherries

1 cup fresh blackberries

Pour all fruit into a large bowl. Gently mix together. To create a patriotic salad complete with reds, white, and blues—and get an extra helping of calcium—add a dollop of whipped cream on top and serve.

Bustling Makes Better Bones

Physical fitness is another key to healthier bones. The more you bustle, the better. Being bedridden, or merely a couch potato, causes calcium to leave the body in massive amounts through the urine. On the other hand, study after study extols exercise, especially early in life, as bones' protector. Even very mild activity among elderly persons slows bone loss and increases skeletal strength.[9]

What's the best exercise for bones? Any activity that increases the load on bone or stresses bone, like jogging or going nowhere on a stair master, builds skeletal power. Yet studies show that even routine walking—a daily 20- to 30-minute walk—builds denser bones, especially when you take your calcium everyday.[2, 10]

■ *Makeover Hint #60—Childproof Exercise*

Exercise sounds great. But how do you fit a regular physical fitness program into a life filled with work and children?

There are several solutions to this problem.

1. Give up and take your chances.
2. Leave the house and conduct your exercise program outside or at a health club—and take your chances (especially if the children are unsupervised).
3. Include the children in your exercise routine. This way you get a workout, and they learn the importance of physical fitness.
4. Get up earlier than everyone and work out alone, in peace and quiet.
5. Let your family know that Mommy and Daddy must exercise everyday or they will not be fit to live with. Stress that working out is not only good for you, but for the mental health of the entire family.

Avoid Stress, Avoid Cavities

Stress is known to cause or add to many health conditions, ranging from tension headaches to indigestion to cancer. But can stress cause holes in your teeth? According to P.R.N. Sutton of Melbourne, Australia, it can. In a 1990 article printed in *Medical Hypotheses,* Sutton discusses how mental stress can cause cavities in less than one month.[27]

It seems that the middle man in this interaction is the immune system. Stress can seriously shake up your defense system, as explained in Chapter 6. This includes the built-in immunity found in your teeth. When your dental defenses are down, bacteria attack without much of a battle. Teeth become unable to defend themselves against cavities.

Too Much Worry Puts Holes in Kelly's Teeth

Kelly discovered firsthand how very real is the connection between stress and cavities. For one whole year, the 35-year-old was working on a big project for her boss. The work involved long hours with little time for relaxation, exercise, or taking care of herself. Kelly knew that the looming deadline of her project, problems that seemed to crop up each day, and general wear and tear on her body were more stress than she was accustomed to handling.

Finally the project ended, and Kelly released a sigh of relief, glad to return to a manageable schedule. One of the first items she took care of was a visit to the dentist. She was shocked to learn that her usually healthy teeth were riddled with four cavities. While Kelly hadn't exercised much in the past 12 months, her usually sound diet hadn't changed. She hadn't indulged in sweets and was careful to floss and brush her teeth regularly. Was it stress that caused so many cavities? Perhaps.

Pick the Right Paste

This next step focuses on your teeth. Did you know that the toothpaste you're using could be undoing your other Bone and Teeth Makeover plans? According to several studies, sodium lauryl sulphate (SLS), the most widely used detergent in toothpastes, hurts the soft tissues in your mouth.[28, 29, 30] This sudsy ingredient does this by stripping away the outer protective covering on gums, increasing permeability here by penetrating the soft tissue surface,[30] and causing general irritation.[31] The higher the concentration of SLS in the toothpaste, the more prevalent are these effects.[31] Scientists found two things helped this situation: 1) using toothpastes containing anti-inflammatory ingredients as well, or 2) using SLS-free toothpaste. I recommend the latter.

Once you start reading labels, you'll find that it's nearly impossible to locate a SLS-free toothpaste. Health food stores carry some brands. The one I recommend is made by Weleda; these very tasty toothpastes come in several flavors. Ask your favorite pharmacy or health food store if it carries these products, or call 800-289-1969 to order them.

As an endnote, I'd like to point out a study that tested several popular mouthwashes. The authors say the "results indicate that the use of some mouth rinses could predispose to excessive tooth substance loss and dentine hypersensitivity, particularly if used prior to toothbrushing."[32] Maybe mouthwash isn't such a good idea either?

Do you listen to your dentist and brush at least twice a day, and practice daily flossing? Proper brushing and flossing techniques are a critical component of tooth care. If you're too tired or busy at the end of the day to floss, pick another time during the day. I always floss and do my "good" brushing after breakfast when I have time and energy. Maybe this or another time works better for you than late evening.

The Silver Versus White Filling Debate

There's a raging debate going on in the alternative health care field about which is better: silver fillings or white. Rather than suggest to you what to do, I'm going to present this information and let you decide. Part of patient responsibility.

The traditional silver or amalgam fillings are composed of half mercury, as well as silver, tin, copper, and sometimes smaller amounts of indium, palladium, or zinc; white fillings are resin-based composites. Other filling alternatives include glass ionomer cements, ceramics, and gold. For more than 150 years, silver amalgams have been used in dentistry; they are still widely used and preferred over other types of fillings. Only costly gold has been used longer.

The advantage of amalgam over other filling types is mainly its longevity in teeth (eight to 12 years), and cost when compared to others. For instance, gold costs four to eight times more, while composite is about one and a half times more expensive. It's also argued that while composite or white fillings have improved considerably over the years, they don't tend to last as long as silver or gold, or aren't as sturdy in high-stress, chomping areas. Some people find that composite fillings temporarily increase sensitivity of the affected tooth; I can personally attest to this. On the other hand, with composites, your teeth look better (can't tell there's a filling there) and even if there's minimal risk having silver fillings, now you have none. Also, composites are better at conserving tooth structure than amalgams.

Now for the heat. Mercury-based amalgams have come under fire in recent years because of their possible adverse health effects. In their 1993 report, scientists and public health experts from the U.S. Public Health Service and Environmental Protection Agency state very clearly that "dental amalgam can release minute amounts of elemental mercury, a heavy metal whose toxicity at high intake levels (such as in industrial exposures) is well-established."[33] They go on to say that a fraction of the mercury in amalgams is absorbed by the body, and that people with silver fillings certainly have higher mercury concentrations in their blood, urine, kidneys and brain than those without these fillings. However, it is the consensus of these experts that while a small number of people respond with allergic reactions to mercury, there are too few studies and it's too difficult to ascertain whether or not mercury in fillings is harmful. Improvements due to removal of silver fillings are mainly anecdotal, they point out. "Although minute amounts of mercury are released from amalgam restorations," they say, "they do not cause demonstrable adverse effects of significance to the general public." Thus this government report concludes that dentists should continue using mercury-based amalgams, and discourages the removal and replacement of silver fillings with other types.[33]

Let's travel to the other side of the world for a different opinion. In Sweden, a similar group—the Department of Environmental Hygiene Karolinska Institute and the National Institute of Environmental Medicine in Stockholm—also researched the amalgam phenomenon. They used autopsies to assess the impact of mercury fillings on health. These scientists found that the more mercury fillings a person had, the higher the concentration of mercury there was in that individual's brain and kidneys.[34] The researchers admit that foods eaten, especially mercury-contaminated fish, smoking, and alcohol can influence these results. However, even taking that into account, they feel their results are valid. Results like these have persuaded the Swedish government to ban mercury fillings in pregnant women and children; it plans to phase out all other silver fillings over the next few years.[35]

Whether or not to use amalgams seems to hinge on how you interpret results. For the Americans, the cup is half full; the Swedes consider it half empty.

Amalgam Removal Proof

Robert L. Siblerud, M.S. from Fort Collins, Colorado wanted to see if silver fillings had an impact on people's happiness. First he sought out volunteers with and without mercury amalgams, and then checked to see if there was evidence of mercury in their bodies. Indeed, he found that urine samples of the amalgam subjects contained 201 percent more mercury than the amalgam-free group. He also found that the amalgam bunch reported more emotional distress; when these individuals had their amalgams removed, 80 percent said they felt better.[36]

Bone-Robbing Medications

The last step to saving your bones is to watch the medicines you take. There are members of both the over-the-counter and prescription medication crowd that actually steal valuable mass from your skeleton. Aspirin, acetaminophen, ibuprofen, and other non-steroidal anti-inflammatory drugs (NSAIDs) interfere with bone repair and cartilage metabolism.[37] This is a frightening thought when you consider how cavalier many are about popping an aspirin or other pain pill for headaches, fevers, or other discomforts. Those with arthritis often take a dozen or more of these pills daily for pain and inflammation. Other medicines linked to osteoporosis risk, particularly when taken long-term, include anticonvulsant drugs, heparin, thyroid hormone, methotrexate, steroids and cortisone, tetracycline, and furosemide.[38]

Bone and Teeth Makeover Checkup

Are your teeth glistening and bones ever so strong? Great! This is what you just completed:

- Ousted some of the calcium robbers—sugar, salt, caffeine, alcohol.
- Incorporated calcium and other important minerals into your diet; made sure they were in your vitamin pill.
- Added important vitamins like D and K.
- Cut down even more on sugar.

- Determined that smoking and alcohol are still on the list of no-nos.
- Discovered the wonder of brightly colored fruits, berries, and cherries.
- Established a regular exercise routine . . . puff, puff.
- Learned to control stress.
- Looked for a detergent-free toothpaste. Gave up mouthwash.
- Thought about and read more about silver fillings.
- Checked the medicine cabinet for drugs that hurt bones.

For Related Problems, See

- Backache
- Sprains and Strains

Laboratory Tests Your Doctor Can Order

- Dual x-ray absorptiometry or DEXA (confirms bone density)
- NTx Bone Loss Assay (indicates amount of bone being lost)

Chapter 12

Secrets of
Beautiful Skin

Your Body's First Line of Defense

To many, skin is merely a canvas to decorate with make-up and clothing. But it is much more. This 20 pounds of body covering encases the rest of the body's tissues—holds everything together, if you will. It is also one of the primary detoxification organs. Fat-soluble poisons like heavy metals and DDT are excreted from the body in sweat. Skin is one of the first lines of defense against germs and poisons. Intact skin is impregnable to infectious agents, though its porous nature does allow outside poisons to enter. When skin is broken, special cells called histiocytes attack and devour intruders.

With the help of blood vessels, skin helps regulate body temperature. When you're too hot, heat is dispersed through sweating. When it cools down, the skin helps conserve heat by shivering.

Last but not least, the skin provides us with sensations like warmth, cold, pressure, touch, itchiness, wetness, tickling, softness, hardness and pain. Some of these feelings are purely pleasurable. Who doesn't enjoy a hug or caress, the soft feel of a pet's fur, the warmth of the sun on a summer's day? On the other hand, skin is also responsible for that itch that drives you crazy, and intolerable pain. Skin is not only a source of enjoyment, but a gauge to determine when something's wrong. If, for example, you had little sensation in your feet—as happens with some people with advanced diabetes—you could cut your feet and not even notice the harm. Pain is a signal that something's wrong, a sign to stop whatever is causing the injury and get help.

When your Skin Screams for a Makeover

The skin constantly renews itself by shedding billions of cells each day. Still, there are times when a makeover is in order. Unlike other body systems, you can physically see when the skin is ready to be made over. As the canvas of the body, the skin displays its needs as an itchy rash, acne, eczema, psoriasis, hives, or other visible marks. Then there are times when the skin speaks to you in whispers about its wants. You may notice that cuts and wounds don't heal as quickly as they should. Perhaps unexplainable bruises appear. Little red spots, called petechiae, gradually show up on your skin. It could be dryness, oiliness, or paleness that calls your attention. Or maybe your mirror says it best with its waxen image.

That's not to say that these troubles are skin-related only. As you've learned by now, all parts of the body are connected in one way or another. So while you can make over your skin superficially with some results, you also need to make over those other organs that contribute to your skin's distress. These include the liver, digestive system, and other body parts.

If your skin changes after starting a new medication, consult with the prescribing physician. Also see your doctor if a skin rash or infection persists, if a mole changes shape, color, or becomes itchy or painful, or if a skin condition is particularly severe or is associated with other symptoms.

Sleep Away the Bags

Your skin, or to be more specific, bags under your eyes are a dead giveaway that you're not sleeping enough. Insufficient sleep also tends to make skin sallow-looking, pale, and generally unhealthy. We also know that during sleep, blood flow increases to your skin;[1] little sleep and it receives less of that nutrient-rich, garbage-removing circulation.

So, wake up when your skin speaks to you, and go to bed.

■ *Makeover Hint #62—Groom Yourself for Bed*

Most adults need eight hours of sleep per night, children even more. It's also important to have a regular bedtime routine that you follow an hour before turning the lights out. I call this grooming yourself for bed. For instance, read a relaxing book (no work), listen to music, have a cup of calming herbal tea or soak in a hot bath. Make sure your bedroom is pleasant. Do the decor and colors appeal to you? Is your bedroom cool enough to sleep comfortably, but not so cold that you stay awake? Would burning a scented candle make it more pleasing? Are your sleeping quarters dark?

Treat Your Skin to Natural Ingredients

Once you've slept away the bags, consider the cosmetics and other skin products you use. This goes for both women and men. As the outside covering for the body, the skin is like a wall upon which a sundry of pollutants, car exhaust, chlorine from treated water, and other airborne chemicals are thrown. That's not to mention what we voluntarily apply to our skin each day.

Make-up may be fine for a beauty makeover, but it could also be behind that acne you still have at 35. Check the ingredients in your cosmetics; use hypo-allergenic, naturally based products instead.

The same goes for soaps and creams. Regular soap removes protective oils and may aggravate sensitive skin. If you have a rash that won't go away, stop using soap for a week and use only warm (not hot) water and a face cloth followed by a cold water splash, and see what happens. Switch to a glycerine-based soap. If dryness is the problem, try a soap with vitamin E, aloe, or chamomile added. Again, check the other ingredients. Be as careful of creams and lotions as you are with soaps. Men, watch your shaving cream and after-shave lotion if skin troubles arise.

Consume Fiber for Clearer Skin

What can a heaping bowl of oatmeal or oat bran each morning do for your Skin Makeover? More than you know.

The skin is one of the major elimination organs. That means the skin helps take out your body's garbage. When internal elimination—the digestive tract, liver, and kidneys—are having problems, the skin's elimination duties increase. So an overwhelmed liver (see Chapter 3), poor digestion or absorption (see Chapter 4), or struggling kidneys (see Chapter 5) push more trash toward the skin. The evidence is in blemishes and other skin problems.

Faulty digestion not only slows the bowels, but leaves the skin looking grayish and aged. Extra oat bran and other fiber also reduce constipation and putrefied compounds made from slow-moving feces; your goal is to prevent these undesirables from being reabsorbed into circulation and out on to the skin.

■ *Makeover Hint #63—How to Make an Oatmeal Mask*

Oatmeal isn't just for eating. You can use it to make a facial mask too.

Puree 1/2 cup of dry, raw oatmeal in a blender or food processor until it's in powder form. Mix this with 1/4 cup of pure water until you have a creamy paste. Gently apply to your face and massage onto your nose, chin, forehead and cheeks using circular movements. Lie down (you might want a towel under your head), close your eyes, and relax for 15 minutes. Imagine your skin coming alive and looking luminous. End by rinsing your skin with lukewarm water. Pat dry.

Wash Your Insides to Help the Outside

Keep drinking that water for shimmering skin. Like fiber, water helps your other elimination organs—the kidneys and digestive tract—work more effectively so that your skin isn't in charge of the trash. Aim for two quarts of pure water daily. If you're not a water drinker, begin with a cup or two and work your way up, by half a glass a day. Clean, filtered water tastes much better than tap.

■ *Makeover Hint #64—How to Ensure You Have Clean Water*

Since water, and plenty of it, is so essential to clear skin and good health, it makes sense to drink the purest water possible. The cleanest water for your money comes from a reverse osmosis unit.

This filtration system is attached directly to your kitchen tap and removes most pollution and minerals. When combined with a carbon filter, almost all contaminants are extracted. If you don't have access to such a system, you can try:

- Bottled water. In most cases this is safe. To be absolutely sure, request a list of ingredients from the company you purchase water from most frequently.
- Distilled water. More expensive than reverse osmosis, but removes more contaminants. May taste flat due to mineral removal as well.
- Sediment filter. This screen removes larger particles like dirt, but not the finer ones that reverse osmosis does.
- Carbon filters. Good for taking out chlorine and organic chemicals. It doesn't, however, eliminate germs or toxic metals.
- Membrane and ceramic filters. These long-lasting filters remove parasites and bacteria.
- Redox filters. This chemical exchange system removes toxic metals, chlorine, and diminishes bacteria.[2]

Fatty Acids for Better Skin

I'm now going to tell you to eat more fat for your skin.

While most Americans are resisting fats of all types, there's a movement within natural health circles to increase essential fatty acids (EFA). It's true that too much of the wrong fats contributes to heart disease, high blood pressure, obesity, some cancers, high cholesterol, and a host of other unpleasant conditions. However, the body needs some fat to operate. Your body uses fat to make hormones, build cell membranes, keep your kidneys humming, govern nerve transmission, fuel your heart, keep inflammation at bay, transport oxygen throughout the body, and perform a host of other vital functions. The trick is to consume beneficial fats—essential fatty acids—and minimize those fats that do more harm than good. Saturated fats, found mainly in animal-based foods like meat, poultry skins, and dairy, and hydrogenated or partially hydrogenated fats, like margarine, are the fats to downplay.

While a shortage of EFAs can become obvious as constipation, aching joints, memory problems, and fatigue, your skin all but shouts its need for this essential nutrient. Dry flaky skin and hair, and cracking nails are also signs of an EFA deficiency.

Adopting a whole-foods diet brimming with whole grains, raw unsalted nuts and seeds, beans and legumes is the best way to go. In the meantime, add one to two tablespoons of flax seed oil to your daily menu (either in homemade salad dressing, or take straight. . . . gulp!). Or try the following Makeover Hint.

■ *Makeover Hint #65—Flax Appeal*

If you have a coffee grinder or blender, and a place to buy flax seeds, then you're ready for the best makeover hint ever. Every day, put one to two tablespoons of flax seeds into your grinder or blender and mash them up into flax meal. Scoop these into a bowl and place them on your kitchen table. Then throughout the day, sprinkle a generous portion of these EFA powerhouses onto your food—cereal, salad, sandwich, stew, casserole—it doesn't matter.

If you're worried about the taste, don't be. When our son's young friend spotted a mysterious bowl of flax meal on our table and asked what it was, my son, Adam, replied, "Oh, that's flax. It's great. And it doesn't taste like anything!" Kid tested; mother approved.

Clear Skin Needs Nutrients

Beautiful skin requires a make-up bag full of nutrients provided by the blood vessels that circulate through dermal tissues. The skin's texture turns first to "goose flesh," and then a dry, rough, scaly "toad skin" (known medically as follicular hyperkeratosis), when vitamin A is very low. EFA deficiency, low vitamin B or insufficient cleansing also add to this condition. Dry skin, or xeroderma, where a fine, dandruff-like layer spreads all over the skin, especially the legs, also results when vitamin A is down.[3] Instigate a vitamin A makeover by turning to foods like yellow, orange, and green vegetables, eggs, and cod liver oil.

Age spots, seen on the hands, are actually cellular debris caused in part by cells damaged by roaming free radical molecules. One way to combat age spots is to eat foods rich in antioxidant nutrients. The red, orange, yellow, and dark green vegetables and fruits like carrots, yams, squash, broccoli and lettuces, are full of antioxidant pigments called carotenoids. Taking a supplement with beta-carotene (just one of hundreds of known carotenoids) or a mixture of carotenoids can help. Vitamins C and E are two other well-known antioxidant vitamins found respectively in citrus fruits, cantaloupe and peppers, eggs and fresh, cold-pressed vegetable oils.

For mysterious bruises, poor healing skin, and funny little red spots called petechiae—these are pinpoint hemorrhages—try taking extra doses of vitamin C and bioflavonoids. In addition to eating all the right foods, pop 1000 mg of each nutrient per meal.

■ *Makeover Hint #66—Watch Your Vitamin A*

Unfortunately, one of the signs of too much vitamin A—dry skin—is similar to a symptom of vitamin A deficiency. Other vitamin A toxicity signs to watch for are brittle nails, hair loss, loss of appetite, fatigue, irritability, and gingivitis. In your zeal to feed your skin, don't take too many vitamin A pills. Concentrate, instead, on vitamin A-rich foods, or get your vitamin A from a well-balanced multiple vitamin/mineral pill. A reasonable daily dose is 5000 IU (equivalent to 1000 mg or RE). Some supplements offer only beta-carotene, the precursor of vitamin A. Make sure your supplement says "natural beta-carotene."

Is the Sun Your Friend or Foe?

The sun is bad for your skin—or is it? With all the warnings we're given about sun exposure, skin cancer, and aging, you'd think that God was playing a cruel trick on us by placing that large, warm, inviting ball in the sky. Actually, sunlight—in moderate, regular doses—is good and even mandatory for good health and healthy skin.

We need sunlight for several reasons. Sun helps the skin produce vitamin D and heightens its absorption. For these reasons, the
bones benefit. In Ayurvedic medicine, the healing tradition from
India, the sun's warm rays are a source of higher consciousness. A
15- to 20-minute daily walk outside—avoid the most intense times
from noon to 3 P.M.—is actually a recommended treatment for some
skin conditions like acne and psoriasis.

For added protection under the sun, take advantage of fresh
fruits and vegetables rich in antioxidants, like carotenoids and
flavonoids, and high in potassium. Be sure to take vitamins E and C,
and if you happen to burn, apply vitamin E oil directly to your skin.
It's been shown to reduce the redness and inflammation caused by
the sun.[4] Other natural ways to cool burning skin include applying
aloe vera juice, zinc oxide, and vitamin A oil.

If you've been inside all winter, begin exposure gradually with
half an hour per day for a week and work up slowly. Remember,
sunburn is your body's warning that you've had too much. Guard
young children with both limited exposure and by placing a hat on
both them and you. (You'll look younger for it.) Be wary if near
water, snow, or metal, as these reflect and absorb rays that cause a
burn more quickly. You can burn just as easily on a gloomy day as
on a sunny one. Take extra care if you have moles, a history of skin
cancer, burn easily, or are taking medication that increases sensitivity to the sun.

Does Sunscreen Increase Your Risk of Skin Cancer?

In a shocking and controversial California study, Drs. Cedric
and Frank Garland report that using—not avoiding—suntan lotions
might be responsible for the rise in skin cancers. The reason, they
state, is because sunscreen interferes with the skin's production of
vitamin D, a nutrient that helps guard against melanoma and other
skin cancers. Also, sunscreens prevent sunburn, our warning that
we've had enough sun. The Garland research team also states that
there's been a direct link between sunscreen sales and skin cancer
incidence.[5]

No Wrinkles? No Smoking!

Here's one more reason to avoid tobacco. It ages you! Female and male smokers age 40 and older are two to three times more likely to have moderate to severe wrinkling compared to nonsmokers.[6]

Sally's Puffing Speeds up Aging

Years ago I had the opportunity to renew an old friendship. A friend of mine from my hometown of Victoria, British Columbia, had moved to Calgary three years previous. During a trip to visit my sister, who also resided in the oil capital of Canada, I decided to look up Sally. I phoned her the day after I arrived in Calgary, and we agreed to meet for lunch.

I arrived at the restaurant first, happy and somewhat nervous to see my friend. Sally was older than me, 28 to my youthful 21, and I was proud of the fact that this mature woman would have me for her friend. Sally's petite frame and easygoing manner gave the impression she was much younger. However, when Sally finally arrived for our luncheon date, I saw that her youngish complexion had aged considerably. She was an avid smoker, and since our last meeting had developed several lines around her eyes and mouth. If ever I was tempted to take up puffing, that moment erased all allure.

Sweat it Out

Perspiration is how we stay cool in hot weather, and how toxins are tossed from the body through the skin. Natural health practitioners take advantage of this innate detoxification process by promoting perspiration. Movement or exercise that makes you perspire is one way to cleanse the body and clear the skin. Done daily in moderate doses, it not only tones muscles (see Chapter 9), but helps elimination.

Another method uses saunas. Finland is their homeland. Dr. J. Perasalo from the Finnish Student Health Service in Helsinki writes a convincing article on the many attributes of this steamy heat in the *Annals of Clinical Research.*[7] With 1.4 million saunas scattered throughout this small country, there's no doubt that the Finns adore this relaxing (and cleansing) pastime. For one, saunas promote per-spiration which effectively clears the skin and its sweat glands of bacteria. This prevents pimples. Finns have also used saunas as a place for childbirth and as a spot to cure a variety of ailments; a sauna to these people is "a holy place."

■ *Makeover Hint #67—The Finnish-ing Touch*

A full hot bath, no longer than 20 minutes, is an easy-at-home way to induce sweating and cleanse the body. Sip on a cup of yarrow or peppermint tea to enhance perspiration as you soak; while you're at it, pour a cup in your bath. Adding catnip, chamomile or lime blossom tea to your bath makes it more relaxing. This method is also useful for relieving muscle spasms and aching joints. Be careful of hot bathing if you're very weak or anemic, tend to bleed, or have a serious illness. Don't offer this technique to very old or very young individuals without professional supervision.

Makeup Herbs

Besides being our original medicines, herbs were our first cosmet-ics. When you run out of beauty products, run to the kitchen or local herb shop for these Skin Makeover aids.

- *Cucumis sativus* or cucumber slices placed over the eyes relieve strain.
- *Achillea millefolium* is yarrow; when made into a tea, it can be used as a wash for oily skin.
- Fresh *Fragaria vesca*—strawberries—rubbed on the skin is refreshing. Fragaria shortcake anyone?
- Blackheads may disappear with a dab of *Lycopersicon esculen-tum*, or tomato.
- A wash of *Arctium lappa*, the common weed called burdock, fights pimples.
- Normal skin enjoys a wash of *Mentha piperita* (peppermint), *Salvia officinalis* (sage) and *Matricaria recutita* (chamomile).

■ *Makeover Hint #68—Oatmeal Bathing*

After you've lathered oatmeal all over your face (see Makeover Hint #63), add it to your bath water for all sorts of skin rashes or irritation. Here's how. Cook one pound of oatmeal in two quarts of water for half an hour on low. When done, strain off excess liquid, and add it to your bath.

If You're Happy and You Know It, Look at Your Skin

The skin is a blabbermouth when it comes to how you're feeling. For instance, itching and sweating are immediate signs that you're stressed; others break out in hives within a few minutes. Fear shows itself with a paling of the skin or goose bumps. Embarrassment may be displayed with blushing; anger can also appear as a reddening of the face. For those with an allergic tendency, the weepy, itchy rash of eczema can emerge. Other skin conditions set off with the pressures of life include herpes, acne, warts, and psoriasis.

If you're just plain happy (and healthy), look for a rosy, vibrant glow.

Skin Makeover Checkup

As you admire your radiant new skin, glance at how you got there:

- Got some sleep, sleep, and more sleep.
- Screened cosmetics and cleansers.
- Remembered again with the fiber.
- Remembered once more, again with the water.
- Added flax seed oil, and other fats.
- Checked food and supplements for skin-happy vitamins.
- Did some sunning—but not too much.
- Stopped smoking.
- Learned to sweat.

- Made some cosmetics in the kitchen.
- Smiled.

For Related Problems, See

- Acne
- Eczema
- Hives
- Psoriasis
- Varicose Veins

Chapter 13

The Keys to Keener Vision

The All-Seeing Eyes

Eyes are the cameras of the body. Through them we receive color photographs of the world, pictures that give us information, memories, and enjoyment. When the eyes fail or weaken, reading or driving can be difficult—both severe detriments in this culture. If sight becomes severely impaired, movement and everyday activities like making a cup of tea or watching television are troublesome, if not impossible. For these reasons alone, it's important to take every Vision Makeover step possible to preserve your precious sight.

The volume of blood that flows through the eye each day is extremely high, relatively speaking, when compared to other body parts. Blood provides nutrients that guard the eyeball from damage caused by sunlight and exposure to free radical molecules. The regular workings of the eye also need nourishment.

Structurally, only one-fifth of the round eyeball is visible; the other four-fifths is encased in the skull's orbital cavity. Tissue and fat pads cushion the very delicate eyeball within this bony socket. The eyelids and fringe of eyelashes protect the outer exposed eye, by automatically blinking whenever dust or other unexpected object lurks near. Watch what happens next time someone's hand gets too close to your face. The transparent cornea and the fibrous "whites" of your eyes also guard sight from injury. Lacrimal or tear glands continuously leak out tears that lubricate and wash away dirt from your eyes; a special enzyme in tears kills unwanted bacteria.

The muscular iris, that part that gives you brown, green, hazel, or baby blue eyes, has in its middle a circular opening called the pupil. Light shines through this pinhole, and then passes through the lens which focuses images onto the retina—like film in a camera—situated at the back of the eye. The macula or "yellow spot" is the central area of the retina where vision is most acute. Photoreceptors—specialized cells called rods and cones—cover the retina where light energy is converted into nerve impulses that travel to the visual areas in the brain so you can see.

At least eight small muscles let you blink, glance sideways, and roll your eyes in disgust. Busy blood vessels rush nutrients and oxygen in, and a complex network of nerves works alongside these muscles to make sight possible.

Protect Your Sight With These Makeover Steps

Like other parts of the body, age and the perils of modern living are wearing on eyes. Problems include eyestrain from squinting at a computer screen all day, to redness caused by pollution or too little sleep. These acute problems are usually solved with a few common-sense steps like taking regular computer breaks and getting enough sleep.

More difficult to treat are the most common eye diseases of old age: cataracts, glaucoma, and macular degeneration. Unfortunately, these conditions develop very slowly, often without notice. When they're apparent, there's often no treatment. So, it's important that you include in your Natural Health Makeover steps to guard your priceless eyesight.

The leading cause of blindness in adults 50 and older is a condition called macular degeneration; almost 20 percent of those over 65 are affected. The number of people with beginning signs of this eye-stealing disease is probably higher. Early symptoms of macular degeneration are subtle. They include decreased central vision—the macula, remember, is in the middle of the retina—difficulty adapting to changes in brightness whether going from dark to light, or vice versa. Someone may experience disturbances while reading, or when looking at color. Contrasts in shades and color might not be as sharp. Very often, a person waits up to 10 years before seeking help because hints that something's wrong are so vague.[1] As of this writing, conventional medicine offers no cure.

Four million Americans are affected by cataracts, another insidious eye problem. Here the normally crystal-clear lens gradually turns murky. Loss of eyesight is gradual and painless. Cataracts begin in middle age, and are egged on by trauma to the eyes, X-rays, systemic diseases like diabetes, or medicines such as steroids. Conventional treatment involves surgery, though special glasses can be worn while the cataract is developing.

The third eye demon to watch for is glaucoma. Here, pressure inside the eye builds to such a point that eyesight is either partially or totally lost. Two million Americans are afflicted, but one quarter of these cases are undetected. Like cataracts and macular degeneration, the chronic open-angle type of glaucoma is slow-moving. A gradual loss of peripheral vision is the first tip-off, though unsuspecting trouble starts much earlier. Unlike the other two eye conditions, there is a kind of glaucoma that is a medical emergency called acute angle-closure glaucoma. It is characterized by eye and head pain—usually one-sided—as well as fleeting visual loss and colorful halos around lights. If this happens to you, call your doctor or go to the nearest hospital immediately.

It's fortunate for us that ophthalmology has been at the forefront of nutrition, compared to other conventional medical specialties. Solid research points to a wholesome diet and lifestyle as prevention against macular degeneration, cataracts, and glaucoma. These same steps can sometimes slow or reverse such conditions. To ensure your eyes are fit, read on.

Smoke Gets in Your Eyes

There's no doubt that smoking, a major free radical promoter, hurts the eyes. Free radicals are volatile molecules that in large amounts age and sicken you. Ironically, the largest source of free radicals is your body, which uses them to neutralize toxins and disarm germs. However, pollution, pesticides, radiation, drugs, alcohol, rancid fats, too much sun, *and* smoking push free radical levels from the useful to the harmful side.

At Harvard Medical School, William Christen, Sc.D. found those who smoked a pack or more daily were two to three times more likely to lose their vision due to macular degeneration than people who never smoked.[2] Smoking not only boosts free radical load, but steals vitamin C[3] and other important free-radical-fighting antioxidant nutrients from the bloodstream. Puffing on a cigarette, pipe, or cigar also impedes blood flow, thus nutrient and oxygen delivery, to the eyes. Some experts consider smoking to be a marker of a generally poor lifestyle.[4]

So, the first step you must take to improve eyesight is to snuff out all tobacco products. If this task seems overwhelming, consider the consequences if you don't. Besides risking blindness later in life, you invite lung and other cancers, emphysema, and overall poor health. While suggestions on how to quit are beyond the scope of this book, begin by locating a natural health practitioner who specializes in addiction treatment. Useful therapies in this area include auricular acupuncture, dietary changes, nutrient supplementation, herbs, and, last but not least, counseling. Stop smoking tip: take extra doses of vitamin C and other antioxidants to replenish body stores.

The Dim Vision Study

American and Australian scientists joined forces to confirm whether smoking played a role in cataract formation. Cataracts are a condition where the normally clear and colorless lenses in your eyes turn cloudy. These researchers printed these results in the *Archives of Ophthalmology* (1995, vol 113): Smokers were more than twice as likely to develop significant opacities of the eyes' lenses as were non- or past smokers. The more they smoked, the worse the problem.[5]

Alcohol Gets in Your Eyes Too

Too much wine, beer, or hard liquor affects eyesight too, both directly and by decreasing nutrient absorption.[6] The National Cancer Institute published a report in the *American Journal of Clinical Nutrition* (1995) stating that lutein and zeaxanthin—compounds important for eye health—are lower among women who drink alcohol versus teetotalers.[7] As with smoking, there's also a direct relationship between the alcohol you consume and your chance of getting cataracts.[8]

Monitor your liquor. If you choose to drink, make it the exception, not the rule. If you feel you have a drinking problem, consult with a practitioner experienced in treating this kind of addiction—whether she uses conventional or natural methods.

Spinach to the Rescue

If you like spinach salad, you're in luck. Spinach is especially high in lutein, a yellow carotene that congregates in your eye's retina. Zeaxanthin, another carotene, is often found beside lutein in the foods you eat; it's also produced by your body from lutein. Steven Pratt, M.D., of Scripps Memorial Hospital in La Jolla, California, and assistant clinical professor of ophthalmology at the University of California-San Diego is sold on the importance of lutein in eye health. "I eat a spinach salad every day," he proudly states.

Dr. Pratt knows that a diet brimming with spinach and other lutein-rich vegetables and fruits pays off. When patients showing early signs of macular degeneration listen to his nutritional advice, Pratt says not only are most healthier within a year, but many are free of this eye condition. Research backs up his observations.[9]

"Lutein in the lens," explains Pratt, "acts as nature's own sunglasses. Lutein and zeaxanthin absorb blue light, the most dangerous type of light for the eye." Ultraviolet light is mostly filtered out by the cornea and lens; yet visible blue light still reaches the retina. As an antioxidant, lutein in the macula helps protect the eye from photochemical damage caused by UV light, high-energy visible light, and other free radical-producing events like smoking and alcohol.

Kale, collard greens, broccoli, and other dark green, leafy vegetables also contain appreciable amounts of this eye-loving nutrient. But there's more. Over 400 carotenes have been identified to date; better-known ones are beta-carotene, in carrots, and lycopene, high in tomatoes. Carotenes give fruits and vegetables—like cantaloupe, yams, and red peppers—their eye-pleasing red, orange, and yellow colors. Like lutein, these pigments please your eyes in other ways too, namely as eye-guarding antioxidants.

Researcher Susan Hankinson led a Harvard study group to watch what over 50,000 nurses ate for eight years. The women who consumed more carotene-rich foods, not just those high in lutein, developed fewer cataracts.[5]

The moral here is to remember your mother's words: Eat all your vegetables (and then some). Diet supplies all the nutrients we need, if we eat a wide variety of high-quality food.

It's said that rabbits never go blind because they eat lots of carrots. Now you can see that there's some truth in that. Use your hunger and this carrot cure to fend off poor eyesight.

Directly prior to dinner (or lunch), before the food's ready and you're starving, pull out the carrot sticks. You can peel and slice them right there, or prepare them ahead of time for those munchie moments. Or if this is too much, buy prepared "baby carrots," bagged and ready to eat. (Not as nutritious, but better than not eating any carrots.) Munch away on this original fat-free, nutrition-packed snack. Guilt not included.

Add Anthocyanidins for Healthy Eyes

If carotenes give fruits and vegetables their autumn colors, then anthocyanidins are the flavonoids that paint produce—cherries, blackberries, grapes—with reds, blues, and purples. Like carotenes, anthocyanidins are antioxidants, instrumental in deactivating eye-harming free radical molecules. However, they keep eyes healthy in other ways too: by raising vitamin C levels in cells and bolstering overall eye strength. The anthocyanidin flavonoids are renowned for reinforcing blood vessels, including those in and connected to the eyeballs. This, in turn, improves blood flow and the delivery of nutrients and oxygen to the eyes.

Bilberry, or *Vaccinium myrtillus*, has a reputation as a sightful remedy. Folk healers have relied on this delicious berry to treat eyes. During World War II, legend has it that British Royal Air Force pilots who spread bilberry jam on their bread saw better during nighttime missions. Modern day science confirms that nontoxic bilberry is high in anthocyanidins, and may ward off cataracts, macular degeneration and glaucoma[10].

For those unable to find bilberries, local favorites like purple grapes, blueberries, and black currants serve just as well.

Some experts claim blueberries contain more anthocyanidins than any other blue, purple, or red fruit. You can strengthen your eyes in the summer with fresh blueberries; add frozen berries to your cereal or yogurt in the winter. Or for a delicious, eye-popping treat, try this recipe for Blueberry Eye Pie.

CRUST

2 cups whole wheat pastry flour (for a lighter crust try 1 cup unbleached white and 1 cup whole wheat; you can also experiment with other flours, such as spelt and barley)

2/3 cup butter

cold water as needed

Sift flour(s) together into a bowl. Cut butter into mixture and crumble into flour with pastry blender or hands until thoroughly mixed. Gradually add water, stirring with a fork, only until you form a ball of dough—not too dry and not too sticky. Put dough in the fridge for 30 minutes. When ready to work with pastry, flour rolling board and rolling pin. Place half of pastry on board and sprinkle a small amount of flour on top to prevent sticking. Roll out to 1/8-inch thickness and place in pie pan. Trim edges. Roll out second piece of pastry; place on top of pie pan after blueberry filling is added to pan.

BLUEBERRY FILLING

4 1/2 cups fresh blueberries

1/2 to 2/3 cup of honey or other sweetener

2 tbsp. cornstarch or arrowroot; mix with 1/4 cup water

1 1/2 tbsp. lemon juice

Mix all above ingredients in a large bowl. Pour into pie crust and top with second sheet of pastry. Trim edges, and cut several one-inch vent holes in top. Bake at 450 degrees for 10 minutes; reduce the heat to 350 degrees and bake an additional 35 to 40 minutes or until golden brown.

Serve warm after a meal of spinach salad, and see how much clearer everything seems.

Use Eye Savers

Protecting your eyes with foods high in lutein—nature's sunglasses—is a good step. But you need to cut down on the sun's glare on the outside too. Steven Pratt, M.D., suggests wearing the wraparound style of sunglasses that fit closely to your face; the larger the lenses, the better. Choose the type that screens out the most harmful rays, in the 450 nm range. Add a wide-brimmed hat to your goggle-type glasses, and not only will you look rather fetching, but you'll reduce UV light by 50 percent. Protecting eyes with this get-up is not only for adults, but for children as well.

Take Vitamins for Clearer Vision

Time to pull your vitamin bottle out again, as the next step in your Vision Makeover. A deficiency of vitamin A can end in night blindness or eventual cataract development. Very severe vitamin A deficiency, common among small children in some parts of Asia, Africa, and South America, sometimes results in a blinding condition called xerophthalmia.[11] In the case of retinitis pigmentosa, a genetic degeneration of the retina, vitamin A treatment helps preserve the retina's rod and cone function, thus slowing visual deterioration.[12]

Vitamin C, known for its ability to strengthen various body tissues by promoting collagen synthesis, appears to strengthen the eyes too. This is especially important for those with glaucoma, though research results in this area are mixed.[13] Other scientific stories attest to vitamin C's ability to preclude the development of macular degeneration[9] and cataracts.[5] Chemical burns to the cornea have also been treated with vitamin C.[14]

The eye uses the mineral zinc as a cofactor in several enzymes necessary for proper visual function. In fact, zinc is the most abundant mineral in the eye, and second most prevalent trace element in the body. Unfortunately, zinc is commonly deficient in standard diets, particularly among the elderly. Simple supplementation can, according to a Louisiana State University Medical Center study, offset macular degeneration. David Newsome, M.D., gave 151 people with this sight-threatening condition either zinc pills or a placebo. Those who took zinc had significantly less visual loss after one to two years of treatment than the group on sugar tablets.[15] Foods high in zinc include pumpkin seeds, sunflower seeds, soybeans and meat.

There are, of course, many other nutrients that feed vision and help prevent the development of degenerative eye diseases. But you can start with the above.

After reading about individual nutrients, it's very tempting to run out, stock up and take those particular vitamins and minerals. Please, don't do this!

As eye insurance, take a high-potency supplement containing a complete assortment of all known vitamins and minerals. To do otherwise invites nutritional upset and potential problems. The nutrients we need work in tandem, and when one is very high or low it can affect the absorption or effectiveness of another. For instance, 250 to 500 mg of vitamin C daily was found to be sufficient to prevent cataracts over a 10-year period.[5] More than 15 mg of zinc each day on a regular basis is too much (to use without professional supervision), and should also be taken with copper. Vitamin A is ample at 5000 IU each day. Higher amounts are fine under special conditions; but to be absolutely safe, consult first with a professional versed in nutrition.

Get Rid of Those Meddling Metals

As eye lenses get older, concentration of heavy metals seems to increase. Heavy metals are those poisonous minerals like cadmium, mercury, nickel, and lead that tend to settle in the body and cause a variety of problems ranging from mental disturbances in children (lead) to fatigue and headaches. These poisons are more prevalent than you might think. Seafood and cosmetic powders may contain arsenic; leaded gasoline releases lead into the air that then settles in the soil. Cigarette smoke spews out cadmium. Anyone who works in a gas station, dentist's office, or as a printer, jeweler, or roofer is at highest risk of heavy metal contamination.

This is all unfortunate because there is a possible link between heavy metals—cadmium in particular—and cataract formation. It's speculated that cadmium pushes out zinc that is necessary for eye function, and/or is just plain toxic.[16]

■ *Makeover Hint #72—Lighten Up on Heavy Metals*

To lighten your load of heavy metals, begin here:

- Begin by avoiding those situations that expose you (see Chapters 3 and 5).
- If you suspect you've been overly exposed, ask your doctor about testing you for these metals with a hair analysis, urine sample, or blood—whatever is appropriate for your situation.
- Take a good, high-potency multiple vitamin and mineral supplement.
- Take some extra vitamin C (1000 mg three times daily).
- Eat lots of sulphur-based foods like garlic, onions, beans, and eggs.
- High-fiber foods like whole grains will help remove some of these toxins.
- Find a physician who performs chelation therapy, and ask if you're a suitable candidate.

Exercise Your Eyes

The small muscles that maneuver your eyeball are no different from the other muscles in your body; all need varied and daily movement to work properly. You might say, "But I move my eyes all day. I blink. I look from side to side. I look up and down." This is true, we do naturally move our eyes as needed throughout the day. But we also live in an age where concentrating on close work, be it paperwork, computers, or books, outweighs eye relaxation.

This combination of focusing in closely and tight eye muscles compromises vision and can cause eyestrain and headaches. The late William Bates, M.D., a New York ophthalmologist, advocated that this combination can be behind why some people need glasses. Glasses, he felt, were a crutch for a problem that could be corrected with certain steps. First, he suggested regular breaks every hour for hardworking eyes. Second, deep breathing improves blood and oxygen flow not only to eyes, but to the rest of your body (see

Makeover Hint #79—The Right Way to Breathe In and Out). Third, stretching exercises that release tension around your eyes, head, neck, and shoulders relieve eyestrain (see Chapter 9).

■ *Makeover Hint #73—Eyeball Push-Ups*

A simple way to give your eyes a workout is with what I call Eyeball Push-Ups. If you've been doing close, concentrated work, begin by staring off into space for a minute or so. This is like a pre-workout warm-up. Next comes the sweat.

- Find an interesting picture or object on a distant wall; hold your gaze for 15 seconds (like a push-up).

- Then focus back on something close, your hands for instance. Hold your gaze for another 15 seconds (like lowering yourself after a push-up).

- Continue doing your Eyeball Push-Ups four times or until your eyes feel relaxed.

Relief for the Dry Eye Blues

If your eyes feel unusually dry, your problem could be Dry Eye Syndrome. For those experiencing other symptoms, like joint pain or fatigue, dry eyes could be just one sign that your health is being affected by rheumatoid arthritis, lupus, Sjogren's syndrome, or some other systemic disease. If you suspect this is the case, visit with your doctor.

Dry Eye Syndrome is also a condition unto itself, caused in part by a "tear" defect. Tears aren't just for crying; they are part of a vital and dynamic structure that protects your delicate eyeball from the irritating and hostile world. Tears are made up of a tear film consisting of three main layers. The outermost layer is oily; it slows down tear evaporation and acts as a seal over the eye. The watery middle layer is what tears are mostly made of. When we cry or get something in our eyes, this watery layer expands and helps clean out our eyes (and emotions). This layer also contains a bacteria-killing protein called lysozyme to protect eyes from infection. Last is the mucous layer nestled up against the eyeball itself. Its stickiness captures dirt and other debris in the eye and pushes it toward the inner corner of the eye—the same place you wipe "sleep" away.[17]

When your not-so-simple tears wash away, due to decreased secretion or increased evaporation, dry eyes can be a problem. While infrequent blinking could be the cause (see Makeover Hint #74—Think and Blink), your dry eyes could also be caused by one of the following:

- Rubbing eyes
- Hay fever or other allergies that cause red, itchy, irritated eyes
- Daily soap use around the eyes (often the case when eyelids are also dry)
- Eye drop overuse
- Contact lenses (usually the hard kind)
- Previous eye surgery
- Any trauma to the surface of the eyeball (physical, chemical exposure, infections).

While there are no substantive cures for dry eyes, knowing the cause and correcting it can help. Avoiding those situations that can injure your eyes and possibly lead to this problem (as listed above) is also wise. Artificial tears can be used, but they come with their own set of problems. Unlike real tears, fake tears don't contain important substances like lysozymes; instead, when overused, they can make dry eyes worse and increase your chance of infection by washing away these protective compounds.

■ Makeover Hint #74—Think and Blink

During a visit to my ophthalmologist, I complained of eye strain and dryness. After ruling out other possible causes, the doctor placed a small amount of fluorescein dye in my eye, and had me blink fully several times. He then instructed me to keep my eyes open for several seconds while he determined how long it took for the tears protecting my eye to disperse. Normal dispersion, or as he called it "tear break-up time," is eight to 10 seconds. My eye dryness, he determined, was in part due to my eye's short dispersion time— five to six seconds.

Not too much we could do about this physiological oddity.

However, he told me that while using computers (something I do every day, hours on end), watching TV, or even reading, many people stare or squint and forget to blink. The average and most comfortable blinking time is every five seconds. So when your eyes feel strained, think, then slowly blink . . . one, two, three . . . times. This will help remoisten parched eyeballs, and relieve some of that achiness. Eye movements help spread tears around too.

Discover the Healing Secret
of Ginkgo Biloba

Ginkgo biloba is a most interesting tree. It lives for as long as a millennium, and because its ancestry can be traced back 200 million years, it's been dubbed by some as the "living fossil." Most people are probably familiar with ginkgo trees as an ornamental addition to their garden. So what has this got to do with eyes?

Because of its ability to scavenge free radical molecules, stabilize the membranes of cells, promote blood circulation and nervous system function, ginkgo plays a significant role in preventing and possibly treating macular degeneration.

Hundreds of studies attest to the advantages of taking ginkgo for other conditions, such as inadequate blood flow to the brain (a risk for stroke), some types of depression, impotence, inner ear troubles like vertigo and ringing, multiple sclerosis, and vascular problems such as Raynaud's and intermittent claudication.[18]

Take this gingko step to better eye health if:

1. You're at risk or in the early stages of macular degeneration or diabetic retinopathy, or

2. If you're affected by one of the other conditions helped by ginkgo listed above.

When All Else Fails, Think Liver

In Traditional Chinese Medicine, how well your liver functions is directly tied to eyesight. Although it's foreign to Western thought to think of the liver affecting vision, when you consider that the liver both stores and filters blood, then the connection to eyes makes perfect sense. Remember, blood flow through the eyes is extremely high. Traditional Chinese healers also view the liver as a regulator of emotions and thoughts. So if you're overly stressed, your liver feels it as do your eyes.[19]

If your eyes feel poorly, take steps to heal your liver (see Chapter 3). This isn't as crazy as it might seem. Even though we're talking about your body in 12 different parts, it's still all joined together.

Vision Makeover Checkup

Doesn't the world seem clearer? This is what you've just done:

- Been reminded one last time of the health consequences of smoking and drinking.
- Feasted on spinach and carrots.
- Added more blueberries to your diet.
- Bought new sunglasses and a wide-brimmed hat.
- Checked that vitamin bottle again for eye nutrients.
- Made a checklist of heavy metals in your life.
- Learned eye exercises.
- Determined if you have dry eyes, and why.
- Were reminded of the importance of the liver.

For Related Problems, See

- Fatigue
- Headaches

Chapter 14

Supercharge
Your Brain

Keeping Your Nervous System
in Tone

We speak of the body-mind as if our head could be easily detached from the rest of us. The head, home to the brain, is very much a member of the body. Perhaps it's our highly developed cognitive abilities and emotions that encourage us to separate physical sensations, complaints, and illness from thoughts and feelings.

At any rate, the nervous system reminds us constantly that the brain is firmly and undeniably attached to the rest of the body. The nervous system is divided roughly into two segments: the sensory and motor portions. The sensory part links each body part to the sensory section in the brain and allows us to feel pain and pleasure, hot and cold, and other sensations. Similarly, the motor portions of the brain and nervous system provide stimuli for walking and keep our internal organs functioning. You understand now why spinal cord injuries are so traumatic and often result in paralysis.

The brain itself is a complex and not entirely charted entity. The largest part is called the cerebrum and is divided into two hemispheres, within which are several lobes. The occipital, or back, lobe is where the vision centers are. Hearing is controlled by the temporal lobe and speech on the far side of the frontal lobe. Also housed in the brain are the hypothalamus and pituitary gland. The hypothalamus has a hand in controlling moods and motivation, as well as endocrine function. The pituitary, or master, gland is divided into two sections: posterior and anterior. The former releases the hormones vasopressin and oxytocin. The larger anterior lobe is ruled by the hypothalamus; in turn, this part of the pituitary sends out special chemicals that tell endocrine glands when to release their hormones.

Making Over the Body-Mind Link

As mentioned in Chapter 6, there's a definite link between your emotions, thoughts, the nervous system, and the rest of your body. Much of this connection occurs by way of the endocrine and immunity systems. What does this mean? Well, unless you pay as much attention to how you feel and think as you do to physical symptoms and sensations, then your Natural Health Makeover will remain incomplete. By looking at all aspects of yourself—physical, mental, emotional, and spiritual—you are practicing whole-person health care.

So what are some signs that you need a Mind Makeover? They might include:

- Fatigue
- Insomnia
- Depression
- Anxiety
- Frustration
- Cloudy thinking
- Memory loss

Food for Thought

Brain food. That's the next topic for discussion. Your brain has a voracious appetite. If you don't feed it right—both quality and quantity of food—it doesn't function and neither do you. Hopefully you know what I'm talking about by now. That's right, fresh vegetables and fruits, whole grains and legumes, lean meats and fish, consumed with diversity in mind.

As the central operator of the body, this hungry organ has to be satisfied at all times. Allow me to explain. Although 100 billion cells comprise the brain, it represents only 1/50th of your total body weight. Yet those cells are extremely active, conducting body business and thinking, and eating up much of what you feed yourself.

For as metabolically active as the brain is, it has very few energy reserves. The brain needs fats, in particular essential fatty acids, for cellular upkeep. Amino acids—the building blocks of protein—provide raw material for neurotransmitters, the chemical messengers of the brain and nervous system. So it seems that you not only *are* what you eat, you also *think* what you eat. For example, eating carbohydrate-type foods increases serotonin, the neurotransmitter that calms and relaxes you.[1]

Besides this, insulin is no help at all. Your body converts most of the food you eat into glucose—a basic form of sugar. Insulin, a hormone secreted by the pancreas, helps most of the body's cells grasp and use glucose. Your brain can't do this. Instead, glucose passes without assistance into the brain and brain cells second-by-second. That's why it's important to keep blood glucose (sugar) levels even at all times. Under ideal dietary circumstances, the body maintains uniform blood sugar for hours on end (see Low Blood Sugar). When it does fall, irritability, headaches, and dizziness are your brain's reactions. In the most severe cases, fainting, convulsions and even coma can result.

■ Makeover Hint #75—Eat a Brainy Breakfast

When I tell patients they must eat breakfast, many turn pale. Breakfast? In the morning? You've got to be kidding, they say. Yet a good breakfast helps kids learn and adults work. Here are a few hints on how to turn your stomach on to morning food.

1. Don't eat anything after dinner.
2. Don't eat dinner later than 6pm.
3. Shower and dress *before* breakfast, not after.
4. Begin your morning repast with a glass of water flavored with a slice of lemon.
5. Take your breakfast to work and eat it during your coffee break.

6. Eat filling, not greasy, foods like oatmeal, whole grain toast and sugarless jam, fruit, whole grain pancakes topped with yogurt and blueberries. If you can stomach eggs, go ahead.

Cognition Nutrition

Now that you're regularly feeding your brain, be sure that all necessary vitamins and minerals are covered. You can use your multiple vitamin/mineral supplement for this in most cases. Certainly the brain cannot develop properly without a generous serving of nutrients each day[2]—that's why obstetricians recommend prenatal vitamins for their pregnant patients. It's also been shown in studies that children improve academically by taking nutritional supplements, especially if they're eating a poor diet.[3] Even adult minds benefit from sound nutrition.[4]

Of course the brain needs a wide assortment of nutrients to get through the day. Calcium, magnesium, and potassium are particularly nourishing minerals. However, it's the B-vitamins that everyone remembers when it comes to the brain. Besides facilitating memory, these nutrients help form neurotransmitters. Pyridoxal phosphate, a B_6 member, is pivotal in the synthesis of the neurotransmitters serotonin, dopamine and gamma-amino butyric acid. When thiamin (B1) is too low, the neurotransmitters glutamine and aspartate also decline. Choline, the vitamin-like cousin of the B-complex, is needed for acetylcholine. Other members of the B-complex family include riboflavin (B_2), niacin (B_3), pantothenic acid (B_5), B_{12}, folic acid, and biotin. Inositol is sometimes grouped here too.

As added protection against free-radical damage, look to the antioxidants like vitamins C and E, selenium, and the carotenoid compounds. (See Poisons to Watch For.)

■ **Makeover Hint #76—Eat Oats to Soothe Jangled Nerves**

Good old-fashioned oatmeal is a brain favorite and nervous system supporter. It's rich in magnesium, and provides some calcium and B-vitamins. Oats taken as a food or in medicinal herbal form are a traditional remedy for nervous debility and exhaustion associated with depression. They are often used during convalescence after a lengthy illness too. So eat a big bowl of oatmeal or oat bran for breakfast (or a snack) topped off with walnuts, raisins, and a scoop of yogurt. While you're at it, soak in an oatmeal bath and spread it on your face (see Chapter 12).

Rev Up Your Brain Power

Your mind needs to "flex its muscle" on a regular basis in order to stay sharp. And like your body, variety is important too. Marian Cleeves Diamond, Ph.D. demonstrated that it's possible to increase both the size and function of the brain through interesting and diverse mental activities. Using rats to make her point, Dr. Diamond showed that keeping her rodents' minds engaged not only enhanced the number and size of connections between brain cells and brain cell size (number wasn't affected), but also increased blood supply to the area.[5]

How you exercise your brain depends on personal taste. Formal education—college or university—certainly keeps the brain busy for at least four years. Some people might choose to continue this trend with night classes at a local community college. My sister Kim, who resides in remote Prince Rupert, British Columbia, used correspondence courses to keep her brain active while raising her two small children. After eight years of reading and writing, her mind was not only sharper but she graduated with a Bachelors degree in English. For others, it might be interesting to:

- Read about something new.
- Play trivia (not trivial) board games.
- Converse (TV must be off).
- Hold discussion groups on a specific topic. You can do this at the dinner table too.
- Do crossword puzzles.
- Play chess.
- Balance your checkbook without a calculator.
- Write letters instead of phoning distant friends.
- Start a new hobby.
- Watch *Jeopardy*.

- Look up words you don't know in the dictionary.
- Help your child with homework.
- Listen to educational tapes in the car.
- Learn all you can about natural health.

Set Aside Alone Time

Having time—just for you—is vital. This might mean several 15-minute breaks spaced liberally throughout the day. If you have young children at home, you might create a "quiet time" when everyone in the household is silently engaged in his or her own activity, like reading or doing a puzzle. As the parent, this gives you semi-alone time. I know many daycare providers in our area that use afternoon nap-time as their recharge time. Alone time could also be an evening alone, or an all-day event every couple of months. Some people even enjoy solo vacations.

While I can't tell you how to spend your alone time, I personally equate it with meditation. By that, I mean this singly spent spell is meant to refresh you mentally and emotionally—thus ultimately physically. Keeping this in mind, the following guidelines might help:

- Don't use this time for work.
- Don't use this time to worry.
- Before you turn on the television or radio, listen to the quiet.

Whatever or however you integrate hours just for you, make it a priority. Let me tell you why. Being alone provides you with:

- Relaxation time
- Thinking time
- Dreaming time
- Breathing time
- Stretching time (physically or mentally)
- Collapsing time
- Unscheduled time
- Responsibility-free time

- Selfish time
- Frivolous time
- Healing time.

■ *Makeover Hint #77—Take a Two-Minute Holiday*

For those times when you have to get away but can't, take two minutes and escape. Places to hide out might be the lunchroom, bathroom, storeroom, the car, or any quiet corner. When you get there, take a cleansing breath—and then another. Close your eyes; if you wish, put in ear plugs. Now indulge in your favorite day-dream and smile.

Don't Fall Into the Too-Tired-To-Think Trap

Get at least eight hours of sleep each night. More if you're sick and embroiled in a stressful situation. Sleep is one of the top factors in maintaining well-being. Yet busy schedules and endless demands for our time shove sleep to the bottom of our priority list. If you want to make over and maintain health, however, you must find the time for eight hours of restful, uninterrupted sleep each and every day.

I know several people who brag about how little sleep they get. Knowing how important nighttime rest is, I really don't understand why this should be an admirable trait. One hundred years ago, people got on average nine hours of sleep each night. Now we try to get by with seven or less—and it shows. Sleep deprivation appears not only as fatigue, but also as body aches, impaired memory, decreased concentration, and increased susceptibility to illness. Those who squeeze by with less sleep are more accident-prone and less apt to think clearly. Children who go to bed too late don't do as well in school and their parents aren't as sharp at work.

It is true that some adults need less than eight hours, and some need more. Use these signs to determine your optimal sleeping time. You may be sleep-deprived if:

- You nod off while sitting down during the day.
- You fall asleep as soon as your head hits the pillow at night.

- You're irritable.
- You have vague body aches, and even stomach upset, that go away after a full night's sleep.
- You have trouble remembering things.
- You can't concentrate.
- You're accident prone.
- You rely on coffee, black tea, soft drinks, or other caffeine beverages to stay alert.

■ *Makeover Hint #78—Six Ways to Recover Lost Sleep*

Didn't get your ZZZs last night? Try these tips to catch up.

1. Go to bed one hour early. If you can't sleep, stay there and read a relaxing book. Even if you do this only one night a week, you'll feel better for it.

2. Sleep in a little. Even an extra 15 minutes will help.

3. Take a 20-minute catnap.

4. If you're not sleeping due to worry, try a cup of valerian root tea half an hour before bedtime.

5. If jet lag has got you down, try a 3 mg capsule of melatonin 90 minutes before the lights go out.

6. If a sick or restless child is keeping you awake, ask your spouse to care for him just this one night—and wear ear plugs.

Air Out Your Brain

Breathe. That's your next task. I don't mean shallow little puffs. I want you to inhale purposefully and deeply. Flood your brain and body with the oxygen it needs. Your very busy brain uses up oxygen almost as fast as it does glucose. And when that lifeline of air is shut off for a short time, disaster can strike. Four to five minutes of circulatory arrest (all blood flow completely stops) causes permanent brain damage in half of all people, and most people after 10 minutes.[6] A dramatic example of this is a stroke. While there are several causes and physiological explanations why a stroke occurs, one is cerebral insufficiency due to transitory disruptions of blood flow to the brain. Atherosclerosis, or clogged arteries in the brain, are often behind this cutoff of oxygen. Symptoms—including neurological—vary depending on what part of the brain is affected. TIAs, or transient ischemic attacks, are mini-strokes and often portend a major stroke. These episodes last anywhere from 2 to 30 minutes with confusion, vertigo, slurred speech, weakness, and tingling as part of the picture.

Sticking to your low-saturated fat and high-fiber diet is a great stroke-preventer (see Chapter 8). You can also take the herb ginkgo to enhance oxygen and glucose usage by the brain.

■ *Makeover Hint #79—The Right Way to Breathe In and Out*

When you're feeling breath-less, use this simple 1-2-3 method to breathe easier and deeper.

1. Sit up straight, close your eyes, and place your hands on your abdomen.
2. Slowly inhale through your nose to the count of seven. Feel your breath fill your chest, rib cage, and expand your upper abdomen. Hold to the count of two.
3. Slowly exhale; gently push on your abdominal muscles to help push the air out. Rest to the count of two. Repeat 5 to 10 times. (Don't hyperventilate, now.)

Poisons to Watch For

Your brain is very susceptible to environmental toxins, be they solvents or heavy metals (poisons, not rock bands—though maybe I should include loud music too). As protector and owner of this delicate organ, you must ensure that you steer clear of harmful substances. See Chapter 3 for a complete discussion about how to "Wash Away the Poisons" at work and at home. Food allergies can also be at work; again see Chapter 3.

Specifically, be mindful of heavy metal contamination. Your best treatment is prevention. But if you suspect you've been over-ly exposed, visit with a physician who can test you through hair analysis, urine or blood samples. He can also treat you for toxici-ty problems.

Lead poisoning, supposedly one factor in the mental decline of the Roman Empire, could be our undoing too. Exposure to this heavy metal is commonplace and neurotoxic. When leaded paint, banned in 1978, crumbles and turns to dust, people can inhale it or consume it if touched. Children are especially susceptible. Drinking water tainted by lead in old plumbing is another hazard, as is breath-ing fumes from leaded gasoline, or exposure to soil contaminated with settled car fumes. Imported pottery, lead crystal glassware and ink on the outside of plastic bread bags are also sources of lead. Fatigue, reduced appetite, decreased intelligence, and neurological disorders are some signs of lead poisoning.

The world's most abundant metal, aluminum, is another brain poison we must look out for. It's in baking powder, antiperspirants, antacids, black tea, drinking water (drink filtered water), cookware, aluminum foil and cans, coffee, bleached flour and soil saturated with acid rain. Alzheimer's has been linked to aluminum toxicity, as has hyperactivity in children. Too little magnesium and calcium can increase its effects.

Cadmium, obtained from cigarettes, coffee, white flour, and zinc and copper smelters, is a toxic nerve-wrenching metal. Accumulation of mercury—in batteries, tuna and other fish, floor polishes, some cosmetics, silver fillings—is brain-unfriendly. Other toxic metals include antimony, arsenic, beryllium, bismuth, nickel, platinum, sil-ver, thallium, thorium, tin, and uranium.

Jim Tosses Canning Pot and Clears his Mind

For over 10 years, Jim owned a very large silver-colored pot. Being an avid gardener, he and his wife relied on this two-gallon container to render down fruits and vegetables for canning. It was the ideal size. It also pleased Jim that such a useful item had come to them so cheaply—50 cents spent at a garage sale. Besides growing and canning his own food, 62-year-old Jim was an avid reader. A couple of years before the pot purchase, he had read about the potential hazards of aluminum. Not wanting to take any risks, Jim cleansed his life of aluminum products—antiperspirant and the like.

One afternoon while talking with his daughter, he described the latest garden harvest, and also mentioned how concerned he was about his failing memory. For several years, Jim's brain seemed to be growing less sharp than it once was. Out of the blue, his daughter asked if he owned any aluminum pots. Jim stopped for a moment; the big, silver, garage sale pot came to mind. Was it aluminum? Immediately following the conversation with his daughter, Jim removed the canning pot from his cupboard. A month or two later, his memory hadn't improved, but it wasn't getting worse either. Was it the big, garage sale pot that was affecting his memory? Possibly. Either way, Jim was happy to be truly aluminum-free.

Dream On

I add this step as part of your Mind Makeover because without it the rest of your makeover can seem empty. Work on turning your dreams into reality. I believe that unrealized goals drag us down emotionally; and as you know, negative feelings have a very definite impact on physical well-being. So I challenge you to mold your life into exactly what you want. It won't necessarily be quick or easy; I know this from experience. But I also know the satisfaction that comes from clarifying desires, then consciously pursuing them. Perhaps the following acronym will help.

D—Dream. You need to fantasize first so your hopes and goals can surface.

A—Acknowledge. Believe and affirm that you can and want to make your dreams come true.

R—Realize. Take steps to realize your dream no matter how small.

E—Envision success. This is vital. If you know in your heart that you'll triumph, you will.

Dare to dream.

■ *Makeover Hint #80—Create the Perfect Day*

Creating the perfect day is an easy and fun way to practice your dream realization. Begin by listing your favorite things. Then invite happiness into your life by planning "Perfect Days" for yourself on a regular basis. Here's how:

1. Pick a day (several months in advance if necessary), circle it on your calendar, and book it like you would any other important event.

2. Make arrangements so you're free—babysitter for the kids, spouse is notified, etc.

3. Save money if necessary.

4. On the day, start early. The hardest part is leaving your house and responsibilities behind. If it helps, go out of town.

5. Now, have fun.

The best Perfect Days are spontaneous when you do what you want as you desire it. Recently, on one of my Perfect Days I began with breakfast at my favorite bistro followed by clothes shopping. I then went for a long walk, and saw not one but two movies. My day ended with visiting a friend I don't see very often, and home—after the children were in bed.

Neil Quits His Job and Finds Happiness

Neil was miserable. At 36 he felt hopelessly trapped in his job as a mental health counselor for a large agency. When he first began, the work was enjoyable and challenging, and he found satisfaction helping the people that came to see him. But eight years of working with distressed people, in an agency that demanded he see 30 clients weekly had sent him reeling into burnout. Every day Neil came home to his wife with the same complaints: headaches, achy neck and shoulders, tight stomach, and exhaustion; many nights he was unable to sleep.

As these physical problems grew worse, Neil looked to his doctor for answers. The doctor prescribed pain medication for Neil's headaches and sleeping pills for nighttime. Next Neil saw a chiropractor who suggested neck exercises and scheduled weekly sessions for spinal manipulation. A holistically-oriented physician gave Neil vitamins and minerals. Another doctor recommended that he be evaluated for depression. While some of these ideas helped slightly, nothing solved all his troubles. Finally Neil's wife told him to quit his job. While Neil knew his counseling work was having a toll on his health and happiness, the thought of quitting—especially when his family needed his paycheck to live—was frightening.

Two years after his wife's suggestion, Neil finally did quit. He had no idea what he would do instead or where he would work. He'd never thought before about what work he'd really enjoy. So Neil decided that his new assignment for the next few months would be to search for his ideal career. As he began exploring the workplace, Neil noticed that all his bothersome symptoms evaporated one by one.

Mind you, both Neil and his wife lost numerous nights of sleep over money and the possibility of failure. This was a tremendous risk he was taking, and without his wife's blessing and a back-up financial plan he would not have attempted it. Timing was another critical consideration. For several years before he resigned, Neil thought of quitting but the time was never right. He waited, instead, until his wife's paycheck was substantial enough to support the family and the children were in school.

Neil's revival in his health and mental outlook not only made him feel better than he had in years, but fueled his creativity. Today, five years later, Neil has started his own business, and is healthier, wealthier, and happier than he's ever been before.

Mind Makeover Checkup

Does your brain feel beautiful? These are the final steps you took in your Natural Health Makeover:

- You now eat breakfast—like it or not.
- You have made another vitamin checkup, this time for brain nutrients.
- You want to be alone.
- You're sleeping so much, you rival Rip Van Winkle.

- You learned how to breathe (so that's how it's done!).
- You made one last sweep for poisons.
- You are reassessing your life, and looking for ways to reshape it.

For Related Problems, See

All conditions listed in Part Two are related to the mind. Specifically, see:

- Anxiety
- Fatigue
- Headaches
- Insomnia

Laboratory Tests Your Doctor Can Order

- Hair Analysis—heavy metals
- Urine Test—heavy metals

How Did You Do? Complete the Before-and-After Chart

Congratulations! You have completed your Natural Health Makeover and have taken a huge step toward better lifelong health. During the past few weeks, you've eaten well, exercised regularly, perhaps used nutrients and herbs, watched out for stress, slept more, discovered new ways of cooking, and learned the importance of taking control of your well-being.

Depending on where you started health-wise, you may feel enormous benefits from this 12-step makeover plan. Or the effects may be more subtle. This is where your Before-and-After Chart comes in. Flip back to Chapter 2, and glance at the initial responses you made regarding your health. Now fill out the After portion of this chart and compare your answers to the Before part. What has changed? Has there been improvement? Have you forgotten how bad you felt when you began?

Most people who complete the Natural Health Makeover will notice at least some positive changes in their health. However, it's been my experience that the longer one sticks with good health-promoting habits, the better one feels. A few weeks or months is often not sufficient to undo years of unhealthy living. For every year of aches and pains, count on it taking one month to recover. In fact, promise yourself that every year you'll devote a few weeks to a touchup, using whatever steps are required from your Natural Health Makeover plan. 'Tis only human to slip off the health wagon once in awhile. Some unhealthy habits are harder to break than others. If you tumble completely off, just dust yourself off and start all over again.

If you're suffering from a more serious ailment, you might require the services of a physician who can tailor treatments specifically for you. But finishing a Natural Health Makeover is a great beginning. Therapies, whether natural or conventional, work better when laid upon a foundation of healthy living.

part two

Natural Remedies for Over Thirty Common Ailments

Getting Started

Now that you've completed (or while you're working through) your Natural Health Makeover, you can use this section when you need practical answers to over thirty common ailments. This information will help you stock a brand-new medicine chest brimming with herbs and vitamins, instead of prescription and over-the-counter medications. Research continues to validate these methods, and every year we're learning what traditional healers have known for thousands of years—that herbs and sound lifestyle choices have a dramatic impact on health and illness.

I begin each part below by describing the condition, then move on with tips on how to prevent it. This is followed by nutritional advice, herbs you can try (listed according to actions), homeopathic remedies that might help (the italics highlight the main symptom to watch for) and lifestyle recommendations. See Appendix A for guidelines on how to use herbs, and when certain ones *should not* be taken. Please read about each herb you want to use before trying it. Appendix B describes the principles behind homeopathy and how to use these remedies effectively.

Where appropriate, I end each section with a Lookout Alert: a list of symptoms or situations that require your physician's attention. Please don't ignore this information. If any illness is ongoing or doesn't improve with the suggested treatments, call your doctor. For suggestions on natural health practitioners, see Appendix D. The nutrients, herbs, and homeopathic remedies I recommend can be found in most health food stores or even drugstores. If you're not sure how to use any of these natural substances, consult with a knowledgeable practitioner.

■ *Makeover Hint #81—Try Natural First*

For mild conditions that you normally self-treat with over-the-counter medicines, try natural treatments first. They are usually safer and often less expensive than most synthetic medications. If you find that natural treatments don't work the first time you try them, there could be many reasons why.

- The products you're using may be of poor quality. For example, packaged herbs vary widely in potency depending on how they were cultivated, harvested, manufactured, and packaged.

211

- Natural products (like medicines) must be used correctly, i.e. in adequate amounts at proper intervals, to be effective.

- Natural treatments often work more slowly and are more subtle than stronger medicines. Give them time.

- Natural (and conventional) medicines tend to work better when you build a firm foundation of health with proper diet, exercise, sleep, and stress control. (This is where your Natural Health Makeover comes in.)

- Natural medicines work best when the principles of natural health are adhered to (see Chapter 1).

- Each person is unique. This means that different herbs, nutrients, and lifestyle steps must be made to fit each individual's needs.

- Self-care is the first level of health care. But if you don't get better using the following suggestions, consult with your doctor or a natural health care professional.

ACNE

At the bottom of each hair follicle is a pouch called the sebaceous gland. When natural oils get trapped in that pouch and bacteria grow, a pimple is born—red and inflamed. Pimples occur mainly on the face, and occasionally on the back, chest and shoulders.

Many things cause this most common skin problem. Hormonal changes, such as during puberty (especially in boys), or just before a period or mid-cycle for women. Various chemicals and pollutants can also aggravate or create acne. Others break out from poor food selections, or a reaction to certain foods. Low levels of nutrients can also aggravate an acne problem. Also see Canker Sores, Eczema, Hives, Psoriasis; refer to Chapter 12 (skin).

How to Prevent Pimples

- Drink water. Make sure it's pure and plentiful.

- Avoid overwashing your face. Once in the morning and once before bed should be adequate.

- Pick plain-jane soaps. Avoid cleansers with perfumes, colorings, and other unnecessary ingredients. Glycerine soaps work well for many; or try a soap with the herb calendula added, or vitamins A or E.
- Take makeup breaks. Leave your face bare at night, on weekends, whenever you don't need to look stunning.
- Be choosy about your cosmetics. Like soap, choose makeup that's free of potentially allergenic materials. Look into natural cosmetics free of skin-annoying ingredients.
- Protect your skin from pollutants. Also look out for machine oils, coal tar derivatives, chlorinated hydrocarbons.
- Use filtered water to wash your face, particularly if your tap water smells like chlorine.

Food and Nutrition for Acne

- Sugar be gone! Also avoid other refined carbohydrates like white flour.
- Stick with whole grains such as whole wheat and brown rice.
- Be careful of fats. Keep saturated fat and overall fat intake down.
- No more margarine or any foods containing trans fatty acids or hydrogenated oils (read labels).
- Add good fats. Your skin does need essential fatty acids found in flax seed oil (take 1 tbsp daily—see Makeover Hint #65—Flax Appeal), raw, unsalted nuts and seeds, fish and whole grains.
- Keep carbohydrates to a dull roar. For some, too many carbohydrate foods (pastas, breads) make acne worse.
- Avoid commercial milk. The hormones added to commercial milk worsen some cases of acne. Drink organic milk instead, or a dairy substitute like soy or rice milk.
- Get enough protein. This means beans and legumes, organic poultry, fish, lean meats, nuts and seeds.
- Pass on the pop. High in sugar and additives, soft drinks do nothing to prevent pimples.
- Caffeine is a no-no, whether it's in pop, coffee, or black tea.
- Make sure your multiple vitamin and mineral supplement contains: vitamin C (1000 mg), vitamin E (400 IU), zinc (50 mg for two months, then 15 mg maintenance), chromium (200 mcg).

- Vitamin A. Very high amounts of this vitamin improve acne. However, if you'd like to try this nutrient, see your doctor for help as high doses taken for a long period are potentially toxic.

Herbal Treatment

- Acne lotion—calendula, chickweed, witch hazel
- Dry skin—burdock, cleavers
- Clear skin through better liver function—blue flag, dandelion
- General skin herbs—red clover, yellow dock

The Homeopathic Difference

Using homeopathic remedies alone will not solve an acne problem—especially if you're taking them in low potency, acute fashion. Most pimples require lifestyle changes. If you have a particularly resistant case of acne and want to try homeopathy, consult with a professional homeopath for constitutional prescribing. In the meantime, you can try one of these remedies for temporary and partial relief.

- Belladonna—*Acne rosacea.* When you think Belladonna, think red alternating with pale skin. Along with pustules, your face may feel dry, red, and hot. This remedy is specific for acne rosacea, a chronic inflammatory skin condition of the mid face that usually begins in middle age or later.

- Hepar sulphuris calcareum—*Teenage acne.* If you or your youngster has moist blemishes, the type prone to forming pus, this may help. Some might also feel a prickly-type pain; others find their acne bleeds easily. Cold, dry, and touching the skin make it worse.

- Ledum—*Forehead pimples.* For those blemishes on the forehead, try Ledum. Some find a sticking pain accompanies this type of acne. Cold makes it better.

- Sulphur—*Unwashable acne.* These blemishes are not only dry and itchy with pustules, but burning as well. There's an unhealthy look to the skin. Scratching the itch makes the acne worse as does washing. For some, these pimples appear after using a topical medication.

Lifestyle Link

- Sunshine. Aim for 15 to 20 minutes daily; avoid the most intense times from noon to 3pm.
- Soap alternatives. Regular soap can make acne worse. Try a calendula-based cleanser instead. For the very sensitive, wash with warm water and pat your skin dry.
- Try a Bentonite clay mask.
- Consider PMS. Acne directly before a menstrual period may be part of premenstrual syndrome. Try taking a B-complex with adequate vitamin B_6.
- Digestive woes. For some, poor digestion of food can aggravate acne. Adopt the eating style recommended under Food and Nutrition. If this doesn't solve the problem, try using hydrochloric acid or digestive enzymes (See Chapter 4).

■ *Makeover Hint #82—Break Out the Tea Tree Oil*

Tea tree oil, also known as *Melaleuca alternifolia*, has bacteria-fighting properties. Apply this oil to acne-affected skin a couple of times each day. Some people are sensitive to full-strength tea tree oil, so dab a small amount on a sample skin area first. If the oil burns or irritates you, dilute it half and half in vegetable oil before applying.

ALLERGIES

See Hay fever.

ANXIETY

Unlike fear, which is directed at a specific person, thing, or situation, anxiety is vague. It's a physical, psychological, and behavioral response to stress. Many things contribute to anxiety: heredity, childhood experiences, health, and lifestyle. Our fast-paced lives—where quick adaptation to change is essential—create stress and anxiety. In addition, pollutants, chemicals, poor food choices and health habits allow anxiety to grow. For more information, see Fatigue, Headaches, Insomnia, Low Blood Sugar. Turn to Chapters 7 (adrenal glands), 8 (the heart), and 14 (the mind) for related topics.

How to Prevent Anxiety

- The balancing act. Try to divide your time equally between physical activity and mental exertion. This will relieve stress and prevent anxiety.

- Delegate. We get anxious when there's too much to do. You can't do it all, so learn what can be delegated (household chores, work duties), what you personally must do, and what activities are not essential and can be tossed.

- The right company. Associate with positive people, ones who will support you, not undermine or doubt you. While you're at it, stick with positive reading material, TV shows (even the news), and other forms of entertainment. (There's no rule that you *have* to watch violence even if everyone else is.)

- Exercise. Physical activity works off tension, floods your body with oxygen, and is generally invigorating.

- Relax. Easier said than done. Nevertheless, make a list of activities that truly calm you down, like walking, reading romance novels, planting flowers. Then take time to do them every day.

- Sleep. Fatigue magnifies most problems, both physical and emotional. So when you feel irritable, go to bed early.

- Chemical alert. The stressors that promote anxiety aren't just mental and emotional—they're also physical. Besides the above, reduce chemicals in your home and workplace, including household cleaners, solvents and pesticides. (See Makeover Hint #3—Less is More).

Food and Nutrition to Calm You

- Downsize caffeine. Caffeine, whether it's in coffee, black tea, chocolate, or soda pop, is a stimulant. It can create insomnia and robs your body of thiamin, vital for proper nervous system function.

- Sugar blues. Coffee's partner in crime is usually a glazed doughnut or other sweet delight. Refined sugar boosts blood sugar and mood temporarily. Soon afterward, both plummet leaving you crabby and anxious.
- Spare the salt. Too much salt depletes potassium, a mineral necessary for proper nerve functioning.
- Eat slowly and moderately. Reasonable portions eaten in a relaxed atmosphere will not only help digestion, but can calm and center you.
- Have a Papa-bowl of oatmeal for breakfast. Oats are well-known for nourishing the nervous system.
- B-complex. This family of vitamins (thiamin, riboflavin, niacin, B_6, folic acid, B_{12}) nourish the nervous system so they help you handle stress better, and keep anxiety down.
- Calcium and magnesium (1000 mg and 500 mg) taken daily are relaxing.

Herbal Treatment

- Calming—linden, oats, passion flower, skullcap, valerian
- Nervous digestion—chamomile, hops, peppermint
- Insomnia—lady's slipper, passion flower, valerian
- Muscle tension—skullcap, valerian

The Homeopathic Difference

- Arsenicum album—*Great fear and anxiety.* A restless nature accompanied by chilliness, fatigue, and weakness is the mark of someone who suits Arsenicum. This anxious type is also a clean freak, striving to control her environment. She's also possessive of things and people because of insecurity.
- Ignatia—*Changeable mood.* Ignatia is known as the grief remedy. It's often appropriate for someone who's suffering from grief or worry. Sighing and weeping are common signs, as are a tendency to be inward and non-communicative. Moods change quickly.

- Lycopodium—*Fear of rejection.* The anxious person who can't function in social gatherings because he worries about what others think fits the Lycopodium mold. A false air of bravado may be used to hide these insecurities, to the point of being overbearing. At the same time, he's afraid to try new things. Lycopodium-types like others around—but not too close.

- Rhus toxicodendron—*On the move.* A restless, anxious person fits the picture of Rhus tox. This need for movement continues on into bedtime, so much so that tossing and turning in bed makes it difficult to sleep. Even his mind won't stop moving when the lights are turned out.

Lifestyle Link

- Stop smoking. A recent study discovered that more women with panic disorders (an extreme form of anxiety) were smokers than were their anxiety-free sisters.[1]

- Eliminate drugs. Stimulating drugs like cocaine and amphetamines feed an anxious mood. If you can't stop on your own, seek help from an addictions expert.

- Take a snooze. While it may be difficult to fall asleep, dozing is imperative. Anxiety climbs when you are sleep-deprived.

- Other problems. If a past trauma or current situations are creating or aggravating your anxiety, seek the help of a counselor.

Lookout Alert

When anxiety grows beyond normal apprehension in intensity or duration and begins interfering with everyday life, it's termed a panic disorder. Here are some signs to watch for.

- Sense of terror for no rational reason
- Inability to catch your breath
- Racing heartbeat, irregular heartbeat, or sharp chest pains
- Trembling, sweating, or dizziness
- Anxiety accompanied by nausea and/or diarrhea
- Connection with reality lost

ARTHRITIS

See Gout.

BACKACHE

Most people suffer from back pain at one time or another. Very often tension underlies stiff or sore muscles. Other common aggravators include poor posture and gait, a "beer" belly, incorrect lifting techniques, and injuries—immediate or past. A herniated or ruptured disc, infection or fracture of the back bone or other more serious afflictions that require medical attention are possibilities too.

Seemingly unrelated conditions can also bring on back pain. Things like a bladder infection, uterine fibroids or cysts or infections, osteoporosis, osteoarthritis, menstrual cramps, and pregnancy can cause you to grasp your back and moan. Knowing exactly what's behind your aching back is important in solving this problem. Also be aware of whether this is an acute (immediate) problem, chronic (long-standing) trouble or a combination of both. Also see Anxiety, Headaches, Sprains & Strains, Urinary Tract Infections. Refer to Chapters 5 (kidneys), 9 (muscles), 11 (bones), and 14 (the mind) as well for more information.

How to Prevent Backaches

- Practice perfect posture. Stand up straight, tilt your pelvis in and your shoulders back. This may feel unnatural, but after awhile it'll become second nature.

- Sit up straight—for all of you who are chained to a desk.

- A gracious gait. When you move improperly, back troubles can arise.

- Lift and separate. When carrying heavy (or even light) objects, use common sense. Bend down with a straight back and lift.

- Help for the heavies. If a load is more than you can carry, ask for help.

- Be flexible. A supple, fluid spine has fewer problems. Use stretching or yoga to gain flexibility and iron out the kinks.

- Plain old exercise. Regular physical activity helps prevent back pain.

- Down with stress. Often backaches aren't so much physical as emotional and mental in origin. (After all, isn't that where most tension begins?) Learn to cope, and your back will love you for it.

- Breathe for your back. Deep and conscious breathing relaxes tension and increases oxygen flow to all your muscles (see Makeover Hint #79—The Right Way to Breathe In and Out).

Food and Nutrition for Healing

- Vitamin C and bioflavonoids. These nutrients, taken in equal amounts (1000 mg each daily), help strengthen connective tissue, and thus your back. If you're a smoker, quit, or at the very least take an extra 3000 mg spread throughout the day; smoking depletes vitamin C levels.

- Antioxidants. Besides vitamin C, add a general antioxidant supplement to your daily regimen, while healing.

- Bromelain or bust. This enzyme from the pineapple stem reduces pain and inflammation when taken between meals. Pancreatic enzymes can also be taken this way.

- Tackle inflammation. For back problems that are red, swollen, and hurting (signs of inflammation), avoid foods that promote swelling. These include saturated fats (in red meat, poultry skin, dairy fat) and turn instead to the essential fatty acids (flax seed oil, fish, nuts and seeds) that diminish inflammation.

- Drink water.

- Manganese. Take 50 to 100 mg of this mineral daily, in divided doses for two weeks.

- Extra calcium and magnesium. Load up on these minerals for awhile if muscle spasm is a problem. Include a dose (300 mg/150 mg) before bed with a snack if you can't sleep. Beware: too much magnesium can cause diarrhea.

Herbal Treatment

- Loosen muscles—skullcap, valerian
- Pain—black willow, Jamaican dogwood, St. John's wort, valerian

- Herbal liniment can include (don't use any of these on broken skin)—peppermint (oil), rosemary (oil), St. John's wort
- Help sleep—passion flower, valerian

■ *Makeover Hint #83—In a Pinch, Use a Pinch of These*

It's late, you've thrown your back out and the stores are closed. Here's a recipe for a homemade liniment.

1/4 tsp of *either* cayenne powder, ginger powder, or mustard powder

1 tsp of KY jelly or cream

Mix the two together and apply to back pain. Do not smear on sensitive or broken skin. And don't leave this mixture on too long. Watch for reddening of the skin or a warm feeling, then wipe off.

The Homeopathic Difference

- Calcarea fluorica—*Low back pain.* When your lower back gives you trouble, and eases up with a little stretching and walking about, think of Calcarea fluorica.
- Phosphorus—*Right between the shoulder blades.* Phosphorus addresses burning backaches, especially between the shoulder blades. Only sleeping in a dark room and lying on your right side feels good. Almost everything else makes it hurt: touch, warm food or drink, weather change, evening, climbing stairs, physical exertion . . . even thinking.
- Rhus toxicodendron—*Worse after a good night's rest.* You know those backaches that feel terrible after lying down for awhile? This is what you take for it. You'll probably find a little movement and heat will limber it up, though.
- Sabina—*I can't move.* This remedy offers help for a very specific type of trouble: paralytic pain in the small of the back. It feels worse with the smallest movement and heat, although cool fresh air brings some relief.

Lifestyle Link

- Ice it. The coolness of an ice pack helps reduce swelling for an acute backache. Do this for 24 hours, then alternate ice with a heating pad for a few days.

- Rest times four. For an immediate injury, don't overdo it and rest for at least four days. Use your pain as a gauge for your activity during the first week following an injury.

- Visit your local back specialist. This could be a massage therapist, chiropractor, osteopathic doctor, naturopathic physician, or physical therapist. The earlier you get help, the better your chances of recovery from an acute problem.

- Try acupuncture. This ancient Oriental art is wonderful for pain control; a series of treatments might help those with chronic back troubles.

- Uneven legs. Some people have one leg longer than the other. Ask your doctor about shoe lifts to correct this problem.

Lookout Alert

If muscular and stress control techniques don't help within a week, see your doctor for a diagnosis of your problem. If you experience these symptoms in addition to your back pain, seek professional help.

- Fever
- Flank pain
- Painful or burning urination
- Frequent or urgent urination, or frequent nighttime urination
- Sudden backache without known cause
- Severe back pain

BLADDER INFECTIONS

See Urinary Tract Infections.

BRONCHITIS (ACUTE)

This usual winter-time affliction is literally an inflammation of the bronchi found in the lungs. It often begins as a cold with runny nose, fever and chills, sore throat and achy muscles. Then it progresses into an upper respiratory infection where a cough develops—first dry and non-productive, then wetter with mucus. Some people experience difficulty breathing and chest pain as well. Pollution, fatigue, and stress, taxing the body with poor eating, and not enough exercise increase your susceptibility to this condition.

Like a cold, the body can heal bronchitis—a generally mild malady—without treatment (though suggestions below will hopefully help you recover more quickly or at least with fewer symptoms). However, older or debilitated people must be wary, or they might end up with pneumonia if not careful. Chronic bronchitis, not covered here, is often caused by smoking. Also see Colds and Flu, Coughing, Ear Infections, Fever, Sore Throat; refer to Chapter 6 (immunity).

How to Prevent Bronchitis

- Avoid bronchial infection by boosting immunity (see Chapter 7). This means get enough sleep, eat right, and avoid overdoing it.
- Prepare for winter. Harsh winters, like those we endure in South Dakota, are hard on everyone no matter how healthy. So I get ready by religiously taking my vitamins and minerals, loading up on vitamin C (1000 mg three times a day), drinking immune boosting teas like echinacea, and watching the sugar and exercise.
- Hibernate. Another resistance-building activity is snoozing. For those who live in colder climates, don't be alarmed if you find you need another hour's worth of sleep each night during winter.
- Avoid exposure to infected individuals.
- Don't smoke. And non-smokers, avoid exposure to second-hand smoke.
- Consider allergic possibilities. Ask your doctor if you can be tested for inhalant or food allergies. Avoid offending substances for at least one month and see what happens.

Food and Nutrition for Your Lungs

- Hot and spicy. Indulge in all your favorite spicy foods like jalapeno and other hot peppers, mustard, horseradish, garlic, and onions.
- Did I mention garlic and onions? These are natural bug slayers.
- No more mucus. Side-stepping sugar, dairy foods, starches, and eggs, as well as other potentially allergenic foods like citrus fruits and high-gluten grains (wheat, oats, barley, and rye) can diminish phlegm.
- Flood yourself with fluids. This means pure water, herbal teas, broths, and fresh vegetable juices. Avoid fruit juices, as the fruit sugar drags down immunity.
- Avoid sugar.
- Take your multi. Be sure it contains vitamin A, E, and zinc—all helpful for bronchitis.
- Don't take iron while sick. This mineral promotes bacterial growth.
- Extra vitamin C and bioflavonoids. Take 500 to 1000 mg of each every two hours. If you experience any gastric problems (diarrhea, gas, cramps), cut back.

Herbal Treatment

- Fight bugs—echinacea, elecampane, garlic, thyme
- Ease coughing—coltsfoot, elecampane, mullein, thyme
- Expectorants—elecampane, hyssop, thyme, white horehound
- Soothe bronchi—elecampane, marshmallow leaf

The Homeopathic Difference

See Coughing for other homeopathic suggestions.

- Antimonium tartaricum—*So much mucus, so little time.* The bronchi feel like they're overloaded with mucus, yet not much is coughed up. There's a rattling sound, too, when you cough, and a burning sensation in the chest. It all feels better sitting up, not so good lying down.

- Bryonia—*Deep chest cough*. This common cough remedy is for painful, dry coughs that have traveled into the chest. When you ask someone with this type of cough if it hurts, he'll reply, "Only when I breathe and move." Ironically, lying on the sore spot feels better. Those with a Bryonia-type cough are thirsty, tired, and irritable.

- Ipecac—*The cough that rattles*. This cough is deep, wet, and rattles because of all the mucus that has settled in the lungs. Breathing out is difficult, and much harder than taking air in. Coughing is so intense at times it may result in gagging or vomiting.

- Kali muriaticum—*Bronchial congestion that's stuck*. There's tenacious mucus in your bronchi, so thick and white that it's difficult to cough up. Like Ipecac, this bronchial cough rattles, but the cough is short and spasmodic, more like a whooping sound. Some hoarseness may result too, as well as a white or gray tongue.

Lifestyle Link

- Avoid smoky rooms. Tobacco fumes only make matters worse.

- Don't drink. Alcohol, caffeine, and pop, that is.

- Get your beauty (and health) sleep. Take naps, go to bed early, stay home from work and watch the soaps, whatever it takes to give your body time to heal.

- Inhale hot steam. Use a vaporizer at night and when you're resting. Add a few drops of eucalyptus oil to the water, or a dash of Vicks Vapor Rub™ (contains eucalyptus) for lung soothing steam.

- Soak in a hot tub. Add eucalyptus oil here too.

- Kick out the pets. If you also have allergies to cats and dogs, and heaven forbid, have one living with you, consider asking it to leave. At the very least, don't sleep with it. (I actually love animals, especially my two cats.)

- Watch for indoor pollution. New carpets, paint, homes, and cars emit poisonous fumes. If you're susceptible to bronchitis, or seem worse in a new home or new car, rethink how you live.

Lookout Alert

If your bronchitis or cough is ongoing and doesn't appear to be infectious, watch for other causes. Various dusts, fumes from strong acids or volatile solvents, cigarette or other smoke might be irritating your lungs and causing inflammation. Other signs to take note of are:

- Fever lasting a week or longer
- Any severe symptoms, or those lasting more than a couple of weeks
- Shortness of breath upon exertion
- A bluish tinge to your skin
- Recurrent bronchial infections
- Unintentional weight loss
- Persistent weakness
- Chronic wheezing that's worse upon lying down

CANKER SORES

Canker sores are small painful sores that range in size from a mere pinpoint to 1/2 inch and appear singly or in groups of two to 15. Doctors call these mini-mouth ulcers aphthous stomatitis or ulcerative stomatitis. While they usually clear up on their own in one to three weeks, they also tend to recur. One in five individuals is cursed, most of them women. These are different from cold sores, which are caused by the herpes virus.

While no one is entirely sure why canker sores develop, some theorize it's a localized immune reaction or possibly an autoimmune (the immune system attacking your mouth) reaction. For some, food sensitivities spark an outbreak. Others find stress a precipitating factor. Nutrient deficiencies have also been implicated. Read Chapter 6 (immunity) for more information.

How to Prevent Canker Sores

- Manage stress. When life becomes overwhelming, it not only breaks your spirit, but your immunity too. For those who are susceptible, canker sores are one way to express stress.

- Stay rested. Sleep deprivation sets some people up for a canker recurrence.
- Pick your dentist well. Dental trauma can lead to canker sores.
- Prepare for heat. Extreme heat—caused by weather, fevers, or exercise—spark canker sores in some.

Food and Nutrition for Your Mouth

- Nutrient deficiencies, especially of folic acid, pantothenic acid, vitamin B_{12}, iron, add to canker sores. Take these as part of a multiple vitamin and mineral pill.
- Fill up on vitamin C. This nutrient helps repair mouth tissue and, if allergies are present, acts as an antihistamine. Take 500 to 1000 mg three times each day.
- Zinc. Known for its wound-repairing abilities, zinc heals canker sores in some people. Try 25 mg (as zinc picolinate) for no longer than two months.
- Food sensitivities. Canker sores can be an allergic reaction to food (dairy, wheat, tomato, pineapple). Try eliminating these for a couple of weeks and see what happens.
- Help digestion. Take acidophilus before bed to help reestablish bowel bugs. (Important if you have a history of antibiotic use.) Also try digestive enzymes with meals.

Herbal Treatment

- Decrease stress—linden, oats, passion flower, skullcap, valerian
- Improve immunity—cleavers, echinacea
- Mouth wash (make a tea with these herbs, rinse and swallow)—chamomile, sage
- Nutritive herbs—alfalfa, dandelion, nettles, oats

■ Makeover Hint #84—Chew on Licorice

Herbal licorice (not the candy) has been proven to help heal canker sores. One of the most effective forms is deglycyrrhizinated licorice (DGL) in chewable tablets, best taken before meals.[2] You can find these at your local health food store.

The Homeopathic Difference

- Borax—*Bitter taste.* For canker sores that are hot and painful to the touch, and cause a bitter taste in your mouth, think Borax. These sores are so tender, they may bleed while eating. This remedy is fitting for those who have a concurrent thrush (mouth yeast) infection going on.
- Kali muriaticum—*A white, gray-coated tongue.* Like Borax, this type of canker sore can accompany thrush, as well as a coated tongue. Also look for swollen glands about the neck and jaw.
- Phosphorus—*Gums that bleed.* These canker sores are found in a mouth with bleeding gums; your mouth feels dry and thirsty, and you yearn for cold water. Like many canker sores, stress only makes Phosphorus sores worse, as does touching the painful area, and indulging in warm food and drink.
- Sulphuricum acidum—*Bad breath!* This canker sore remedy also includes gums that bleed easily, and possibly sores with pus. Poor digestion may be a contributing cause. No wonder your breath is bad.

Lifestyle Link

- Allergies. Possibly an allergic reaction . . . are you worse during pollen season or other times? Do you have other allergic reactions? Keep track of your outbreaks and see if you can pinpoint sores to a particular time, place, or exposure to, for example, pets or food.

Lookout Alert

- Sore that doesn't heal
- Severe pain
- Sores that are white, gray, yellowish, or brownish in color
- Persistent sores on the tongue
- Facial swelling
- Seek help if you're a long-term smoker

COLDS AND FLU

There is a respiratory tract condition that occurs so frequently, it's been dubbed the common cold. Most are familiar with its runny nose, sneezing, sore throat, headache, fever, and general ill feeling. Slightly less common, but still a winter regular, is influenza or the flu. It is often difficult to distinguish this illness from a cold, but it differs in its abrupt onset, shorter duration and more pronounced fever, chills, muscle aches, and fatigue. Also see Bronchitis, Coughing, Ear Infections, Fever, and Sore Throat. Read Chapter 6 (immunity).

How to Prevent a Cold or Flu

- Avoid exposure to infected individuals.
- Don't strain your brain. Mental fatigue, emotional distress, and physical exhaustion all invite colds and the flu.
- Get enough sleep. Eight hours per night on average; more if you need it. This is more important than you think.
- Eat plenty of fresh fruits and vegetables (this is your mother talking); don't forget whole grains.
- A daily dose of essential fatty acids (see Makeover Hint #65— Flax Appeal).
- If the air is dry where you live, use a humidifier.

Food and Nutrition for Colds and Flu

- Don't eat sugar. This means white sugar, brown sugar, maple syrup, honey, fructose and anything else masquerading as sugar. Ginger ale and 7-up are no-no's too. You can have some when you're better, but not when you're sick.
- Stay away from alcohol and caffeine (coffee, black tea, chocolate and cocoa, soft drinks).
- If you must drink fruit juices, dilute them half and half with water. Contrary to what we've been told, gallons of orange juice don't cure a cold—they make it worse.
- Drink lots of fluids like water, herbal teas, and homemade vegetable broth.

- Eat only to appetite. If you're not hungry, it's simple—don't eat. (Listen to your body.)
- Load up on vitamin C-packed foods such as broccoli, green peppers, tomatoes, and alfalfa sprouts. Or supplement with 1000 mg vitamin C every two hours. If you develop stomach cramps or diarrhea while taking vitamin C pills, cut back on the dosage. This vitamin C treatment is even more effective if taken with the same amount of bioflavonoids, also found in fresh fruits and vegetables.
- Avoid iron while ill.
- Go for the gold and orange and yellow and dark green vegetables—all packed with beta-carotene. Or use pills, about 200,000 IU daily while ill.
- Lace your breath with garlic and onions. So smelly, they keep the germs away.

■ Makeover Hint #85—Help From the Kitchen

Mix these common kitchen ingredients together in a mug to make a cold-fighting herbal tea or choose just one (up to 2–3 tsp. of total dried herb). Add boiling water, cover with a saucer, and steep for 15 minutes. Strain and drink.

1 tsp ginger (root or powder)

1 tsp sage (dried or powder)

1 bag of peppermint tea

Herbal Treatment

- Achy joints and headache—black willow, meadow sweet
- Coughing—elecampane, grindelia, mullein
- Fever—elder, feverfew, yarrow
- Runny nose—ephedra
- Bug battlers—astragalus, echinacea, goldenseal

The Homeopathic Difference

- Aconite—*Sudden symptoms.* If someone touches you, you're going to scream! Your head hurts, you're burning up, and bright red blood is seeping from your nose. You feel like a caged cat, restless and anxious. Use this remedy for the first 24 hours of your illness, particularly for that cold or flu that appears abruptly.

- Allium cepa—*A cold like an onion.* Those same symptoms caused by dicing an onion—burning eyes, nose, and lips, along with profuse, searing, clear discharge—is the Allium cold. Look for thirst, minimal fever, and symptoms that are better in the open air.

- Bryonia—*Chest cold.* You sound like a seal—dry, spasmodic, hacking cough. Everything seems to ache—your head, muscles and joints. What's left? To make matters worse, your mouth feels like the Sahara Desert; more water please! You "want to be alone" in the dark and feel cranky. All this feels worse when you move about.

- Gelsemium—*The three "Ds"—drowsy, droopy eyelids, dull.* You've had this type of downer cold before. It may start with a tickle in your throat and drop in energy. Pretty soon, moving, or even thinking, is asking too much. Your nose is running with watery stuff, but you don't feel like drinking anything. You feel chilly, stiff, and have a headache along your upper back and nape of the neck; all this sends you hibernating to the bedroom.

- Nux vomica—*Your cold is the fault of a cold, dry winter.* Aaaahhhhh. . . . choo!! You can't stop sneezing. And to make things worse, your nose can't make up its mind if it's stuffed up or running. Your throat is sore and raw with a feather-duster tickle of a cough. The light hurts your eyes, your tummy is queasy and you're constipated. You are definitely crabby. The morning is your worst time; eating doesn't help either.

- Pulsatilla—*Chilly crybaby.* Thick yellowish, green stuff is oozing from your nose—thank goodness it's bland, not burning. To top off your aching head is a case of diarrhea and nausea. You feel like a little baby, happy one minute, crying the next. Food and drink don't interest you.

Lifestyle Link

- Take naps—it's very European. Sleep longer at night too. Rest is vital to healing.
- Only exercise if you feel up to it. This is no time to train for a marathon; reserve your energy for getting better.
- Practice being lazy. Keep your work load to a minimum and delegate extra tasks so you can take it easy. Better yet, stay home and watch *Oprah*.
- Vaporize your air if coughing, a dry throat, or stuffed-up nose are keeping you awake. Add four drops of eucalyptus oil, a glob of Vicks™ or other chest rub containing eucalyptus to a vaporizer. Not only will the warm steam ease you, but the exotic smell of eucalyptus will help breathing (and announce to the rest of the household that you're sick).

Lookout Alert

- Yellow eyes or skin
- Very light-colored stools
- Dark looking urine
- Stiff neck, especially if it's painful upon bending
- Extremely painful headache
- Convulsions
- Severe symptoms, especially fatigue, weakness, irritability or confusion
- Extreme breathing problems, chest pain and wheezing (critical in infants)
- Sudden or unrelenting vomiting or diarrhea (most critical in children)
- If your illness lasts one week without noticeable improvement

CONSTIPATION

Constipation is a common problem, often due to poor food choices. Little or no roughage, provided by fruits, vegetables, and whole grains, slows food's trip through the intestines. The result is infrequent, incomplete bowel movements that are difficult to evacuate. Faulty health habits are the most frequent reasons for constipation, as well as a "sluggish" liver (see Chapter 3); other more critical conditions such as hypothyroidism or diverticulosis can also be the cause. In persons over 50, constipation lasting more than a week may be a sign of a more serious health problem. Also see Hemorrhoids and Indigestion; refer to Chapter 4 (digestion).

How to Prevent Constipation

Since most cases of constipation are caused by slips in diet and exercise, preventive measures are much the same as the Lifestyle Links it takes to correct this problem. Also consider . . .

- New medicines. If you become constipated after starting a new medication, mention it to your doctor. Many common medicines can plug up bowels. These include antipsychotics, muscle relaxants, antidepressants, and blood pressure medications.
- Beware of laxatives and enemas. How ironic that these very same medicines and techniques we use to correct constipation can eventually exacerbate the problem. This is because after a while the body relies on these aids, and is unable to go on its own.
- Plan for travel. Unfamiliar bathrooms are well-known constipation makers. Before a trip, remember to drink lots of water, eat lots of fiber, breathe frequently and, just to be safe, carry some herbal laxatives for temporary relief.

Food and Nutrition for Constipation

- Fluids, fluids, and more fluids. Water is your best bet here.
- Fill up on fiber. Once again, those foods are vegetables, fruit, whole grains, beans, and legumes.
- Is it your iron supplement? Some iron supplements (sulfate, gluconate) can plug up bowels. If you need extra iron (and most people don't), try iron picolinate, succinate, or fumarate.

Herbal Treatment

Just because a laxative is herbal and "natural" doesn't make it the solution to stalled bowels. I occasionally recommend herbal laxatives as a step toward normalizing bowel movements for patients who have used laxatives chronically. After switching to an herbal laxative tea, I have them gradually decrease the amount they drink (e.g., one cup daily the first week, 1/2 cup daily the second week) while making dietary and lifestyle changes.

- To bulk up stools—flax, oat bran, psyllium
- Laxatives—aloe, barberry, cascara, dandelion, rhubarb root, senna, yellow dock
- Liver/gallbladder help—barberry, blue flag, dandelion, milk thistle, yellow dock
- Tonify the colon—rhubarb root

The Homeopathic Difference

- Alumina—*Soft, sticky stools.* This remedy works best for hard and dry stools. There's no desire for a bowel movement, yet the rectum is sore, maybe bleeding and possibly itchy and burning. When you do go to the bathroom, great straining is involved.
- Bryonia—*The child's remedy.* For children who have great difficulty passing dry, dark stools.
- Graphites—*Large and smelly.* Graphites is for a type of constipation where stools are large, smelly, and made up of many lumps stuck together with mucus.
- Silicea—*Bashful stools.* The so-called bashful stools, those that may slip back when partially expelled, and in this case are large and hard, are best treated with Silicea.

Lifestyle Link

- Move that body. Regular physical activity helps move bowels too.
- Stress release. Tension, be it emotional or mental, creates tight intestines too.
- Intolerant foods. Food allergies can be the cause of chronic constipation.

- Leave laxatives alone. Reliance on these medicines (including herbs) can add to constipation problems.
- Correct digestion problems. Try taking acidophilus, 1/8 teaspoon two times daily, to re-seed the good bugs in your colon, especially if your problem began after antibiotic use.

Lookout Alert

- Constipation that alternates with diarrhea
- Blood in the stool
- Mucus or pus in the stool
- Black tarry stools
- Severe and/or unrelenting stomach pain or cramps
- Constipation that accompanies fatigue, cold intolerance, weight gain, and dry skin

COUGHING

To cough or not to cough is your body's way of cleaning out the lungs. The cough reflex is set off when something stimulates the airways. That something ranges from a virus to cigarette smoke.

If you wake up with a cough and fever, and your nose is running, no doubt your cough is due to a cold or other upper respiratory infection such as bronchitis. Smokers frequently wake in the morning hacking; long-term smokers develop "smoker's cough." Don't forget that living with a smoker, even if you don't indulge, can create a similar reaction.

Coughing in the absence of an infection or smoking may indicate an allergic reaction. If you cough only certain times of the year, this may be a reaction to pollen or other seasonal material. Watch if you only cough in particular environments, like at work—you may be reacting to noxious chemicals. Never ignore a persistent cough. It could indicate a more serious condition like emphysema or lung cancer. If your cough doesn't go away after using the following suggestions, visit your doctor. Also see Bronchitis, Colds and Flu, Ear Infections, Fever, Sore Throat; refer to Chapter 7 (immunity).

How to Prevent Coughing

- The reason is? To prevent a cough, you need to know what causes it.
- Avoid a cough due to infection by boosting immunity (see Chapter 7). This means get enough sleep, eat right, and avoid overdoing it.
- Avoid exposure to infected individuals.
- Don't smoke. Non-smokers, avoid exposure to second-hand smoke.
- Avoid or minimize exposure to toxic fumes. This means paints, solvents, and other poisonous chemicals. Use a face filter when exposure is unavoidable.
- Consider allergic possibilities. Ask your doctor if you can be tested for inhalant or food allergies. If possible, try avoiding the offending substance and see what happens.

Food and Nutrition for Coughs

- Drink water. Fluids like water, broth, and vegetable juices help break up lung congestion.
- No sugar.
- Avoid mucus-producing foods like milk and other dairy foods (cheese, butter, yogurt, ice cream), starches, eggs, and wheat.
- Aniseed, caraway, and fennel. These spices also have medicinal qualities, specifically, as expectorants and in calming respiratory spasms—in other words, cough. The pleasing taste of aniseed and fennel are also used to flavor cough medicines.
- Take time for thyme. Use this spice on food, make a tea, or take as an herbal remedy for irritating coughs.
- Food-based poultice. Applying different foods to the chest in order to help clear it out, or cause expectoration, is an old-time trick and one still used by naturopathic doctors. If you have mustard powder or horseradish in your cupboards, try making a poultice to relieve that nasty cough.
- Hot honey and lemon mixed together in a mug help soothe the throat and calm a cough.

- Avoid iron if cough is infectious.

■ *Makeover Hint #86—How to Make a Poultice*

A poultice is basically a pad, often containing healing ingredients, that is placed on an ailing body part. In this case, we're talking about a chest poultice specifically designed to open the airways for easier breathing and less coughing. Choose one of the following recipes for your cough. Do not use mustard or horseradish on very young children (under three) or those with sensitive skin.

MUSTARD POULTICE

3 Tbsp mustard powder

Water

Clean pillow case

Towel

Put mustard powder in a soup bowl. Add enough water to make a paste and stir. Spoon paste inside pillow case. Have patient lie down. Place pillow case on the patient's chest. Spread paste around inside case so it covers chest. (Note: Mustard paste is *inside* case, and not directly on patient's chest.) Place towel, and then blanket on top of the patient's pillow case poultice. Leave poultice on patient's chest until skin turns pink, or patient tells you that skin is warm. Be careful that the poultice doesn't burn the skin. Remove poultice. Patient may lean over edge of bed and expectorate into basin afterward.

HORSERADISH POULTICE

3 Tbsp horseradish

Clean pillow case

Towel

Follow same directions as for mustard poultice, but substitute horseradish for mustard powder paste. As with mustard poultice, don't leave horseradish on chest too long or skin will blister and burn.

■ *Makeover Hint #87—Homemade Cough Syrup*

1 large onion, cut up

3/4 cup honey

3 cloves garlic, diced

Mix onion, garlic, and honey in a large pot. Simmer over low heat for two to three hours. You can use a crockpot instead, if you like; cook for five to six hours on low. Take one teaspoon of onion/garlic syrup every hour or as needed for cough.

Herbal Treatment

Herbs work well for coughs, but you need to discover the underlying cause too. I suggest using herbal cough remedies only when your cough interferes with sleep or rest. Remember, a cough is your body's way of cleansing the lungs and healing. Also, don't ignore a cough that won't go away.

- Acute dry cough, soothing—marshmallow leaf, slippery elm
- Expectorant—angelica, coltsfoot, daisy, senega
- Bronchitis—mullein, pleurisy root, sundew, white horehound
- Catarrh—elecampane, elder flowers
- Pneumonia (See your doctor)—pleurisy root
- Respiratory relaxant—grindelia
- Whooping cough—mouse ear, sundew, white horehound
- General coughs; flavoring—licorice

The Homeopathic Difference

- Belladonna—*The crying cough.* When your throat is so red and raw that it makes you (or your child) weep when you cough, think of Belladonna.
- Bryonia—*Deep chest cough.* This common cough remedy is for painful, dry coughs that have traveled into the chest. When you ask someone with this type of cough if it hurts, he'll reply, "Only when I breathe and move." Ironically, lying on the sore

spot feels better. Those with a Bryonia-type cough are thirsty, tired, and irritable.

- Ipecac—*The cough that rattles.* This cough is deep, wet, and rattles because of all the mucus that has settled in the lungs. Breathing out is difficult, and much harder than taking air in. Coughing is so intense at times it may result in gagging or vomiting.
- Lachesis—*Choking cough.* A characteristic of Lachesis is that the slightest constriction around the throat is intolerable; this same feature makes coughing worse. Even swallowing water is hard. That tickle in the throat that bursts forth into a short, dry cough is typical for this remedy. It's worse around or during sleep-time.
- Spongia—*Sounds like a saw blade.* This harsh, croupy cough is dry, and may wake the afflicted early in the evening. Drinking liquids that are not ice cold makes the cough better, though talking, excitement, lying down, and alcohol bring it on.

Lifestyle Link

- Cough up phlegm and blow your nose one nostril at a time. Doing this helps keep your lungs clean and clear. Remember, a cough is how your body cleans out the lungs.
- If the air is dry where you live, use a humidifier; if needed, use a vaporizer at night.
- Apply a hot water bottle or heating pad on your chest for 20 minutes. Then lie on a bed, and hang your head over a pan. Cough out any loose phlegm.
- Avoid respiratory irritants, smoke, dust, or chemicals.
- Avoid environments that are too hot or too cold. Stay in places that have Mama-Bear temperatures—just right.

Lookout Alert

- Lingering cough
- Coughing up blood
- Swallowing something that blocks your air passages
- Coughing up a gritty-like substance
- Chest pain.

- Problems breathing
- Cough getting progressively worse
- Painful cough
- Cough is consistently worse after exercise or cold exposure
- Sudden or marked wheezing, vomiting, headaches, weakness, seizures or neck stiffness
- Accompanying symptoms persist or are severe

DIARRHEA

One way the body expels germs, toxins, and other irritants is through diarrhea—loose, watery, frequent stools. Stomach flu or other intestinal infections are its most common causes, followed by food poisoning. Emotional distress also creates fast-moving bowels. Dehydration from diarrhea, especially among children, is a major risk. Also see Anxiety, Food Poisoning, Indigestion; refer to Chapter 4 (digestion).

How to Prevent Diarrhea

- Cut back on caffeine. Too much coffee can cause diarrhea.
- Stay calm. Nerves, for some people, cause diarrhea.
- Careful of the water. When you travel or camp, carry bottled water with you.

Food and Nutrition for Digestion

- Eat yogurt. The culture, or good bugs, in this food can help tame infectious diarrhea.
- Alternately, you can take a *Lactobacillus acidophilus* or probiotic pill after the diarrhea is done to replace bugs lost from your colon.
- Avoid milk. Those who are lactose intolerant may experience diarrhea when they drink milk.
- Cut out the diet pop. Artificial sweeteners, especially in large amounts, can create diarrhea in some.

- Drink plenty of fluids, especially liquids with electrolytes like fruit and vegetable juices.

- Avoid eating for a while.

- After the worst has past, dine on soft foods: soup, cooked fruit, and yogurt.

- Eat apples, bananas, tomatoes, potatoes, and carrots, which might stop the diarrhea.

- Are you taking too much C? Overdosing on vitamin C can cause diarrhea, gas, bloating, and abdominal cramps. If that happens, stop taking it for awhile, then take smaller amounts.

- Is it magnesium? Loading up on magnesium can also lead to diarrhea. More than 500 to 600 mg daily is the laxative point for many people.

- Gorging on fresh fruit? If it's summer and you've eaten one too many peaches or other fruit, that might be the cause.

- If ongoing or recurrent, ask your doctor to check out food allergies.

■ *Makeover Hint #88—Natural Fluid Replacement*

Try this to restore lost fluids and electrolytes after a bout of diarrhea: mix equal amounts of tomato juice and cabbage juice together, and sip.

Herbal Treatment

- Astringent—agrimony, American cranesbill, greater plantain

- Chronic diarrhea (see your doctor)—black catechu

- Healing—agrimony, greater plantain

- Infectious—golden seal, Oregon grape

- In children—agrimony, meadow sweet, thyme

- Nervous diarrhea—tormentil

The Homeopathic Difference

A study conducted by Seattle physician and homeopath Jennifer Jacobs, M.D., M.P.H., proved once and for all that homeopathy helps diarrhea. She treated several children from Nicaragua, ages six months to five years, suffering from acute diarrhea. Each remedy was prescribed based on individual symptoms; a second group of children was given fake pills. After five days, the homeopathically treated children improved noticeably more than the others.[3] You too can use homeopathic remedies to ease diarrhea.

- Gelsemium—*Nervous diarrhea*. If you've ever had diarrhea because of fear, anxiety, or worry, this is the remedy for you. It'll help calm both you and your bowels.

- Phosphorus—*For that empty feeling*. When copious amounts of green stool leave you weak and empty-feeling—no pain, though—and keep you awake at night, think of Phosphorus.

- Podophyllum—*Painful and profuse*. Try this remedy for diarrhea involving a colicky pain and bad-smelling, watery green or yellow stools. This gushing and profuse diarrhea may alternate with a headache and is worse after eating, drinking, or moving about.

Lifestyle Link
- Rest.

Lookout Alert
- Diarrhea lasting more than a few days
- Alternates with constipation
- Fever, stomach cramps, blood or mucus in stool
- If person not drinking or eating (can lead to dehydration)
- Be particularly cautious in young children (they dehydrate more quickly)

EAR INFECTIONS

Many parents think ear infections during childhood are to be expected. It ain't necessarily so. The most common ear illness among kids three months to three years is acute otitis media, a bacterial or viral infection of the middle ear. This ailment often begins as a chest cold, though the first sign will probably be your child complaining of an earache. Very young children are often irritable or pull at their affected ear—which may look red. Nausea, vomiting, fever, and even diarrhea are other symptoms to watch for. Some kids suffer from temporary hearing loss.

A child's very anatomy contributes to this condition. That is, his winding ear tube allows mucus and germs to congregate and multiply—a perfect infection setup. According to Chinese Medicine, young children are natural mucus producers, hence those chronic runny noses you're forever wiping. However, like adults, we must look at a child's lifestyle, too, for causative clues. Food sensitivities and poor diet certainly contribute to chronic ear infections. Babies who are fed mother's milk versus formula are less apt to be affected. Exposure to second-hand smoke also increases a child's susceptibility to illness. Be especially aware of these factors if your child (or you) suffers from chronic or recurrent infections. Antibiotics and surgery (ear tubes) are not the only solutions.

Although adults do get ear infections and can use the following treatments, I'm focusing my suggestions on children since they're the most frequent victims. Also see Bronchitis, Colds and Flu, Coughing, Fever, Sore Throat; refer to Chapter 6 (immunity).

How to Prevent Ear Infections

- Breast feed. Nursing your infant exclusively until she's at least six months old is one of the best ways I know to avoid ear infections. Mother's milk is full of infection-fighting compounds, prevents food allergies from developing (one cause of ear infections), and is the perfect food for a new baby's developing gut.
- Stay away from the bottle. Babies fed formula in a bottle are at higher risk of ear infections than breast-fed children. If you do use a bottle, it's best to sit with your baby and hold him so his head is slightly elevated; don't lay him on his back with a propped bottle.

- Introducing baby to food. The premature introduction (before five or six months) of solid foods can damage a child's intestinal lining. The result is an increased risk of developing food allergies—which can contribute to ear infections.
- Delay certain foods. Introducing foods high on the allergy scale (wheat, dairy, corn, soy, tomatoes, citrus fruits, eggs, chocolate, peanuts) prematurely can create health problems later on . . . like ear infections.
- Groom defenses. Follow general immune-boosting ideas as outlined in Chapter 6.

Food and Nutrition for Earaches

- Sugar ban. All types of sugar (white, brown, honey—also glucose, dextrose, corn syrup, maltose). Read labels if you're not sure what has sugar.
- Dodge fruit juice. Young children often live on this sweet liquid. However, the fruit sugars in juice not only kill appetite for other foods and contribute to obesity, but can diminish your child's immunity. Avoid during illness (it really makes a difference); use as a treat other times. Best bet is to dilute fruit juice half and half with water.
- Boost fluids. Teach your children to love water. Also broths and fresh vegetable juices are fine.
- Push the veggies. A child does better with plenty of fresh vegetables and fruits, and whole grains. The younger they are when you offer them these foods, the more likely they are to eat them.
- Phase out fatty foods. Kids' fast food is often laden with fat. Cut this out, and their ears might feel better.
- Food sensitivities. During an acute infection, eliminate dairy foods. If there's no improvement, also cut out wheat, corn, and oranges. When the child is better, have a food allergy panel done by your doctor if ear infections keep coming back.
- Vitamin C. Decide the dose by multiplying their age × 100 mg up to 1000 mg; give every two hours while ill. Discontinue if child experiences diarrhea. (See Diarrhea)

- Beef up on carotenes. This is the orange-yellow-dark green color in vegetables. Eat extra servings, and take a supplement.
- Children's multi. During and as a precaution, give your child a multiple vitamin/mineral pill.
- Push probiotics. If you or your child has used antibiotics, or relied on them extensively in the past, supplement with acidophilus and other "probiotics" to replenish the good bacteria in the colon.
- Too little, too late. Specific nutrient deficiencies have been implicated in recurrent ear infections. If the above measures don't work, consult a knowledgeable nutritionist or naturopathic doctor on how to supplement. Nutrients to watch for include vitamin A, zinc, and iron. Note: iron shouldn't be given during an infection.

Herbal Treatment

- Ear drops (put in ear only; don't take by mouth)—aconite, garlic, golden seal, mullein, pasque flower, pennywort
- Bug killers—echinacea, garlic, golden seal, wild indigo
- Immune builders—echinacea, garlic, golden seal
- Increase circulation around ear—ginkgo
- Sleeping aids—chamomile, passion flower, skullcap, valerian

The Homeopathic Difference

- Belladonna—*Throbbing hot ear.* This is a great remedy for acute ear infections in children. The child might be sensitive to loud noises and touch, and cry out in her sleep from pain. The earache is worse in the afternoon and from lying down.
- Chamomila—*Whining and aching.* Another great child's remedy, Chamomile, fits children whose sore ears are ringing. Ears might feel stopped up, sometimes with a stitching pain. These earaches make the child hot and thirsty. The guiding symptom for this remedy is irritability that only a hug can calm.
- Kali muriaticum—*Chronic ear infection.* This remedy is most suitable for chronic conditions of the middle ear. Often the glands around the ear are also swollen, and the child hears snapping noises. Eating fatty foods makes it worse.

- Pulsatilla—*Stuffed-up ears*. Pulsatilla ears are red on the out-side, and feel full on the inside. A thick, smelly discharge might leak from the ears. The pain is worse at night, and when your child doesn't answer you it's probably because he can't hear.

Lifestyle Link

- Antibiotic myth. Studies show that antibiotics have been overused for children's ear infections.[4] Work with your doctor, and ask if you can try natural methods first with his guidance. If antibiotics are needed, see if you can decrease the dose and/or duration of treatment. (Be sure to follow up with pro-biotics. See Food and Nutrition for Earaches.)
- Hot and cold. Hydrotherapy, or water treatment, is an old-fashioned but effective natural therapy. For ear infections, place a comfortably hot washcloth to your child's sore ear for about five minutes. Alternate this with a comfortably cold cloth for a minute or so. Repeat this three times.
- Sleep and rest.
- Cover those ears. Especially when outside on cold winter days, wear a hat or scarf.

Lookout Alert

Most ear infections heal without complications. However, if your child displays any of the following signs, seek help from your physician. Also, if you suspect your child's hearing has declined and not returned after the infection clears, be sure to have her checked. This is critical for very small children, under the age of one.

- Sudden profound hearing loss
- Vertigo
- Chills and fever
- Headache
- Ear drainage
- Stiff neck
- Persistent vomiting or diarrhea
- Other ongoing and/or severe symptoms

ECZEMA

It's difficult to stop scratching and rubbing this very itchy skin rash called eczema. If you take a close look, you'll notice your skin is red, dry, and swollen with little blisters that eventually pop and ooze. Areas that are scratched become scaly and crusty, with thicker than normal skin. Elbow and knee creases are often affected, although other areas like the eyelids, neck, and wrists are also stricken. Doctors call this rash atopic dermatitis; atopic refers to eczema's allergic tendency. That is, people with this chronic rash often have a family history of allergies including eczema, hay fever, and asthma. About one out of every 20 people has it, and for many it begins in childhood and comes and goes throughout life. See related topics, Acne and Psoriasis. Read Chapter 12 (skin).

How to Prevent Eczema

- Pick the right parents. Those with eczema usually have a family history of this or other allergic-type conditions. You can't do anything about the genetics, but you can use natural treatments to minimize their effects.
- Moisturize skin. Especially in winter months, drink plenty of water and use moisturizing creams.
- Avoid skin irritants. This includes harsh soaps, household cleaners, and chemicals. I had one young patient whose eczema got considerably worse if her father didn't filter out the chlorine in her bath water.
- Eat right. See below.

Food and Nutrition for the Skin

- Eliminate allergic foods. Cow's milk, eggs, wheat, and tomatoes most commonly aggravate eczema—start by avoiding these for a month.
- Get rid of food additives. Shun foods with artificial colorings, flavorings, and preservatives. This is best done by sticking with whole, natural foods.
- Face the fats. Use essential fatty acids that quiet inflammation, rather than feed it. Begin with evening primrose oil (EPO), 1000

mg three times daily (for an adult) for at least two months. Then try switching to less expensive flax seed oil (1–2 Tbsp daily).

- Rub EPO directly on the sore spots.
- Eat fish. The fat in fish works as an anti-inflammatory.
- Kick out the steak and wine. Red meat and alcohol tend to make eczema worse by promoting inflammation.
- Zinc. This mineral is often low in those with eczema, a critical loss since it helps decrease inflammation and aids healing of the skin. Try 30 mg daily for a month, then switch to a more moderate 15 mg dose.
- Itch attack. For symptomatic relief, apply zinc oxide cream (see Zinc above).
- Multiple. Make sure your daily supplement contains vitamins A and E.

Herbal Treatment

- Skin cream—aloe, calendula, chamomile, chickweed, golden seal, St. John's wort
- Dry eczema—burdock, cleavers
- In children—nettles, red clover
- Itching (also see skin cream)—figwort
- Nervous eczema—nettles

■ *Makeover Hint #89—A Weedy Wash*

Can't stand that itch anymore? Look no farther than your backyard for an herb that'll help—chickweed. Pick the flowers and leaves, cut up and steep 1 Tbsp in a cup of hot water. Let sit until lukewarm, then wash your itchy skin with it. Repeat as needed.

The Homeopathic Difference

- Calcarea sulphurica—*Dry eczema.* For eczema with those yellow scabs that sometimes ooze a pus-like discharge, think Calc sulphurica. If your child has this, the eczema is more likely dry.

- Ledum—*Facial eczema*. If you have this kind of eczema, and it's itchy at night in bed, try Ledum.
- Lycopodium—*Heated eczema*. This extremely itchy form of eczema bleeds easily when scratched. The skin may look thick, and frequently has cracks or fissures. Heat from a warm room or bed can bring it on; it feels much better when cold.
- Sulphur—*Settles in skin folds*. Itchy! Burning! Dry! Scaly! That describes the Sulphur-brand of eczema. Scratching makes it ooze, and you may find it settles in skin folds. The itchiness gets even itchier with dampness, like wet weather or bathing.

Lifestyle Link

- Control stress. (See Chapter 7).
- Wash clothes with mild detergents. Eczematous skin is sensitive skin that is easily irritated from chemicals or soaps.
- Avoid rough-feeling clothes, like wool.
- Apply a hot compress to the affected area.
- Seek counseling for unresolved issues. If you find certain situations trigger an outbreak, it may be time to talk to a counselor for help dealing with it.

Lookout Alert

- Fuzzy vision. People with long-standing eczema may develop cataracts in their 20s and 30s. Have your eyes checked regularly.
- High fever during an outbreak.
- Unrelenting or severe rash.

FATIGUE

Because fatigue is a symptom and not a disease, there are many causes. Like constipation, persistent tiredness is best resolved by first determining the reason. Inadequate sleep is the number one cause of fatigue in this country. Stress, lack of exercise, and even poor eating habits also contribute to feeling wrung out. There are, of course, medical reasons too. A chronic, undetected infection anywhere in the body can make you tired, as well as anemia, cancer, heart disease, or an array of other ailments. If taking the following simple steps don't wake you up, enlist your doctor's help in rooting out the cause of your fatigue. If standard laboratory tests are unsuccessful, consider visiting with a naturopathic physician to explore less conventional reasons like Chronic Fatigue Syndrome, food allergies, digestive disorders, environmental sensitivities, or subclinical hypothyroidism (also called Wilson's Syndrome). Look up Anxiety and Insomnia, and refer to Chapter 7 (adrenals) for more information.

How to Prevent Fatigue

- Get enough sleep.
- Stay well. In other words, use healthy practices to avoid chronic infections and other illnesses that drain energy.

Food and Nutrition for Exhaustion

- No caffeine. This pick-me-up eventually lets you down. Used chronically or in large amounts, caffeine can wear your adrenal glands down (see Chapter 7).
- Beware of sugar. Like caffeine, sweet foods give you a burst of energy—only to let you down a short time later. Consider eliminating sugar altogether. (Note: The first two to seven sugar-free days will be draining.)
- Slow down on fat. Fat takes time to digest, making you feel sluggish.
- Drink water by the quart.
- Nutrient shortage. Whether due to insufficient intake, malabsorption, or an inability to utilize vitamins and minerals, this is a definite fatigue-promoter.
- Watch your weight. Carrying extra pounds can be tiring.
- Iron-deficiency anemia. Have your blood checked. Low vitamin B_{12}, chronic disease, and other causes can also lead to anemia or "tired blood."
- Food allergies. Have them checked.

Herbal Treatment

There are many herbs that can be used to combat fatigue—depending on the cause. Below I offer a short list of plants useful for mainly anxiety-provoked fatigue, insomnia, and infections.

- Relax—linden, oats, passion flower, skullcap, valerian
- Promote sleep—lady's slipper, passion flower, valerian
- Untie knotty muscles—skullcap, valerian
- Fight infection—echinacea, garlic, golden seal

The Homeopathic Difference

- Arsenicum album—*Fearful fatigue.* Have you ever been worn out from worrying or being scared? If so, think of Arsenicum. Other signs that point to this remedy are exhaustion from the slightest effort, restless pacing, and for some, despair. Many are also chilly and feel better with fresh air.
- Echinacea—*Achy tired.* For that profound prostration that makes you ache, this homeopathic version of the herb echinacea is worth a try. Some also feel dizzy, confused, or depressed.
- Gelsemium—*A kind of daze.* This fatigue is best described as apathetic or listless. Not only does this remedy fit someone who is dull and drowsy, but also lacks coordination and wants to be alone. Bad news and excitement make this type of fatigue worse, or may bring it on.
- Phosphorus—*Tired brain.* When you feel low and your memory is shot, think of Phosphorus. It's not so much that your body's tired, it's your brain. A tendency to fidget and become easily startled also describe this remedy.

Lifestyle Link

- Aim for eight. Hours of sleep nightly, that is. Without sleep, immunity suffers.
- Snooze for stress. When times are tough—mental, emotional or physical—take time for extra sleep; you need it.

- Delegate. A fast-paced life can be energizing, but like caffeine has a let-down aftereffect.
- Medicine check. For some people, fatigue is a side effect of medication, like Accutane®, Prozac®, and Zoloft®. If you suspect this is your case, check with your doctor.
- Allergic to the world? Environmental sensitivity is becoming more frequent. If you react to a number of chemicals (in addition to being tired), seek the help of a doctor skilled in this area.
- Depressed? If you've experienced past or current psychological trauma, ask for professional help.

Lookout Alert

- Incapacitating fatigue
- Continuous fatigue (even after following above guidelines)
- High fever
- Other symptoms too, like flank pain, painful urination, earache, sore throat, aching muscles

FEVER

When your body temperature rises above 100 degrees F, you officially have a fever. The fever symptom is usually a reaction to an infection from a virus or bacteria, though it's your body that actually creates the fever. When white blood cells detect germs, they release a special protein called a pyrogen which tells the brain's temperature control center to crank it up. It's speculated that high temperatures help activate the immune system, decrease bacterial growth, decrease iron levels (needed by bugs to grow) and shift the body from running on glucose (another favorite bacterial food) over to fat and protein instead.[5]

Chills help increase a fever and can indicate a more hardy infection like the flu or pneumonia; taking aspirin or other anti-fever medicines can also spark the chills. If you have sweats, it means your fever is dropping. Night sweats occur in the early morning as your body temperature (and fever) is on its natural downward slope.

Many bodily functions, including temperature, follow a daily pattern. Fever (and body temperature), for instance, are highest in the late afternoon into early evening. Know too that fevers tend to be higher in childhood (perfectly normal), and decline with age.

Other fever promoters include adverse reaction, to medication, certain non-infectious illnesses like rheumatoid arthritis, heart attacks, cancer. Heatstroke can also bring on a fever; and sometimes we don't know why a fever appears. See related topics: Bronchitis, Colds and Flu, Ear Infections, Food Poisoning, Sore Throats, and Urinary Tract Infections. Read Chapter 6 (immunity) for more information.

How to Prevent Fevers

- Infections. Stay healthy. See Chapter 6 for tips.

- Use medications cautiously. Discuss side effects with your doctor before taking.

- Have fun in the sun—but be careful. Heatstroke is serious. Use sense when outside on a sunny day; drink plenty of fluids (including juices if you're perspiring), wear a hat, and if possible, go inside periodically.

Food and Nutrition for Fever

- A cup of tea. Both peppermint and ginger teas are natural fever fighters. They reduce hot brows by promoting perspiration.

- Treat the cause. If it's infection that's warming you up, take measures to enhance immunity and fight the responsible bug rather than reduce temperature.

- Drink fluids. Replace lost fluid with water, herbal teas, diluted fruit juice, and vegetable juices.

Herbal Treatment

(Also see Bronchitis, Colds and Flu, Ear Infections, Food Poisoning, UTIs)

In general, if anyone is experiencing a "safe" fever (see Lookout Alert below), then reducing a fever is unnecessary and may, in fact, hamper immunity. However, for comfort's sake, you can try one of the following herbs if you wish.

- Cool off with perspiration promoters—boneset, catnip, cayenne, chamomile, elder (flowers or berries), ginger, linden, vervain, yarrow
- Infection erasers—echinacea, garlic, golden seal, peppermint
- Reduce fever (these herbs contain aspirin-like compounds)—black willow, meadow sweet

■ *Makeover Hint #90—Horseradish Tea*

This stimulating herb is an old-time remedy for fevers and the flu. In a pinch, make your own medicine using horseradish root.

1 tsp powdered or chopped horseradish root

Steep in one cup of boiling water for five minutes.

Sip on this brew several times in a day while burning up with a fever.

The Homeopathic Difference

- Belladonna—*Burning desire*. Belladonna is for that fever that burns so hot that every little noise, motion, and light makes you cringe. The odd part of this remedy is that even with all that heat, you're not thirsty.
- Eupatorium perfoliatum—*Fevers AND the chills*. People with this type of fever are typically thirsty before it hits. The muscles in their arms and legs hurt, and they alternate between a fever and the chills.
- Ferrum phosphoricum—*Pale face*. Ferrum phos works well for the beginning stages of a fever, especially one that brings on exhaustion and a pale appearance.
- Gelsemium—*I ache all over*. When a fever makes you tremble with weakness, feel dull with fatigue, and ache all over, think of Gelsemium.

Lifestyle Link

- Rest.
- Cool down with cool compresses. Apply these to your brow or chest.
- Peppermint breath. Inhale the cool fragrance of peppermint oil (placed in warm water or a bath) to both cool a hot fever, or raise a low one (works both ways).

■ *Makeover Hint #91—Keep a Fever, Stop a Cold*

Contrary to conventional medical wisdom, natural health physicians won't tell you to take pills (or herbs) to decrease a fever. A fever, like many symptoms, is the way your body gets well. So if your fever is below 104 F, lasts less than three days, and isn't too uncomfortable, grin, sweat, and bear it. (Follow cautions below for very young children.)

Lookout Alert

- A fever over 104 F
- Any fever in a baby six months or younger
- A fever lasting more than three days or more than 24 hours in a child two years old or younger
- Fever that appears after extended time in the sun
- Fevers that occur after taking medication, especially if newly prescribed or purchased
- Fevers with unusual symptoms, like stiff joints

FOOD POISONING

If you've eaten bad food, you usually know it within a few hours. The symptoms, their severity, and onset vary depending on what you ate, how much, what bug infected your food, and how sensitive your digestive tract is. Symptoms occur anywhere from one to 48 hours after eating contaminated food. Many people mistakenly refer to food poisoning as the "24-hour flu." (There is no such thing.)

It often begins with nausea, gas, and bloating followed by vomiting, diarrhea, and stomach cramps. Your muscles might ache and your temperature can rise. You're weak and feel terrible. Ongoing vomiting and diarrhea can create dehydration and shock, if not remedied. *Staphylococcus* is the most common culprit, and likes to infiltrate custard, fish, and processed meat—especially when left out at room temperature.

Use clues to determine if you truly are suffering from food poisoning. Are others that you dined with also ill? Did you recently eat at a restaurant or did you consume questionable leftovers? Other circumstances mimic food poisoning—like travelers' diarrhea, immediate food allergies (versus delayed), ulcerative colitis, lactose intolerance, heavy metal poisoning, a drug reaction, and plant poisons (e.g., mushrooms). Also see Diarrhea, Fever, Heartburn, Indigestion, Motion Sickness; refer to Chapter 4 (digestion).

How to Prevent Food Poisoning

- Be meticulous about food storage. Don't let perishable food sit out for more than an hour.
- Cook poultry and eggs well.
- Give up sushi. This raw fish dish is a common cause of food poisoning.
- Toss questionable leftovers.
- Don't feed honey to children under one year old. Some honey contains *Botulism* spores, harmful to babies but not adults.

Food and Nutrition for Poisoning

- Careful of the water. When you travel or camp, carry bottled water with you.
- Eat yogurt. Once the worst of it is over, the good bugs in this food replace some of those lost.
- Alternately, you can take a *Lactobacillus acidophilus* or probiotic pill after the diarrhea is done to replace lost bugs from your colon.
- Drink fluids as able, especially liquids with electrolytes, like fruit and vegetable juices.

- Avoid eating for awhile.
- After the first stage is done, dine on soft foods: soup, cooked fruit, and yogurt. Avoid raw fruits and vegetables.
- Dine on garlic. This will help kill any offending bugs.

Herbal Treatment

During acute food poisoning, I would not recommend taking any herbs, except perhaps garlic and citrus seed extract. Instead rely on homeopathic remedies, and follow the above nutritional suggestions.

The Homeopathic Difference

The remedies under Diarrhea might also be useful.

- Arsenicum album—*Even the sight of food makes me sick.* This is a classic remedy for eating spoiled food. It comes complete with nausea, vomiting, and retching, not to mention burning pain in the pit of the stomach. Another sign to look for is great thirst that is quenched with tiny sips.
- Carbo vegetabilis—*Bloating and belching.* This is a remedy for distress after eating that's not quite as severe as Arsenicum. Sour burping (and some gas) is frequent and relieves the bloating and pain temporarily. Cramps that extend to the back and chest force one to bend over, and lying down doesn't help.
- Colchicum—*Cold stomach.* As is typical of food poisoning, this remedy helps with nausea (even to point of fainting, it's so bad) and vomiting up of food, bile, and mucus. Thirst is great, and though you may crave various foods, the very smell makes you sick. The peculiar sign to watch for with Colchicum is a burning or icy sensation in the abdomen.
- Ipecac—*Nausea and vomiting.* Although all the above remedies address the nausea and vomiting of food poisoning, Ipecac (yes, derived from the very same bottle you use in case of poisoning) is the star. Its guiding symptom is queasiness—the kind that is unrelenting. It differs, however, because the stomach feels relaxed, like it's hanging down, though the body is rigid. There's little thirst, and the pain is worst around the navel.

Lifestyle Link

- Take charcoal. That's right! Visit your local health food or drug store for these; take six to start, and then a couple every hour. They help soak up toxins. Don't be alarmed when your stools turn black.
- Bed rest.
- Check with fellow diners. If they're also sick, you might be able to track down the source of your poisoning.
- Throw out suspect food.
- Was it a restaurant? Once you're well, alert the restaurant and possibly the Department of Health so steps can be taken to prevent this from happening to others.

■ *Makeover Hint #92—Eat Burnt Toast*

When in a crunch (or should we say crust), and you're too sick to head out the door for charcoal pills, just burn some toast. The crispy bits are similar to charcoal and help sop up food poisons. (My mother used to make me eat burnt toast by saying it'd give me curly hair. Ha!)

Lookout Alert

- Diarrhea that lasts more than a few days
- If person not drinking or eating (can lead to dehydration)
- Be particularly cautious in young children (they dehydrate more quickly)
- Paralysis or weakness that travels down the body
- Dry mouth or visual disturbances
- Breathing problems
- Symptoms that appear after taking medication
- Symptoms that appear after eating "wild" mushrooms
- Symptoms that appear after eating home-canned food

GOUT

About one million Americans suffer from gout, a type of arthritis caused by high amounts of uric acid in the blood. When too many of these needle-like crystals form, they can settle in the kidneys, causing painful stones; joints, like the big toe, knees, and hips, are also affected. Gout is one of the most agonizing forms of arthritis, characterized by stabbing pain, inflammation, and occasionally scarring.

We've known about gout for over 2000 years, but it's only been since 1981 that we've understood exactly how this condition evolves. Gout develops when uric acid crystals flake off joints and float around the surrounding synovial fluid. The immune system sees these crystals as the enemy and sends out its battalion of white blood cells. The pain begins when the pointy edges of the uric acid crystals puncture large white blood cells called phagocytes. Powerful enzymes are released from the lysosome sacs in the phagocytes and inflammation begins. This inflammation, of course, is merely the body trying to heal itself. However, the end results are joints that are red, swollen, hot, and very, very tender.

This is a condition that tends to run in families, though typically gout hits overweight, sedentary men. A genetic inability to properly metabolize purines in food is one contributing factor. Another is overindulgence in rich meals and alcohol. Also see Backache, Fatigue, Sprains and Strains; read Chapters 4 (digestion) and 9 (muscles).

How to Prevent Gout

- Does Dad have it? If anyone in your family is gout-prone (especially the men), follow a gout-free diet.
- Stay on your toes. In other words, stay active.
- Watch what you eat. You don't necessarily have to avoid foods high in purines, but at the very least keep fatty foods down.

Food and Nutrition for Gout

- Purine foods. Since purines are what uric acid is made from, sticking to a low-purine diet helps immensely. Foods to avoid include anchovies, beef tongue, bouillon, brains, caviar, consomme, duck, goose, gravies, herring, kidneys, liver, mackerel, meat broth or soup, mussels, oysters, sardines, sausage, squab, and sweetbreads. Foods with a moderate amount of purine, and ones you can eat occasionally, are clams, pork, shellfish, and shrimp.

- Pour out the alcohol. Alcohol can increase uric acid production.
- Eat a bowl of cherries. According to the research of Dr. Ludwig N. Blair in the 1940s, eating half a pound or more of fresh cherries helps decrease uric acid levels. Cherry juice is another option.
- Coffee and sugar. Minimizing these foods seems to help; sugar increases uric acid.
- Drink plenty of clean water. This will flush out excess uric acid and decrease kidney stone risk.
- Eat plenty of fatty fish. The oils in fish act as natural anti-inflammatory agents. Warning: Avoid those fish that are high in purines (mackerel, herring, and sardines).

Herbal Treatment

- Reduce uric acid—bilberry, devil's claw
- Decrease pain—devil's claw, thuja
- Diminish inflammation—bilberry
- Keep water gain down—burdock root, celery seed, yarrow

The Homeopathic Difference

- Colchicum—*Red, hot, and swollen.* This is an easy gout remedy to remember because Colchicum (meadow saffron) is the plant that colchicine is made from: the medication used to treat gout. However, unlike colchicine, homeopathic Colchicum is without toxic side effects. Use this remedy for gout of the big toe and heel, especially when you can't bear touch or movement.
- Ledum—*For that shooting pain.* When gouty pains shoot throughout your small joints, especially in the foot and legs, and are hot, swollen and pale, this is your remedy. The soles of your feet are so painful, it's hard to walk. Placing your feet in cold water feels great; heat feels terrible.

- Lycopodium—*One foot hot, one foot cold.* For chronic gout where deposits have accumulated in the joints, this remedy could be the one. The heel is particularly painful, as if treading on a pebble. But most peculiar is that one foot feels cold, while the other one is hot.
- Urtica urens—*All in the family.* When joint pain is associated with a hives-like rash, particularly on the ankles and wrists, think of Urtica urens (see Hives). Sometimes the gout pain and hives will alternate. Coolness makes symptoms worse. This type of gout typically runs in the family.

Lifestyle Link

- Exercise that body for the health of your joints.
- Lose weight if needed. People with extra pounds tend to have higher uric acid levels than those who are svelte.
- Consider lead toxicity. If none of the above steps works, consider getting tested for lead toxicity. An unusual type of gout referred to as *saturnine gout* can occur because of too much lead in the body.[6]

Lookout Alert

- Don't take large amounts of vitamin C. This increases uric acid levels in some people.[7]
- Avoid large quantities of niacin, that is, more than 50 mg daily. Niacin competes with uric acid for excretion from the body—this in turn keeps uric acid levels high.[8]

HAY FEVER

This is an allergic condition that appears at a certain time each year. Those who react to tree pollens begin sneezing in the spring; the grass and weed pollens create summertime misery for some, and good ol' ragweed is sure to start autumn hay fever. The important thing to remember here is that hay fever frequency and severity all depend on where you live and what's floating in the air. Mold, animals, dust, and dust mites are also common culprits.

The symptoms are characteristic enough: first your nose begins to itch, then your eyes, even the roof of your mouth begins to itch and AACHOO!! You sneeze. And sneeze. Red, tearing, itchy eyes are part of the package, and for some, coughing and wheezing develop after a time. Depending on your symptoms, sleeping is difficult, eating impossible, headaches a bother, not to mention irritability (who wouldn't be), depression and fatigue. Because of the constant drain on immune reserves, many hay fever sufferers also find themselves victim to more colds and other upper respiratory infections. Remember, too, that hay fever is an immunity disorder unto its own. The body is pulling out all resources to fight nasty pollen; kind of like attacking an ant with a machine gun. For more information, turn to Bronchitis, Colds and Flu, Coughing, Ear Infections, Eczema, Fatigue, Headaches, Insomnia, and Sore Throat. See Chapters 6 (immunity) and 13 (eyes).

How to Prevent a Hay Fever Attack

- Pick the right parents. Hay fever is usually genetic.
- Move. Because this is an allergic response, often to outside influences like pollens and grasses, living in a different region might help (might not).
- Be a Felix. Keep your home clean to cut down on dust and dust mites.
- Cover up. Place hypoallergenic covers on your pillows and mattress to reduce contact with dust mites.
- Clean hidden allergy makers. This includes humidifiers, air conditioners, furnaces, the drip pans in refrigerators, and mildew anywhere in the house, especially around leaky windows.
- Be like a table. I explain the table analogy to allergic patients in this way: the four legs of the table are your habits of diet, exercise, sleep and stress control. When these are strong, like sturdy legs of a table, they support the load of allergies that sit on top of the table.

Using the following nutritional, herbal, and homeopathic advice a month or two before symptoms hit can lessen your hay fever misery.

Food and Nutrition for Hay Fever

- Eat well; skip the junk. See table analogy above.
- Can the sugar. This only adds to already diminished defenses during hay fever season.
- That goes for the caffeine and alcohol too.
- Keep water up. Hay fever is very dehydrating.
- Extra C. Take 500 to 1000 mg of vitamin C three times daily.
- Multiple protection. Take a high-potency vitamin and mineral pill with adequate vitamin A, B vitamins, calcium, potassium, and manganese.
- Eat cold water fish. They provide essential fats to battle nasal inflammation.
- EPO to the rescue. Evening primrose oil works for some. You can also try flax seed oil.

Herbal Treatment

- Decongestants—ephedra, nettles
- Eye soothers—eyebright
- Clear nasal passages—elder flowers, golden seal, licorice
- Immune builders—echinacea, golden seal

The Homeopathic Difference

- Allium cepa—*Symptoms like peeling an onion.* This remedy is derived from red onion, and is fitting for symptoms such as profuse tearing, red burning eyes, clear, irritating nasal discharge, frequent sneezing and thirst; worse in the evening and indoors.
- Euphrasia—*Onion's opposite.* Euphrasia's symptoms are the flip-side of Allium's: bland nasal discharge and burning tears, grogginess, and a sinus headache.
- Nux vomica—*Easily agitated.* Noise! Light! Odors! They all irritate you and make your maddening symptoms—watery nose that can't decide if it should run or keep you stuffed up—even worse.

- Sabadilla—*Non-stop sneezing.* Aaaaahhhh . . . choo!!! Aaaahhh. . . . The inside of your nose itches, and a copious, watery mucus drains from your nose. Even your red eyes are runny. Stepping outside into the open air eases symptoms a little.

Lifestyle Link

- Skin prick test. Get tested so you know your allergies, and are prepared to battle them.
- Pollen sufferers. Close your windows during pollen season, particularly in the morning (when pollen counts tend to be higher) and on windy days.
- Say good-bye to Rover. If cats, dogs, or other residential pets are causing you grief, consider saying farewell. At the very least, don't let them sleep on your bed.
- Raise the head of your bed. This allows for better breathing (and sleeping) at night.
- Investigate contributing allergies. Medications, foods, or other chemicals, including cigarette smoke or perfume, could be adding to the problem.
- Quit smoking.
- Try acupuncture. As a long-time hay fever sufferer, I know this works. It may require several sessions.

Lookout Alert

- Cough up blood.
- Chest pains.
- Severe or prolonged symptoms.

HEADACHES

A favorite teacher of mine in naturopathic medical school told us, "A headache is not an aspirin deficiency." What he meant by that was there are many reasons we get headaches and, although we regularly turn to aspirin and other painkillers for relief, there are safer and equally effective cures.

Headaches are so common we tend to dismiss them as annoyances rather than accept them as conditions that need treatment. A headache, like any pain, is the body's way of telling you something's wrong. It is a symptom of a larger problem.

Headaches occur for many reasons. Daily tension explains many aching temples; most of my suggestions here address this problem. I also include a few tips for migraines, a one-sided pounding, usually recurring headache that often annoys women in their 20s and 30s. A migraine is not merely a very bad headache, but rather a condition with very definite characteristics. Some see an aura—a veil of light—before the pain hits; others experience different visual disturbances as well as sweet cravings, weakness, depression, or slurred speech. Nausea, vomiting, abdominal distress, or even dizziness can be part of the headache package. Most migraine sufferers prefer to be alone in a dark, quiet room while the two-hour to days-long pain lasts.

Head injuries, infections such as the flu, sun exposure, secondhand tobacco smoke, breathing chemicals or pollutants, high blood pressure, low blood pressure, constipation, brain tumors, or conditions of the ears, nose or teeth can also lead to headaches. Menstrual headaches, especially among women with premenstrual syndrome (PMS), might accompany food cravings, fatigue, and dizziness. Or you can suffer from cluster headaches (intense, one-sided pain) that begin during sleep, causing the eye on the affected side to redden and tear. Also see Anxiety, Backache, Colds and Flu, Constipation, Ear Infections, Fatigue, Fever, Hay Fever, Low Blood Sugar; refer to Chapters 4 (digestion), 7 (adrenals), 9 (muscles), and 13 (eyes).

How to Prevent Headaches

- Rest. Fatigue is a common headache trigger. Get enough sleep every night; take extra care to rest and sleep when you're overtaxed emotionally, mentally, or physically.

- Relax every day. Contrary to what you've been told, rest breaks are a sign of health, not laziness. Spaced out during a busy day, they deter an aching head.

- A change is as good as a rest. Mixing your day up with physical movement and thinking reduces stress (and headaches).

- Even temperatures. Abrupt changes in temperature, for example going from an air-conditioned office out to a sweltering summer's afternoon, or from a snuggly warm home to a frost-bitten winter's day, taxes your body and invites head pain.

Food and Nutrition for Headaches

- Stressed out on food. Stress isn't just emotional and mental; incorrect foods can put undue pressure on your body too. This is especially true for refined foods, caffeine, greasy meals, and sugary treats. Irregular meal times add to the strain.
- Focus on whole foods: vegetables, fruits, whole grains, nuts, seeds, and beans.
- Dine on fish, especially the fatty ones like salmon, halibut, and mackerel. Again, these essential fats help decrease inflammation, sometimes part of a headache.
- Flax instead of fish. If you live in fish-less country, turn to flax seed oil, raw nuts, and seeds.
- Add protein. If you get irritable between meals, low blood sugar or insulin resistance could be the cause of your headaches. Eat protein with each meal and snack.
- Drink water.
- Cayenne. The capsaicin in hot peppers decreases head pain by depleting the body's substance P, a chemical that creates pain.
- Food sensitivities. This is especially true for migraines, where studies indicate that 85 to 93 percent of the headache-prone recover by eliminating allergic foods.[9, 10] Most common causes are cow's milk, wheat, chocolate, eggs, and oranges.
- Good-bye chocolate. Some foods, like chocolate, alcohol, and cheese (all your favorites, wouldn't you know it?) contain chemicals that cause blood vessels in your head to constrict. This can lead to a migraine headache.
- Coffee headache. Those who drink coffee daily risk getting a caffeine withdrawal headache if they skip a day. This is one reason why many are reluctant to quit. When you do stop, do so gradually. If you end cold turkey, allow one week before withdrawal signs are done.

- Magnesium helps those headaches—including migraines—where the sufferer is low in this mineral.[11]
- Add vitamin C. 1000 mg three times daily acts as an antihistamine, helpful if your headache is allergy-provoked.

Herbal Treatment

- Pain—black willow (this plant contains aspirin-like compounds good for pain; however, a headache is *not* a black willow deficiency); ginger; bromelain (take between meals)
- With digestive troubles—chamomile, peppermint, rue
- Menstrual headache—rue
- Migraines—chamomile, feverfew
- Tension headaches—chamomile, feverfew, passion flower, valerian

■ *Makeover Hint #93—Tiger in a Bottle*

An easy and natural treatment for any headache is tiger balm, that same smelly stuff you were rubbing on your aching muscles 20 years ago. A recent study found that this fragrant liniment massaged into temples every 30 minutes or so worked as well or better than Tylenol®.[12] I use the colorless form, and notice that the camphor, menthol, cajeput, and clove oils provide a warming sensation coupled with almost immediate relief. No need to wear perfume either.

The Homeopathic Difference

Acute homeopathic remedies are fine for mild to moderate headaches. However, if those headaches are an ongoing concern seek professional help (constitutional homeopathy may be appropriate). If you know the cause, for instance stress, you need to take care of that. Essential oils like lavender, marjoram, or Tiger Balm are great headache fighters, but avoid them if you want to use one of these homeopathic remedies.

- Belladonna—*Throbbing headache.* For intense pounding pain that makes you sensitive to light, noise, touch, smell, and movement, this could help. These sorts of headaches hit you like a ton of bricks. They often settle in your forehead (though they can be anywhere), and your face feels flushed and hot. This headache feels better sitting up and with firm pressure applied to the painful area.

- Bryonia—*Don't move, it hurts.* This type of headache is aggravated by any movement. While a hug is fine for some, any touch is unwelcome for this person whose head aches constantly, left eye hurts, is nauseated or constipated, feels irritable and wants to be alone.

- Gelsemium—*Migraines.* This remedy fits many of the classic migraine signs such as pain preceded by dim vision or visual disturbances, and a worsening with light, noise, or jarring motion. What characterizes a Gelsemium headache is that it tends to be right-sided. If you (or someone you're helping) look dull and tired with droopy eyes, think of this remedy.

- Nux vomica—*Party now, suffer tomorrow.* This is a good remedy for hangover headaches, and other party activities—eating rich foods, taking drugs, staying up late. It involves an overall sick feeling, tummy upset, bitter taste in the mouth, nausea, and vomiting. (Aren't parties fun?)

- Pulsatilla—*Menstrual headache.* For throbbing headaches before or during a period that are one-sided or sit in the forehead, try Pulsatilla. The telltale sign for this remedy is emotional sensitivity where you crave company and cry easily, in this case from head pain.

■ *Makeover Hint #94—The Comfort Makeover*

Slight discomforts are a fact of life and easily dealt with. But too much heat, noise, or other annoyance is stressful. Listen to your body. When it complains, do spot checks on your environment. Are your clothes or shoes too tight? How are you sitting? Do you live or work in a place that's too noisy, cold, hot, bright, or dark? If so, make the necessary comfort changes.

Lifestyle Link

- Hot and cold. Try an ice pack on your head and put your feet in a tub of hot water. A quiet hot bath with a few drops of lavender oil added can be soothing too.
- Stress management. There are lots of ways to hold tension down. Take a brisk walk during lunch; trade neck and shoulder massages with a friend; listen to music or comedy tapes during rush hour. (See Chapter 7).
- Stand up straight! Check your posture.
- Visit the chiropractor. Manipulation of neck or spine (it's all connected) can relieve chronic headaches for some people.
- Get a massage. A soothing rub helps reduce overall tension, increases blood flow (full of oxygen and nutrients) and lymphatic flow (removes toxins).
- See your dentist. Headache and jaw pain could indicate a problem with your temporomandibular joint, a condition called TMJ. Other teeth problems cause more widespread head pain.
- Eye checkup. Straining eyes can lead to fatigue, nausea, and headache. (See Chapter 13).
- Acupuncture. This is a great pain fighter, and can address more body-wide problems.

Lookout Alert

There are many conditions, some extremely serious, that come with a headache. If your headache is associated with any of the following symptoms or conditions, see your doctor.

- Fever
- Stiff neck
- Convulsions
- Loss of consciousness
- Localized pain, for example in the eye or ear
- Visual problems
- Weakness on one part of your body

- Impaired speech
- Dizziness
- After head trauma
- After taking medicine (including herbs or vitamins)
- Long-lasting or unusual headache

HEARTBURN

Heartburn is just what it sounds like—a burning pain in the heart (mid-chest bone) area. In reality it's a digestive complaint where regurgitated stomach acid mimics heart pain that can radiate to the neck, throat, and even face. It usually happens after eating, and is worse upon lying down or at bedtime. The muscle that normally prevents stomach contents from reentering the esophagus, or tube that connects the mouth to the stomach, can weaken and is a common cause of this uncomfortable condition. Ulcers can also cause a heartburn-like pain. See Indigestion and Ulcers; read Chapters 4 (digestion) and 8 (heart).

How to Prevent Heartburn

- Establish regular meal times.
- Don't overeat.
- Eat slowly.
- Dine in peace.

Food and Nutrition for Heartburn

Many of the suggestions below are designed to minimize stomach acid output—cause of your heartburn—while other healing measures are put into play.

- Partake of Nature's bounty. Add those many fresh vegetables and fruits, whole grains, legumes, nuts and seeds to your meals.
- Eat when relaxed.

- Eat smaller meals.
- Don't eat directly before going to bed.
- Identify the acid provokers. These are alcohol, coffee, citrus fruits, tomato, chocolate, carbonated drinks like pop, spicy foods, black tea, peppers and onions.
- No more fat. Fried foods, whipping cream, milk shakes, and other delectable fatty drinks and foods make matters worse.
- Refrain from gassy foods. This could be individual items or combinations that cause you to belch.

Herbal Treatment

Note: Avoid carminative herbs like peppermint and spearmint. They make matters worse for some.

- Decrease acid—meadow sweet
- Healing—cabbage, comfrey, licorice root, marshmallow root
- Soothing herbs—marshmallow root, slippery elm

The Homeopathic Difference

- Cinchona officinalis—*Sour burps.* For that oh-so-bloated feeling, try Cinchona. Along with this acid, gassy stomach comes burping of bitter belches and liquid. Unfortunately they don't spell R-E-L-I-E-F. Only moving around helps.
- Echinacea angustifolia—*Just let me lie down.* Echinacea is a well-known herb, but homeopathically it also works for heartburn with nausea that feels worse in the cold air. This kind of heartburn makes you exhausted; lying down makes everything feel better.
- Nux vomica—*The workaholic.* Nux vomica is for the person who does everything in excess, including work. And when fatigue hits, he turns to coffee, drugs, or alcohol to keep going. These overindulgences in turn invite headaches, irritability, drowsiness, and *heartburn* that's usually worse in the morning.
- Pulsatilla—*Night-time pain.* For heartburn that strikes at night, Pulsatilla might ease your pain. A thick yellow or white tongue and queasiness that leaves your mouth tasting bad points to this remedy. Rich fatty foods aggravate this kind of heartburn.

Lifestyle Link

• Overdoing it. For those occasional times when you overindulge, don't lie down or bend over. This will surely create a heartburn episode.

• Prop your bed. To relieve nighttime burn, elevate the headboard side of your bed a few inches.

• Quit smoking. This habit relaxes the band of muscle separating the stomach and esophagus.

• Breathe. Many of my heartburn patients are worse during periods of stress. Learn to prepare for those times, or develop methods of handling tension to lessen or prevent a heartburn attack (see Chapter 7).

• Esophageal manipulation. Ask a chiropractor or osteopathic doctor you know about techniques that will help release tension in the area surrounding the esophagus.

Lookout Alert

Also see Ulcer.

• Chest pains not related to eating
• Chest pain that extends to the left arm, shoulders, or neck
• Shortness of breath—especially upon exertion
• Crushing sensation on the chest
• Nighttime pain accompanied by increased heart rate
• Nighttime pain accompanied by rapid breathing
• Intense or unrelenting symptoms

HEMORRHOIDS

Hemorrhoids are very common among the "civilized" in industrialized nations. In fact, half of those people age 50 and above have them, while one third of Americans have hemorrhoids to some degree. Simply stated, hemorrhoids, or piles, are like varicose veins, only in the anal region. There are many different versions: internal, external, combined internal and external.

The most frequent first sign of hemorrhoids is bright red blood on the toilet paper or in the toilet bowl. Other symptoms that can (but not always) indicate hemorrhoids are itching, burning, or irritation in the rectal region, seepage, or swelling. Hemorrhoids are usually painless. Some prolapse or sag outside of the anus and must be pushed back into the rectum after a bowel movement. Pregnancy can cause hemorrhoids. Among the non-pregnant, anything that increases congestion of blood in the anus is a contributory factor—things like straining to defecate (constipation), sneezing and coughing, physical exertion, prolonged standing or sitting. Also see Constipation, Varicose Veins; refer to Chapters 3 (liver) and 4 (digestion).

How to Prevent Hemorrhoids

- Move about. Standing or sitting for a long time invites hemorrhoids. So get up and move about (see Chapter 9).
- Fill up on fiber. Less roughage creates hard-to-pass stools. This means more straining during bowel movements, an ideal way to weaken veins in that region.
- Drink lots of water, at least one quart a day. This prevents constipation.
- Exercise regularly.

Food and Nutrition for Hemorrhoids

- Hurray for fiber. Concentrate on raw vegetables and fruits.
- Water, water, water.
- Flax seed oil. 1 tbsp. daily
- Citrus fruits. Here's where oranges and grapefruit are very helpful, especially the white rind; it contains tissue-healing bioflavonoids.
- Eat the red, purple, and blue. These deep-colored fruits (cherries, berries) contain special flavonoids called proanthocyanidins and anthocyanidins that strengthen veins.
- Take your supplements. Vitamins A, B-complex and E, and zinc aid recovery.

- Vitamin C plus bioflavonoids. An equal dose of each (500 mg to 3000 mg per day in divided doses) essential for tissue repair.
- Zinc oxide. Apply directly to affected region.
- Vitamin E oil. A good topical therapy.

Herbal Treatment

- Astringents—horse chestnut, witch hazel (topical)
- Circulation—ginkgo
- Constipation fighters—flax seed, psyllium seed
- Less swelling—Butcher's broom
- Soothing—aloe, slippery elm
- Tissue healers—aloe, comfrey, yarrow (topical)
- Vessel toners—Butcher's broom, gotu kola, horse chestnut, yarrow

■ *Makeover Hint #95—Direct Herbal Support*

Ointments, pads, or suppositories can offer a soothing and healing quality. However, if dietary and lifestyle changes aren't made these effects will most likely be temporary. Look for products containing one or more of these: witch hazel, aloe vera, plantain, St. John's wort, yarrow, golden seal, comfrey, vitamins A and E.

The Homeopathic Difference

- Aesculus hipposcastanum—*Sitting on pins and needles.* This is the homeopathic version of horse chestnut, and like many homeopathic remedies, it works for hemorrhoids just like the herbal form. This kind of hemorrhoid leaves the rectum feeling full. The area is dry, burning, and excoriating. It's like sitting on a pin cushion.
- Collinsonia canadensis—*And constipation too.* As one homeopathic textbook so graphically put it, these hemorrhoids have the "sensation of sharp sticks in the rectum." Bleeding, itching, aching, and obstinate constipation are also part of the picture. Heat makes it feel better, cold does not.

- Lachesis—*A choking sensation.* There's a throbbing pain and feeling of tightness in the anal region from this kind of hemorrhoids that actually feels better when the rectum bleeds. The hemorrhoids protrude and are purple in color. Sneezing and coughing increase pain, as does heat.
- Muriaticum acidum—*Hurts from toilet paper.* These hemorrhoids are swollen, itchy, dark blue, protruding, and very sensitive, so sensitive that even wiping oneself with toilet paper is agonizing. Women who get hemorrhoids during pregnancy are often helped by this remedy. One characteristic that separates Muriaticum from the others is that urination makes the itching and protrusion worse, and may even initiate involuntary stool evacuation.

Lifestyle Link

- Develop regular toilet habits. This means using the bathroom the same time each day to empty your bowels; avoid straining; give yourself enough time to have a bowel movement.
- Warm Sitz bath. Sit in a warm bath (bottom only), followed by a short cold one. Add witch hazel if you please.

Lookout Alert

- Black stools
- Blood in the stool. Bright red blood is often hemorrhoid related. However, any rectal blood should be investigated.
- Mucus or pus in the stool
- Alternating constipation and diarrhea

HIVES

If little red, swollen, intensely itchy circles (called wheals or welts) arise suddenly on your skin, you have urticaria—commonly known as hives. One in five people have them at one time or another, and because they're caused by so many things it's often impossible to track down their cause. Hives appear because of insect bites, the cold or the heat, physical exercise (usually after a heavy meal), rubbing, scratching or vibrating the skin, water or light, mental anguish or infection, penicillin or aspirin, food or food additives. They may happen once and last anywhere from hours to days, or they can be long-lasting. Also see Acne, Anxiety, Canker Sores, Eczema, Food Poisoning, Psoriasis, Yeast Infections; refer to Chapters 4 (digestion), 7 (adrenals), and 14 (the mind).

How to Prevent Hives

This is often a mysterious condition that comes once and disappears before its cause is known. Pretty hard to prevent, I'd say.

Food and Nutrition for Hives

• Vitamin C. This natural antihistamine may reduce hives.

• Subtract food additives. Choose foods without artificial colorings, flavorings, and other synthetic chemicals. (See Chapter 3.)

• Food allergies. Sensitivity to certain foods can create a host of problems, including hives. Check it out.

• Vasoactive amines. Those same foods that trigger migraine headaches can cause hives (see Headaches).

Herbal Treatment

• Bitters for better digestion—barberry, chamomile, gentian, golden seal

• Mellow out—chamomile, passion flower, skullcap, valerian

The Homeopathic Difference

• Apis mellifica—*Ouch, that stings!* To remember when Apis works, think of a hot, red, swollen bee sting—that's how your hives should feel. Cool compresses make it better, warm (and nighttime) worse. This kind of hives erupts when you sweat or get hot. If no other remedy sticks out, try Apis first.

• Rhus toxicodendron—*The unscratchable itch.* These welts form during cold or wet weather from scratching or perspiring, and are red, swollen, and very, very itchy. Walking makes these hives better, rest worse.

- Urtica urens—*A stinging nettles-type of hives.* If you've ever fallen into a patch of stinging nettles, you know what kind of hives is helped by Urtica urens—itchy, red, stinging, burning blotches. That's because Urtica is stinging nettles, or rather the homeopathic version. This type of hives often appears after vigorous exercise, bathing, or warmth, and feels better from lying down.

Lifestyle Link

Solving hives takes a detective. There are so many things that cause this itchy rash that to truly cure it, you need to figure out what caused it in the first place. If this is a one-time case, the hives might disappear before you figure it out. If hives keep pestering you, keep a diary of your dietary habits (see Chapter 4), activities, medicines and supplements, and emotional state, and see if you can find a correlation.

- Cold cloth. Like all swellings, hives feel better and improve slightly with a cold cloth applied to the area. (Unless, of course, the hives are caused by cold.)
- Feelings. For many, emotions play a part in hives.
- A dash of sun. For those who get hives from the cold, firmly touching the skin, after taking certain medicines, during a skin infection or other disorder, a daily 15-minute dose of sunlight might help.
- Lie back and relax. Practice daily relaxation techniques, like deep breathing, listening to soothing music or tapes with "relaxation talk," meditation, prayer—whatever it takes.
- Put oatmeal in your bath. See Makeover Hint #68.

Lookout Alert

Most cases of hives disappear before you know what caused them. But occasionally this swelling also includes the respiratory passages. When this allergic reaction is severe, the throat may be blocked and breathing difficult. If your throat feels tight or breathing is harder, call your doctor immediately or go to the nearest Emergency Room.

INDIGESTION

Indigestion is a general term for uncomfortable and gaseous feelings that occur in the abdomen after eating. It's caused by a variety of problems such as malabsorption, decreased stomach acid, or diminished digestive enzymes. Also see Anxiety, Constipation, Diarrhea, Food Poisoning, Heartburn, Ulcer. Read Chapters 3 (liver) and 4 (digestion).

How to Prevent Indigestion

- Chew your food. This is where digestion begins.
- Don't rush. Avoid eating in the car, while doing chores, or anything else. Instead, allow your body time to accept and properly digest the food you serve it.
- Laugh at dinner. Relaxed eating, prayer, and company also improve digestion.
- Regulate your repast. Predictable mealtimes let your digestive system work better.

Food and Nutrition for Digesting

See prevention tips above; also:

- Eliminate milk. You might be lactose intolerant.
- Keep eating wholesome. Fresh vegetables and fruits, whole grains, legumes, nuts and seeds.
- Don't eat refined. Processed foods lack enzymes that help you digest.
- Cut back on grains. For some, these foods cause problems.
- Stop at 6:30 P.M. Break the night-snack habit. If you must, some fruit or toast only.
- Simplify. Eat one to three different foods at a time only. Complex food mixtures make more work for your gut.
- Lemon tip. Sip on a glass of water spiked with a wedge of lemon before each meal.
- Green digestion. Eat a large, dark green salad with spinach, radicchio, endive, dandelion greens.

- Nibble. Dine on several small meals throughout the day, rather than three large squares.
- Liquids first, then food. For some people, it helps to drink beverages away from food. If you're used to sipping with meals, do so first, then eat. Or only drink what's required to eat comfortably.
- Digestive help. Try digestive enzymes and hydrochloric acid supplements; take throughout the meal.

Herbal Treatment

- Better bile—balmony, barberry, dandelion root, golden seal, wild yam
- Nervous stomach—chamomile, hops, skullcap, valerian
- No more gas—chamomile, ginger, peppermint
- Power-up digestion—barberry, chamomile, gentian root, golden seal

---

■ *Makeover Hint #96—Use Spices to Reduce Gas*

Many of our culinary herbs and spices are, interestingly enough, also helpful for digestion. Specifically, the following spices help curtail painful gas caused by eating: allspice, aniseed, caraway, cardamon, cayenne, cinnamon, coriander, dill, fennel, ginger.

The Homeopathic Difference

- Carbo vegetabilis—*The food just sits there.* When your stomach is heavy, full, and taut with gassy pain this remedy may help. You feel sleepy, yet the gas gets worse as evening nears and when you lie down. Sour burps and passing gas make it slightly better.
- Chamomilla—*Angry indigestion.* For a crampy, gassy indigestion that hits you after an angry outburst, Chamomilla might help. This remedy is useful for indigestion that leaves your cheeks flushed and a bitter taste in your mouth.
- Lycopodium—*There's a rumbly in my tumbly.* Weak digestion best describes the person who needs Lycopodium. Yet warm drinks and food do make it better. And there's a noticeable noise and rumbling in the stomach.

- Nux vomica—*I can't believe I ate the whole thing.* This is the remedy of overindulgence, be it food, alcohol, drugs, or work. Indigestion of this type makes you impatient and irascible. Flatulence is a problem, as are a bloated abdomen and stomach cramps.

Lifestyle Link

- Upset mood leads to an upset stomach. Avoid eating when you are distressed.

Lookout Alert

- Symptoms that worsen with exertion
- Alternating constipation and diarrhea
- Abdominal pain not related to eating
- Intense abdominal pain
- Bloody or tarry stools
- Mucus or pus in the stools
- Vomiting, especially blood or "coffee-ground" material
- Trouble swallowing
- Unusual weight loss
- Fever
- Jaundice (the whites of the eyes look yellowish)
- Change in symptoms
- Severe or unrelenting symptoms

INSOMNIA

If you have trouble falling asleep, wake up in the middle of the night and can't go back to sleep, or arise too early in the morning, you have insomnia. An astounding one third of Americans can't sleep on a regular basis. Daily pressures make sleeping difficult, as do other emotional difficulties. But how you live—caffeine intake for one—can also keep you awake long past bedtime. Refer to Anxiety, Fatigue, and Heartburn. See Chapters 7 (adrenals) and 14 (the mind).

How to Prevent Insomnia

- Calm down. Anxiety is a frequent cause of insomnia. (See Anxiety.)

- Caffeine be gone. This stimulant, found in coffee, black tea, chocolate, soft drinks, and some medications, creates sleeping problems in more than a few people. Decrease what you consume, or stop using it earlier in the day.

- Avoid alcohol. A glass of wine at the end of a busy day can unwind you, and then leave you wide-eyed later in bed.

- Short naps only. Too much daytime sleep may leave you wide awake at night. Nap for 20 minutes tops.

- Bedroom makeover. An uncomfortable bedroom, whether from temperature, noise, smell, or aesthetics, can rob you of zzz's. Make sure your sleeping chamber is pleasing and used only for sleep and sex—no working, no TV, no eating.

- Bedtime hygiene. Children go to bed better when they have a routine. Adults need a bedtime ritual too. Doctors call this sleeping hygiene. Start with a regular bedtime. Then one hour before that, follow a set routine—brush your teeth, make a cup of herbal tea, put on your PJs, read a happy book, and turn out the lights when sleepy.

■ *Makeover Hint #97—Create the Middle of the Night in the Middle of the Day*

You need to sleep during the day because you're working a graveyard shift or need to catch up on your rest. Your body is bone-tired, but the light streaming in from the window, yelling children, and insensitive lawnmowers are keeping you awake. Follow these ideas for more restful (and successful) slumber:

- Wear ear plugs. Get the snug-fitting kind that blocks most noise.

- Cover your eyes. Use a sleeping mask or T-shirt wrapped over your eyes.

- Keep the room cool. Turn off the heating vent (if winter), and crack the window open. Or if summer, use a fan or air conditioning.
- Do Not Disturb. Turn on the answering machine, take the children to a sitter, and take care of anything else that may interrupt your dozing.

Food and Nutrition for Sleeping

- Calcium/magnesium. These minerals have a soothing effect on your nervous system and muscles, especially if taken before bed with a snack or with your evening meal. (Always take calcium with food.)
- Skimp on nighttime snacks. If you must nibble before bed, keep your snack light and easy to digest. Pick fresh fruit or toast, not a ham sandwich.
- "Sweet" dreams. Avoid sugary foods prior to lights out. After a few hours, a sweet snack leaves your blood sugar low—a surefire wake-up call. (See Low Blood Sugar.) If no food before bed wakes you up, try a small, protein snack like yogurt.
- To B or not to B? Make sure you're getting adequate amounts of the B-complex vitamins in your multiple pill. Also dine on whole grains and dark, leafy greens.

■ *Makeover Hint #98—Be Still, Restless Legs*

A fairly common cause of insomnia is restless leg syndrome, a condition where you wake up from the irresistible urge to move your legs. Taking a calcium and magnesium supplement can help. Vitamin E, 400 IU twice daily, also works for some.

Herbal Treatment

Many different herbs with sedative actions are used for insomnia. They can be used alone, especially valerian or passion flower, or you may find them combined as teas or other herbal products. While these plants certainly don't carry the hazards of sleeping pills, use them only for occasional insomnia or as an adjunct to a more comprehensive sleeping program.

- Indigestion insomnia—chamomile, hops, peppermint
- Restless legs—ginkgo
- Sedatives—passion flower, skullcap, valerian

The Homeopathic Difference

- Coffea cruda—*Can't turn my mind off.* Think of how coffee makes you feel—nervous, agitated, restless—and you'll know when to use Coffea (or homeopathic coffee) for a sleepless night. Coffea is the remedy for a wide-awake mind, but a sleepy body.
- Ignatia—*Emotional insomnia.* If your emotions are keeping you awake, think of Ignatia. It might be shock, grief, sadness, or disappointment that prevents you from falling asleep. Sighing often accompanies this type of insomnia, and you probably don't feel like talking about it.
- Kali phosphoricum—*Nervous exhaustion; no sleep.* Anxiety and lethargy go hand in hand with this remedy. While you feel weak and tired, there's still a sense of irritability and "brain-fag" due to overwork, excitement, or worry.
- Nux vomica—*Early morning waking.* The person who fits this remedy can fall asleep all right, even feels sleepy after eating and early in the evening, but can't sleep after 3am. Waking this early makes the Nux person feel terrible. And even when he does sleep, his dreams are full of hustle and bustle.

Lifestyle Link

- Exercise. Regular activity not only improves overall health, but is a beautiful makeover step for sleeping. Hint: exercising three hours or less before bed has more of a wake-up than a good-night effect.
- Is your bedroom dark? Light filtering in from the street or other rooms disturbs sleep.
- Bathroom break. Don't turn on the light if you get up to urinate at night. It not only wakens you, but disrupts melatonin—the sleeping hormone.

- Avoid ibuprofen. This also interferes with melatonin.
- Low blood sugar. For those prone to low blood sugar, night-time awakenings may be a problem. When glucose drops too low, the brain gets hungry and you wake up.
- Sex. This is a wonderful, natural sleeping aid (see Chapter 10).
- Don't clock-watch. Looking at the time while falling asleep or during the night can make dozing difficult.
- Stay clear of drugs. Like alcohol, these can create sleeping problems.

Lookout Alert

- After starting new medication—prescription or over-the-counter. This includes herbs and vitamins.
- Accompanied by other symptoms, like aching joints.

LOW BLOOD SUGAR

This is a controversial condition. Medically speaking, there are two types of hypoglycemia (low blood sugar). There's spontaneous hypoglycemia, a rare kind of low blood sugar usually caused by severe disease like a tumor in the pancreas or liver. Reactive hypoglycemia, the other kind, is more common and occurs two to four hours after eating or in response to specific drugs like insulin. Low blood sugar is also common among pregnant women, after extended periods of exercise or during fever. For a select few, hypoglycemia is the first warning sign of impending diabetes.

The controversy among doctors and nutritionists surrounds low blood sugar that follows a meal, particularly one high in simple carbohydrates. People who claim to have this condition commonly complain of headaches, irritability, weakness, fatigue, trembling, poor vision, memory problems, and food cravings. Mid-afternoon is a common time for these symptoms to occur.

Jonathan Wright, M.D., calls this "refined carbohydrate disease," meaning it's the processed and refined foods we eat—low in fiber and nutrients—that create unstable blood sugar levels; caffeine and alcohol do the same. Past studies suggest that poor insulin response is responsible,[13] and is referred to as insulin resistance or hyper-insulinemia. Exhausted adrenal glands can also be at hand, as can a malfunctioning liver. Anna MacIntosh, Ph.D., N.D., proposes that we call this condition dysglycemia (literally bad blood sugar) rather than low blood sugar because many people have troubles regulating blood sugar, be it up or down.[14] Other names describing this condition include glucose intolerance, Syndrome X, and carbohydrate intolerance. There's even evidence that low blood sugar is related to high blood pressure.[15] So if other measures (dietary, nutrients, herbs, medication) don't help your hypertension, consider following a low blood sugar regimen.

If you suspect you're prone to this condition, follow the suggestions below. If they don't help, visit with your doctor for a more thorough evaluation. Related topics include Anxiety, Fatigue, Headaches, Indigestion. Also glance at Chapters 3 (liver), 4 (digestion), 7 (adrenals), and 14 (the mind).

How to Prevent Low Blood Sugar

- Steer clear of sugar. Sweet things and refined carbohydrates contribute to this state.
- Eat breakfast. This doesn't mean coffee and a Danish. Feast on oatmeal with fruit and nuts, or an egg alongside whole grain toast or bran muffin.
- Nutritious nibbling. After a wholesome breakfast, keep your body humming with more fiber-filled, nutritious foods.
- All in the family. If low blood sugar signs or alcoholism run in your family, you may be more prone. Take steps early to prevent greater troubles down the road.

Food and Nutrition for Low Blood Sugar

Follow prevention tips, as well as the ideas below.

- The more often you eat, the better you feel. Maintain even blood sugar levels with three small meals interjected with two to three snacks.
- Carry snacks. If it's difficult to stop and eat every couple of hours, carry a bag of raw almonds, walnuts, and raisins to munch on.

- Pour out the alcohol. This adds to the blood sugar roller coaster.
- Eat a little protein with every meal. Help prop up blood sugar with lean meats and poultry, beans, low-fat and cultured dairy, nuts and seeds at each seating.
- Get your chromium. This blood sugar-regulating mineral, in 200 to 300 mcg divided doses daily, helps those who are chromium-deficient.
- Other nutrients. The B vitamins, vitamin C, flavonoids, calcium, magnesium, and zinc are also important for pancreas and adrenal function. Begin with a good multivitamin/mineral.
- Lipotropics. If the liver's at fault, try liver-hungry nutrients (choline, folic acid, vitamin B_{12}, methionine, betaine and carnitine).
- The digestion connection. If gas, bloating, heartburn are also problems, consider indigestion as a factor. See Indigestion and Chapter 4.
- Consider food allergies. If the above steps don't help much, try avoiding suspected food allergies for one to two weeks and see if it helps.

Herbal Treatment

- Adrenal support—licorice
- Improve glucose tolerance—bitter melon, fenugreek, goat's rue, gymnema
- Liver help for more even blood sugar—dandelion, milk thistle

The Homeopathic Difference

A blood sugar dysfunction has such a strong lifestyle and dietary connection that I hesitate suggesting any homeopathic remedies for it. After all, using homeopathy in acute fashion is only a temporary fix. And blood sugar needs permanent nutritional and dietary attention. If you're having troubles getting your wild, modern ways under control, read up on Nux vomica (see Appendix B). This may help. Otherwise, seek the help of a practitioner expert in constitutional homeopathic prescribing. In the meantime, change your diet and see what happens.

Lifestyle Link

- Stop smoking. There's a strong link between cigarette smoking and malfunctioning insulin (called insulin resistance).[16]
- Testing. Ask your doctor for a Glucose-Insulin Tolerance Test if you want confirmation that hypoglycemia is causing you distress.

Lookout Alert

- If you're diabetic and have these symptoms
- If you're taking insulin
- Began a new medication prior to onset of symptoms
- Have a history of alcohol use or abuse
- Convulsion or loss of consciousness occurs
- Chest pain
- Chronic or severe symptoms

MOTION SICKNESS

That queasy feeling, and occasional vomiting, that come with travel is familiar to many. Cold sweats, sleepiness, hyperventilation, weakness, and a pale complexion, dizziness, headache, and fatigue can also occur. For unknown reasons, some of us are susceptible to movement whether by sea, air, car, or train. Some even become ill on a swing. We do know that motion sickness is the result of overstimulation of certain nerves, and that particular things like looking out the window (especially from the back seat), poor ventilation, cigarette smoke, fear and anxiety all make this miserable condition worse. Taking measures to prevent or minimize motion symptoms is much more effective than treating full-blown motion sickness. Refer to Anxiety, Fatigue, Headaches, Insomnia, Low Blood Sugar.

How to Prevent Motion Sickness

- Best seat in the house (or car). Whatever your mode of transportation, sit where you feel the least motion—usually in the middle—over the wings of an airplane, center seat in a car, or mid-ship if on a boat.

- Don't read while traveling.
- Lie down or semi-erect with your head stationary or braced.
- Don't watch the scenery go by; it only makes matters worse.
- Don't travel with smokers. Or ask them to extinguish their cigarettes.
- Get lots of fresh air.

Food and Nutrition for Motion Sickness

- Avoid eating. And drinking, if traveling a short distance.
- Eat lightly. Drink fresh lemon or lime juice, if going on an extended trip.
- Sip on green tea.
- Avoid alcohol.

Herbal Treatment

- Calm down with—passion flower, skullcap, valerian
- Nausea—ginger
- Nervous stomach—chamomile, peppermint (teas work well)

■ *Makeover Hint #99—The Three-Day Ginger Cure*

To avoid the nausea (and sometimes vomiting) of travel, begin sipping three cups of ginger tea three days before you depart. Continue drinking it on the day of your trip (every hour if possible. All this liquid also keeps you hydrated—good for plane rides). To make tea, purchase tea bags or brew this homemade version:

1 tsp powdered or chopped up ginger root

1 cup boiling water

Steep ginger in water for 10 minutes, strain (if needed) and drink.

If you prefer, take capsules: 1000 mg of ginger equals one cup of tea. This plan works well for extensive travel, like plane trips.

The Homeopathic Difference

- Cocculus indicus—*Oh so dizzy!* Nausea marks this motion sickness remedy, as well as an ache in the back of the head and eyes. Along with the vertigo is a weakness that makes it difficult to speak out. (In Dr. William Boericke's 1927 edition of *Materia Medica*, still a standard reference for homeopaths, he emphasizes that these symptoms are worse when riding in a carriage or by ship. I assume we can extrapolate and say this is also true for modern-day car and plane travelers.)

- Nux vomica—*A sensitive, dizzy type.* This remedy fits those who feel irritable and oversensitive with a pounding headache. Dizziness is part of the Nux picture; but the sign to watch for is nausea with dry heaves.

- Petroleum—*I feel like I'm inebriated.* This is another remedy that eases dizziness, especially when upon standing. Also, the back of the head feels very heavy and irritability is apparent. All of this feels better when lying back with the head held up. The sign to watch for most is a "drunk-like" feeling.

- Tabacum—*The moving vomit.* If you're traveling with a smoker, and the smell of tobacco makes your travel sickness worse, think of Tabacum—homeopathic tobacco. This nausea is incessant, and moving makes you vomit. A terrible sinking feeling lies in the pit of your stomach, and your head aches horribly. Open your eyes, and the room (or car) spins.

Lifestyle Link

- Breathe deeply. May help with the nausea and relax you at the same time.

- Fresh air versus stale fumes. Clean air certainly clears one's head and relieves nausea to a point. However, if you're traveling in the city during rush hour, roll up your window and keep auto exhaust out.

Lookout Alert

- Watch for dehydration if prolonged vomiting

PSORIASIS

This is a tough condition to treat both naturally and conventionally. It's fairly common, found in about three of every 100 Americans. All ages are affected, though it usually begins around age 10. Psoriasis tends to run in the family, and is caused by overzealous skin cell production. What results is thick, scaly, dry, sometimes reddish skin that has a silvery sheen to it and isn't itchy. Symptoms come and go. For some, psoriasis isn't too bad with only one or two rashes apparent, usually on the scalp, elbows, knees, back, and buttocks. More severe, widespread cases are also possible, with some people developing joint pain called psoriatic arthritis. Also see Acne and Eczema; read Chapters 3 (liver), 4 (digestion), 12 (skin), and 14 (the mind).

How to Prevent Psoriasis

- Reduce the rays. Moderate sunlight helps psoriasis, but avoid sunburn.

- Guard your skin. Local skin injuries can bring on psoriasis, as well as other irritations.

- Watch your health. Some people, particularly children, have an outbreak after a chest cold, bronchitis, or other upper respiratory infection.

- Avoid topical medications unless absolutely necessary.

- Be cautious of cortisone medications. Withdrawing from these medicines can also bring on psoriasis. If you need such medication, explore other alternatives with your doctor's help.

Food and Nutrition for the Skin

- Saturated fats. Step away from fatty animal-based foods like red meat and whole-fat dairy.

- Feast on fish. Eat plenty of fish like mackerel, halibut, and salmon.

- Eat up essentials. Ensure you're getting plenty of essential fatty acids from raw, unsalted nuts and seeds, whole grains and flax seed (or flax seed oil).

- Give caffeine the boot. Cut the coffee and other caffeine pleasures down or out.

- Eliminate alcohol, and see what happens.
- Enjoy fresh fruits and vegetables.
- Load up on whole grains. These are brown rice, barley, and whole wheat bread.
- Drink water.
- Use a high-potency multiple vitamin and mineral. Make sure it has at least 400 IU of vitamin E, as well as B-complex.
- Add some C. Extra vitamin C, 500 to 1000 mg thrice daily, might also help.
- Zinc. For three months, and no more, take 45 mg of this mineral. Then decrease to 15 mg daily.
- Digestive help. Try digestive enzymes or hydrochloric acid.
- Ask your doctor to test you for food allergies. If you suspect you're reacting to a food(s), eliminate it for one month. Wheat and citrus are common culprits.

■ *Makeover Hint #100—Give Up Pop*

Avoiding sugar is a common natural health suggestion for psoriasis. One afternoon, a fellow in his 50s came to visit me in my office wanting to know how to cure his psoriasis. I mentioned the above ideas, as well as the one about eliminating sugar. Turns out this gentleman drank two quarts of cola each day. "Ya know," he said to me, "when I was hospitalized a few years back, the nurses wouldn't let me have any soft drinks. Come to think of it, my psoriasis cleared up totally." Sounded to me like he already knew what to do, if he so chose.

Herbal Treatment

Many of the following herbs work best for psoriasis if taken long-term. Ask a skilled herbalist to guide you.

- Balancing/nutritive—burdock, nettles, sarsaparilla
- For irritation—sarsaparilla
- Less stress—linden, skullcap, valerian

- Reduce inflammation—licorice
- Scaly skin—burdock, cleavers

■ *Makeover Hint #101—Soothing Cream*

If you're searching for an herbal cream to ease psoriatic irritation, read labels and look for these ingredients: comfrey, chickweed, and marshmallow.

The Homeopathic Difference

- Arsenicum—*It burns.* Look for itchy, swollen, scaly, rough, dry skin, if you want to try Arsenicum. Often the right side is worse than the left, and a flare-up can make you restless. The odd thing about this remedy, though, is that the pain is burning, but cold makes it feel bad.
- Borax—*THE psoriasis remedy.* If confused, choose Borax for your psoriasis first. The back of finger joints are particularly affected, as well as the hands. Symptoms are often better in the evening and worse when the weather gets warm.
- Lycopodium—*Offensive odor.* For this type of psoriasis, there's violent itching and dry skin. Scratching makes the skin bleed, and any secretions—including perspiration—smell bad.
- Sulphur—*Don't wash.* This general skin remedy also helps when your psoriasis burns and itches. It's specific for psoriasis in the folds of skin, like elbow creases and behind the knees. But the distinguishing sign is that it's worse after bathing.

Lifestyle Link

- Move and sweat. Daily exercise is helpful, especially the type that makes you perspire (See Chapter 9).
- Breathe and relax every day (See Chapter 6).

Lookout Alert

- Sores that don't heal
- Accompanying joint pain

SORE THROAT

This is a common wintertime, cold-related symptom. Runny nose, fever, fatigue are some of the signs that a sore throat is infectious in nature. A virus is frequently responsible, though more serious *Streptococcus* (strep throat) can also be the villain. Besides throat pain, swallowing can be irksome. Tonsillitis, more often a bacterial—like strep—infection, has the added symptom of swallowing pain that shoots out to the ears, as well as high fever and vomiting. Laryngitis is key when your voice drops to a whisper. A sore throat is often a sign that an infection is on its way. This is your opportunity to take action and halt it in its tracks. Natural therapies tend to work better when used early.

Because a sore throat is a symptom and not a disease, there are many other causes. If you've been talking, screaming, or singing a lot, you might develop a pained throat. Allergies or inhaling irritating substances (including cigarette smoke) can hurt your throat. Tumors in that area (benign and cancerous) are unusual, but possible, causes. If the following suggestions don't help within a couple of days, see your doctor to rule out the possibility of strep throat. If your throat aches and doesn't seem to be part of a cold or infection, also seek help. See Bronchitis, Colds and Flu, Coughing, Hay Fever, and Heartburn; also refer to Chapter 6 (immunity).

How to Prevent a Sore Throat

- Guard your immunity to fight infection. (See Chapter 6.)
- Avoid cigarette smoke, your own and others'.
- Don't breathe paint. If working around any solvents, including house paint, wear a mask, make sure the area is well ventilated, and take frequent breaks.
- Protect your voice. Overuse can injure it.
- Change toothbrushes every month. Bacteria grow here and may contribute to an infection.

Food and Nutrition for the Throat

- Stay away from sweets. They keep an infection brewing.
- Drink up. The more fluids the better: water, herbal tea, soup, and fresh, raw vegetable juices are best.

- Avoid fruit juices. It's the fruit sugar.
- Homemade gargle. Add 1/4 tsp turmeric and a pinch of salt to warm water, gargle, and spit out.
- Lemon and honey mixed in warm water. Sip slowly.
- Suck on zinc lozenges. See Makeover Hint #102 following.
- Oh, say can you C? Take 500–1000 mg of vitamin C every two hours. Optional: add a similar amount of bioflavonoids.
- Extra carotenes.
- Consider food allergies. A chronic tickle that doesn't appear infectious might be food-related. Key question: if you're stuffed up, is the resulting mucus clear? If so, it's probably not infectious, but allergic.

Herbal Treatment

For teas made with the following herbs, gargle first, then swallow for maximum effectiveness.

- Drying herbs for mucus-filled throats—bayberry, sage, sumac
- Infection reducers—echinacea, garlic, golden seal, osha root, sage
- Soothing—slippery elm, marshmallow root

The Homeopathic Difference

- Belladonna—*Dry as the desert*. As is typical for Belladonna, this sore throat is red and dry. Your throat feels tight and even worse when you drink liquids.
- Drosera rotundifolia—*I can barely talk*. When spit seems to fill your mouth, yet your throat is dry and rough think Drosera. And you're so hoarse, the words don't come out right. Lying down makes your throat feel bad.
- Lachesis—*That choking feeling*. The most notable feature of this sore throat remedy is the sensation of constriction, especially when swallowing. The left side, for some reason, feels the worst.
- Lycopodium—*Better with a cup of tea*. This is a kind of moving sore throat; it may settle on the right, or hop back and forth from right to left. Warm beverages ease it a bit.

Lifestyle Link

A sore throat can be part of inhalant allergies. See Hay fever.

- Indulge in sleep.
- Don't overdo it.
- Give up smoking.
- Ditto for alcohol.
- Question antibiotics. If your doctor prescribes this medicine, first ask for a throat culture to confirm that you indeed have a bacterial infection. Viruses, which cause most sore throats, don't respond to antibiotics.

Lookout Alert

- Severe pain upon swallowing
- Pain that extends to the ear on the same side—especially if the only complaint
- Difficulty breathing
- Spitting up blood
- Pain with talking
- Hoarseness that lasts two weeks or more
- Severe or unrelenting symptoms

■ *Makeover Hint #102—Gargle With Killer Zinc*

According to studies,[17] zinc kills viruses on contact. This means if you want to attack the bugs that are causing your sore throat, you need to suck on a zinc lozenge, not merely swallow a zinc pill. If you can't find zinc lozenges at your local health food store, here's a quick health trick you can try.

Empty one capsule of zinc powder into half a cup of warm water.

Add 1/2 tsp of salt and mix.

Gargle and spit out.

The secret to this remedy is to gargle as often as humanly possible. (Warning, this mixture tastes like metallic dirt.)

SPRAINS AND STRAINS

The body's framework isn't just made up of bones and muscles. Ligaments act as the fasteners between neighboring bones, and tendons are the bridges across muscles and bones. All of these structures are prone to injury. More specifically, a strain occurs when a ligament or muscle is overstretched. Sprains, frequent in the ankle, are a slightly more serious injury where a ligament is either severely stretched or partially torn. Symptoms to watch for are pain (both on movement and at ease), swelling, redness, and heat in the affected joint—especially after a spill or accident. For related information, see Backache, and read Chapters 9 (muscles) and 11 (bones).

How to Prevent Sprains and Strains

- Ease in and out. Warm up before you exercise and cool down afterward.
- Don't overdo it. Especially for intense or prolonged exercise you're not used to.
- Be careful. If you're sick, tired, or recently injured, you're more likely to hurt yourself during these vulnerable times.
- Think before you move. Prior to an exercise regimen, consider your age, health, the environmental factors, your current fitness level. For instance, don't run a marathon if you've never run before.
- Visit with your doctor or a knowledgeable practitioner to help you determine an effective and safe exercise plan.
- Start slow and easy.

Food and Nutrition for Injuries

- Vitamin C and bioflavonoids. Repair damaged tendons and ligaments with these nutrients, taken in equal amounts (1000 mg each daily).

- Other antioxidants. In addition to vitamin C, take other antioxidant nutrients like E and glutathione—look for an antioxidant formula in one supplement.
- Fruit enzymes. Bromelain, made from the pineapple stem, douses pain and inflammation when taken between meals.
- Digestive enzymes. Take extra amounts of pancreatin (pancreatic enzymes) *between* meals to heal injuries. Note: If you experience stomach upset, cut the amount you're taking down or out.
- Eat to douse inflammation. Saturated fats (in red meat, poultry skin, dairy fat) may be swell, but they also enhance swelling. Avoid these while healing.
- Turn to essential fatty acids. Flax seed oil, fish, nuts and seeds, on the other hand, calm inflammation.
- Spice it up. Ginger and turmeric added liberally to food help combat swelling. (See Herbs below.)
- Extra calcium and magnesium. Load up on these minerals for awhile if muscle spasm is a problem. Include a dose (300 mg/150 mg) before bed with a small snack if you can't sleep.
- Manganese. Between 50 and 100 mg in divided doses for two weeks, followed by a maintenance amount (whatever is in your multiple).

■ *Makeover Hint #103—It's Thyme for a Bath*

Speed healing by immersing your injured body part into a hot bath (or basin) spiked with a tea made from dried thyme or rosemary (use one ounce of herb for every two cups of water). Not only will you feel better faster, but you'll also smell wonderful—lasagna anyone?

Herbal Treatment

- Healing—horsetail, nettles
- Pain—black willow, meadow sweet, tiger balm (see Headaches)
- Swelling—feverfew, ginger, turmeric

The Homeopathic Difference

■ **Makeover Hint #104—Homeopathic Enemies**

Smelly, warming liniments that contain camphor and menthol, like Tiger Balm or eucalyptus, feel glorious on sore, stiff muscles. However, avoid these treatments if you plan to use homeopathic remedies. The two don't mix. In fact, such strong-smelling liniments will undo a remedy.

- Arnica—*First-line "owie" defense.* This remedy is designed for all types of injuries, be they sprains, strains, bruises, pain, swelling, and even shock. Known as a muscular tonic, Arnica should be taken by mouth and/or applied in cream form to the injured area immediately and continually for 24 hours.
- Bellis perennis—*For that deep, deep pain.* This is a remedy when you feel sore and bruised, and the strain you've just acquired is deep.
- Rhus toxicodendron—*The follow-up remedy.* After a day's worth of Arnica, switch to Rhus tox for achy sprains and strains that loosen up and feel better with a little motion.
- Ruta graveolens—*The pain keeps going and going.* For post-injury pain that *doesn't* abate with movement, try Ruta, a popular alternative to Rhus tox.

Lifestyle Link

Immediate first aid attention is imperative after an injury. Follow the RICE procedure for best results.

- R—Rest the limb or body part that's been hurt. This prevents additional injury.
- I—Ice the aching area. This reduces swelling.
- C—Compress the region with an elastic bandage. This calms swelling.
- E—Elevate the injured part above heart level. One more way to diminish fluid accumulation.

Lookout Alert

- Have an X-ray done for severe injuries to rule out fractures.
- Pinpoint pain.
- Swelling and pain that occurs without injury (see Gout).
- Injury with fever or other unusual symptom.

ULCERS

An ulcer is basically an open sore. It can pop up on many parts of the body—skin, mouth, eyelid, genitals—but the ones we're going to address are the peptic kind that infiltrate the digestive tract. The most common types occur in the first part of the small intestine, called the duodenum, and the stomach. These areas are bathed in enzymes and stomach acid, which serve to aggravate the situation when protective mucus thins and the underlying tissue is open to injury. Kind of like putting salt in a wound. Other vulnerable areas are the esophagus and further down the small intestine.

Some ulcers are silent and don't cause problems until something more dramatic develops, like bleeding. Others cause a burning, aching, soreness or gnawing-like pain that's steady and confined to one spot. Some ulcers feel better after eating, drinking milk, or taking antacids. Others might awaken you in the middle of the night with pain. Occasionally the pain disappears on its own, only to return.

No longer do we point a finger at stress as the cause of ulcer, although it does make matters worse. In 1983, gastroenterologist, Barry Marshall, from Royal Perth Hospital in Australia, and his colleague Robin Warren discovered that a bacteria called Helicobacter pylori is most likely behind many ulcers. They estimated that 70 percent of gastric (stomach) ulcers and 90 percent of peptic ulcers[18] were caused by this bug. This infection is easily detected with a simple blood test and the results confirmed by an X-ray or endoscopy. For related conditions see Constipation, Diarrhea, Food Poisoning, Heartburn, and Indigestion. Also scan Chapter 4 (digestion).

How to Prevent Ulcers

If you've had ulcers before, or the digestive tract is your weak point, be cautious about your diet, stress level, and other factors that invite ulcers. See suggestions below.

Food and Nutrition for Ulcers

- Avoid alcohol and caffeine.
- Pass on the spices. Cayenne and other spicy foods can aggravate an active ulcer. However, once an ulcer is healed, hot peppers may actually be preventive.
- Reduce saturated fats. These are found mainly in animal foods, like meat and dairy.
- Reduce acid. Pulverize cardamom, cinnamon, and cloves in a coffee grinder; mix 1 tsp in a cup of hot water, steep for 10 to 15 minutes, strain and sip.
- Eat bananas to speed healing.
- Dine on cabbage too.
- Check out food allergies.
- Eat more fiber.
- Increase essential fatty acids. Do this with flax seed oil (1 tbsp. daily in food) or flax meal.
- Check your multi for vitamins A and E, and zinc. These help with recuperation.

■ *Makeover Hint #105—A Little Cabbage with Your Tomato Juice?*

An old naturopathic cure for ulcers involves two common kitchen ingredients: tomato juice and cabbage or sauerkraut. Try it, you'll like it.

Herbal Treatment

- Antacid—meadow sweet
- Antibacterial—echinacea, golden seal

- Healing—cabbage, calendula, comfrey, licorice
- Relaxing—linden, passion flower, skullcap, valerian
- Soothing—comfrey, marshmallow root, slippery elm

The Homeopathic Difference

- Argenitum nitricum—*Radiating pain.* Ulcers of this kind often begin with a gnawing pain that shoots out to all abdominal parts. Belching and gas are other common signs that fit Argenitum. You might crave sweets (though they only make matters worse), as well as salt and cheese.

- Arsensicum album—*Raw stomach.* The burning, gnawing pain that comes with this ulcer may also be accompanied by vomiting of blood and/or bile. Your stomach is extremely raw and hurts from any food or drink; watch for acid-like belches. Your ulcer feels worse with cold foods like ice cream and drink such as ice water. A milk craving is possible.

- Kali bichromicum—*No more beer.* Although stomach pain stops after eating with this kind of ulcer, it feels like food just sits there. The upper left and right regions of your abdomen feel like stitches are running from there through to the backbone. And even though you yearn for beer, it only makes matters worse with nausea and vomiting.

- Uranium nitricum—*Boring pain.* This unusual remedy is specific for both gastric and duodenal ulcers. Excessive thirst and a ravenous appetite set it apart from other ulcer remedies. Other distinguishing signs to take note of are nausea, vomiting, burning in the stomach and a boring (not tedious) pain in a bloated abdomen.

Lifestyle Link

- Stop smoking.
- Avoid taking aspirin, especially if smoking.
- Eliminate antacids.
- Control stress.

Lookout Alert

- If no relief in three weeks
- Continuous nausea, headache and weakness
- Sweating and dizziness
- Fever
- Vomiting of fresh blood
- Vomiting of a "coffee ground" substance
- Blood in the stools
- Black, tarry stools
- Intense, persistent abdominal pain—especially if it extends beyond this area, for example, to the back
- Sudden, intense, steady pain that begins at the bottom of the breast bone. It might spread quickly, and extend to the right, lower section of the abdomen, and possibly to one or both shoulders. This is a MEDICAL EMERGENCY and suggests that the ulcer has perforated.

URINARY TRACT INFECTIONS (UTI)

Lower urinary tract infections (UTI) are very common, and are usually bacterial in origin. Women are hit with UTIs 10 times as often as men, though symptoms are similar: burning on urination, an urgent need to urinate, frequent urination, and getting up at night. Men with UTIs might notice the end of their penis is red and inflamed. Males 40 and older who notice these symptoms, without the burning or inflamed penis, but also with difficulty in starting and stopping urination and a weak urine stream, might have an enlarged prostate (have the doctor perform a prostate exam). When low back or lower abdominal pain accompany these symptoms, a bladder infection might be present. For conditions with similar symptoms, see Backache and Fatigue. Also refer to Chapter 5 (kidneys).

How to Prevent UTIs

These tips can also be used during UTI treatment.

- Women, wipe yourself from the front to the back. This prevents fecal material from contaminating the urinary tract opening (urethra).
- Urinate after intercourse.
- Drink plenty of filtered or bottled water, one to two quarts daily.
- Keep sugar intake down.
- Drink at least six ounces of unsweetened cranberry juice every day (especially if you're prone to UTIs or bladder infections).
- Do your Kegel exercises (see Makeover Hint #51).

Food and Nutrition for the Urinary Tract

- Cranberry juice. This hastens healing from infection. Drink 16 ounces of unsweetened juice each day until clear—usually two weeks; then decrease amount to six ounces daily.
- Blueberries or blueberry juice. Acts like cranberries, maybe even better.
- Vitamin C, 500–1000 mg every two hours during infection. If you experience bowel intolerance (diarrhea, gas, bloating, cramps) stop for the day, and resume taking C in smaller amounts.
- Eat plenty of garlic and onions. They fight the bugs.
- Beta-carotene (100,000 IU each day during infection), and yellow, orange, and dark green vegetables.
- Zinc it. Use 30 mg each day (total, including what's in your multi) until infection is finished, then resume with maintenance dose (15 mg) or what's in your daily multiple vitamin/mineral pills.
- Add good bugs. Take a probiotic supplement to reestablish the good germs in your system. This is vital if you're currently taking or have taken antibiotics to combat a UTI.
- Yogurt is a probiotic. If you like and can tolerate dairy, eat a cup of plain, culture-rich yogurt a day.
- Bladder irritants. Caffeine, artificial sweeteners, and tomatoes can do this.

Herbal Treatment

- Diuretic—cleavers, dandelion, uva ursi
- Soothing—corn silk, couchgrass, marshmallow leaf
- Infection fighters—echinacea, garlic, golden seal, uva ursi

The Homeopathic Difference

- Aconite—*Hot urine.* Urine is retained in the bladder with this type of UTI. You might feel a spasm in that region and fret about urinating because it's so painful and hot.
- Apis mellifica—*It stings.* Apis is suitable for infections where urination is frequent, and even involuntary. Your urine has a deep color, and it leaves you feeling burned, sore, and stung (like a bee invaded you there).
- Cantharis—*Want to, but can't.* This is homeopathic Spanish fly: the infamous aphrodisiac that excites by irritating both genital and urinary systems. If you have a constant urge to urinate or pain in that area—with little result—try Cantharis. Urine might burn, or be bloody.
- Equisetum—*A full bladder feeling.* If you're experiencing a dull, but intense, pain in the bladder, think of Equisetum. Some find incontinence a problem. Although you need to urinate often, it comes out in drips with extreme pain when done. The bladder feels full all the time—even after urination.

Lifestyle Link

- If you use a diaphragm, consider switching to a different form of birth control, as this type can contribute to UTI and bladder infections in some women.
- Kegel exercises (see Makeover Hint #51).
- No smoking.
- Rest. You need it; you're fighting an infection.

Lookout Alert

- Severe pain, especially higher up the back

- Flank or abdominal pain
- Chills, fever, nausea and/or vomiting (which may indicate a more serious kidney infection)
- Bloody urine
- Men: a whitish mucus-like discharge or pus from the penis
- Get a checkup, if you or your family has a history of kidney disease

VAGINITIS

See Yeast Infections.

VARICOSE VEINS

Unfortunately, varicose veins are usually the bane of women and half of those middle-aged because their veins are quite frail and, when the vein wall is hurt, it can balloon. In cases where the valves that control blood flow in the veins are injured, varicose veins result as blood pools. At first, there's a slight swelling or bulging where the vein is affected, but no visible vessel. That may be all, with no symptoms to speak of. Or you might feel more tired with achy, hot, tight legs, and the skin over the veins may swell and turn purple and red. Worst-case scenario—skin ulcers develop. They usually appear on the calves and along the inner leg, top and bottom. Also see Constipation, Fatigue, Hemorrhoids; refer to Chapters 3 (liver), 4 (digestion) and 9 (muscles).

How to Prevent Varicose Veins

Like a garden hose, your veins weaken with time. This, combined with increased pressure inside your veins, is what creates varicose veins. Obviously, the weaker your veins (caused, for example, by aging) and the more pressure exerted inside the veins, the greater the chance of trouble.

- Choose the right family. Varicose veins runs in families.
- Sit down. Excessive standing increases vein pressure—especially when accompanied by carrying heavy loads. So sit down and give your legs a rest.

- Exercise too. Sedentary lifestyle increases your chances of varicosities. So strike a balance between activity and rest.
- Be cautious about lifting. Increased vein pressure again.
- Support hose. Those elastic, tight fitting stockings or socks can ease tired legs. Fashionable too.
- Weight control. Obesity is another major risk factor.
- Toned muscles. As we age, muscle and vein tone drop. Biking, swimming, and walking keep your muscles (and veins) in shape, and push pooled blood back into circulation (see Chapter 9).

Food and Nutrition for Legs

- Roughage roundup. As for many conditions, a high-fiber diet is the most important step to prevent and treat varicose veins. The reason is that straining due to constipation increases the pressure inside your leg's veins. High-fiber foods, like vegetables and legumes, are also nutritional powerhouses.
- Berry up! All those wonderful red, blue, and purple berries you love—blackberries, blueberries, cherries—are full of vein-building flavonoids. Eating them helps treat and prevent varicose veins.
- Fill up on fish and other good fats too, like flaxseed oil, nuts and seeds.
- Keep that blood flowing and those veins healthy. This means cutting down on saturated animal fats, sugar, salt, alcohol, and refined carbohydrate foods.
- Vitamins and minerals. A good multiple containing vitamins A, B-complex, and E as well as zinc help nourish varicose-ridden legs.
- Vitamin C and collagen. This nutrient heals tissue like collagen in doses ranging from 500 mg to 3000 mg daily in divided doses; an equal amount of bioflavonoids helps too.

Herbal Treatment

- Bulk up—flax seed, oat bran or meal, psyllium seed
- Diuretics—hawthorn, horse tail, stone root

- Enhance blood flow—ginkgo, gotu kola
- Strengthen veins—gotu kola, hawthorn, horse chestnut
- Curb swelling (see Diuretics)—Butcher's broom, horse chestnut

■ *Makeover Hint #106—Topical Relief*

To ease aching legs, apply a cream, lotion, or ointment with these herbs: Butcher's broom, calendula, horse chestnut, and witch hazel.

The Homeopathic Difference

- Calcarea fluorica—*Start here.* Calcarea fluorica is considered *the* remedy for varicose veins, especially when vessels are bulging. To make sure this is for you, ask yourself this. Do your legs feel worse during rest and better with warmth? If so, Calcarea is a good fit.
- Hamamelis virginica—*Homeopathic witch hazel.* Here's a case where both the herb and its homeopathic cousin help the same condition. Hamamelis is homeopathic witch hazel, and is particularly good when legs feel tired, and muscles and joints are sore. Sometimes there's a chilliness too, that begins in the back or hips and travels down the legs.
- Pulsatilla—*Heavy and weary.* Another remedy for varicose veins is Pulsatilla, especially when they're restless, cold, and feel tired, in a heavy sort of way.
- Zincum—*Can't sit still.* Zincum works well for large varicose veins of the legs that feel weak, tremble, and twitch. You might find your soles are sensitive too. But most important, you're constantly moving your feet and legs. For women, menstruation makes it worse.

Lifestyle Link

- Menstrual period. For women, varicose veins can be worse during this time, so take extra care.
- Support hose. They ease tired, aching legs.

- Put your feet up. This gives varicose veins a rest.
- Get a leg massage. Rubbing your legs with fragrant almond oil is soothing and helps circulation. Add a little vitamin E oil if you like.

Lookout Alert

Superficial varicose veins are generally harmless, though unsightly. It's when the deep veins are affected that potential problems occur—like blood clots in the lungs (pulmonary embolism), heart attack, and stroke. Watch for these signs:

- Painful skin ulcers or sores in the area of varicose veins
- Fever
- Reddish-brown veins

YEAST INFECTIONS

While they are normal residents in our bodies, when yeast grow beyond normal limits, an infection occurs. The most commonly known yeast infection happens in the genital area, especially among women. Itching and irritation, as well as a cheesy, white discharge are signs yeast has invaded. Men are often symptom-less, though genital irritation may be a complaint. Antibiotics, birth control pills, cortisone medication, pregnancy, and diabetes all contribute to this problem.

Another frequent, though less admitted, area prone to yeast infection is the gastrointestinal tract. Like genital yeast, increasing antibiotic use has made yeast infection an up-and-coming disease. The reason for this is simple. Normally, there is a happy existence between the bacteria and yeast that live in both the genital and digestive tracts. The job of antibiotics is to kill disease-causing bacteria. However, their action is not well directed and the "good" bacteria in our bodies that help keep yeast populations in check are also destroyed. The result is more room for yeast to grow and create an infection. In fact, it is not uncommon for patients taking antibiotics chronically to also be prescribed anti-yeast medicine. *Candida albicans* is one of the most common yeast found in infections, though others appear too.

Yeast infections spring up in other areas as well, such as the throat, skin, and less commonly, the bloodstream. Many of the treatments below are also used for GI yeast. Using this approach for vaginal yeast is more effective and will help prevent recurrence. For related topics see Constipation, Diarrhea, Eczema, Headaches, Indigestion, Low Blood Sugar, and Psoriasis; read Chapters 4 (digestion) and 6 (immunity).

How to Prevent Yeast (and its Recurrence)

- Avoid antibiotics unless absolutely necessary.
- Find alternatives to birth control pills, for example, natural family planning. (Read Toni Weschler's very comprehensive work, *Taking Charge of Your Fertility*, for more information.)
- Limit use of steroid hormone medication. For example, cortisone creams, prednisone.
- Find substitutes for ulcer medicines.
- Tame your sweet tooth. Lots of sugar over time can contribute to this problem.
- Get tested. Ask your doctor to run a stool culture for *Candida* and other yeast. Some women with vaginal yeast also have it in their GI tracts.

Food and Nutrition for Yeast

I'm giving you tips not only for fighting vaginal yeast, but intestinal yeast as well because sometimes both infections are present. I typically tell patients to initially avoid sugary foods, refined carbohydrates, and alcohol. If this doesn't work, follow a stricter diet as outlined below. Once the problem has cleared up, you can reintroduce some of these foods, but try to stick with a wholesome menu to prevent future troubles.

- Avoid sugars and foods high in them. This means table sugar, fructose, corn syrup. These are yeast's favorite foods.
- Eliminate refined carbohydrates. These are foods with white flour and refined grains.
- Don't drink. Liquor makes you sicker quicker.

- If the above three tips don't help, also stop eating milk (it contains lactose or milk sugar), starchy foods (potatoes), and fruits (berries, cherries, apples, and pears are OK).

- Take acidophilus and other probiotics. They contain the good bacteria you want.

- Douche with yogurt. Or insert an acidophilus capsule vaginally.

- Eat garlic.

- Nutrients to include (look to your multi first): Vitamins A, B complex, C and E, bioflavonoids.

- Topical E. Vitamin E oil or cream may relieve itching.

- Is it a yeast allergy? Many yeast diets recommend avoiding all foods with a high amount of yeast or fungi and mold like peanuts, cheese, dried fruit, bread, baked goods, vinegar, grapes, mushrooms, and alcohol. However, this may only be necessary if you have a sensitivity to yeast. Try eliminating these foods for one week, then reintroduce them one at a time. If you get worse, then yeast or mold may be at fault.

- Avoid other allergenic foods.

- There's nothing to eat! Feel free to munch on all vegetables (here's your chance to reach your goal of seven a day), beans and legumes, fish, poultry, lean meats and whole grains (wheat, barley, oats, rice, rye, etc.).

- Go organic. This is especially important for poultry, meats, and dairy, to avoid additional antibiotic exposure.

■ *Makeover Hint #107—The Italian Dressing Douche*

There are two ways to kill yeast. One, make their environment acidic; two, put a killer in their midst. Using common kitchen ingredients, you can make a vaginal douche with 2 tbsp. apple cider vinegar (the acid) and crushed garlic or liquid garlic (the yeast killer) mixed in one quart of water. The only side effect is smelling like a Caesar salad.

Herbal Treatment

These herbs are best used in a vaginal douche; however, the "yeast slayers" can also be taken orally.

- Yeast slayers—black walnut, calendula, echinacea, garlic, golden seal, pau d'arco, St. John's wort, tea tree
- Healing—calendula, comfrey
- Reduce redness—calendula, licorice
- Soothing—comfrey, self-heal

The Homeopathic Difference

- Natrum phosphoricum—*After antibiotics*. A creamy or honey-colored and sour-smelling discharge is apparent with this type of infection; sometimes it's watery. This (like Pulsatilla and Thuja) is a good remedy for yeast infections caused by antibiotic use.
- Pulsatilla—*Backache too*. A creamy white discharge that burns sets Pulsatilla apart from other yeast remedies. You may feel cold, tired, and have a backache.
- Sepia—*Bearing down sensation*. This remedy works for yellow or green discharge with plenty of itching. The vagina is very sore, particularly after intercourse. And there is a strange feeling as if the pelvis is being pulled down toward the vagina.
- Thuja—*Very sensitive*. Signs to look for when considering Thuja are a profuse, thick, white discharge (could be greenish too) and a very sensitive vagina. Symptoms increase at night while in bed and after drinking coffee or eating fatty foods.

Lifestyle Link

- Part of the relationship. If you have a genital yeast infection, have your partner checked and treated if indicated. Use condoms until both of your infections have cleared up.
- Avoid intercourse if possible. Besides decreasing chances of re-infection, this allows red, inflamed tissues to heal properly.
- Wear cotton underpants.

- Sit in a warm bath laced with Epsom salts (one cup).
- Wet basement syndrome. If moist places like damp basements make you feel worse, you may have a mold sensitivity. See above for yeast-containing foods to avoid while getting well.
- Other signs of yeast? Have your doctor check other areas, like the digestive tract, for a yeast infection.

Lookout Alert

The most serious form of yeast infection is systemic or body-wide. Usually this type of condition takes a long time to develop, and is more apt to appear in persons with limited reserves, for instance after radiation treatment, after using corticosteroids or immuno-suppressive medications, in people with diabetes, emphysema, tuberculosis, some types of cancer, severe burns, and AIDS. Also be aware of these circumstances:

- Foreign travel.
- Fever, chills, night sweats, loss of appetite, weight loss, malaise, and depression.
- Usual yeast symptoms don't respond to standard therapy.
- Symptoms are severe.

Appendix A

Over One Hundred Common Herbs and How to Use Them

Before using any of the herbs listed in this book, please read this section. Be a wise herbal consumer by following these steps:

- Know what you're taking. Before you take any herb, educate yourself about its actions on the body, and what it's usually used for.

- Know if there's any reason why you shouldn't take a certain herb. Since some herbs shouldn't be taken in particular situations, watch out for herbs that are contraindicated (shouldn't be taken):

    1. With some medications.
    2. If you have a particular health condition.
    3. If you have a history of a particular health condition.
    4. If you're pregnant. *As a precaution, never take any herbs unless prescribed by your midwife or obstetrician.*
    5. If you're nursing. *Most substances you ingest are passed along to your baby through breast milk.*

- Know why you're taking an herb. Don't take them just because. Whenever you take an herb in moderate to large amounts over a period of time, understand its actions and why it is indicated for your particular condition.

- Know the quality of the herbal products you're taking. Herbs are plants. As such, their potency changes according to when and where they're grown, when they're harvested, how they're prepared, and how long they're been sitting on the shelf. Quiz your herbal vendor or call the herbal company directly with questions. Last, ask others what products work best and try them for yourself.

Herbal Preparation and Usage

Herbs come in a variety of forms—teas, tinctures or alcohol preparations, pills and others. For our purposes here, I'll describe how to prepare herbal tea. As a general rule, if you're taking a tincture 1/4 to 1 teaspoon three times per day should suffice. Many pill products have directions written on the bottle. For more information on exact dosing, refer to the following works:

The Complete Illustrated Holistic Herbal by David Hoffmann, Element Books, 1996.

Herbal Prescriptions for Better Health by Donald J. Brown, ND, Prima, 1996.

The Healing Power of Herbs by Michael T. Murray, ND, Prima, 1995.

A Field Guide to Medicinal Plants by Steven Foster & James A Duke, Ph.D., Houghton Mifflin Co., 1990.

The Green Pharmacy by James A. Duke, Ph.D., Rodale Press, 1997.

TEAS   If you ever drank a cup of herbal tea, you know how to make the medicinal version as well. There are two basic methods to preparing herbal teas. The first is called an infusion and is very much like making a cup of ordinary tea. Place the dried herb or tea bag in a mug, pour boiling water over it, cover with a small plate or plastic lid and let infuse (steep) for 10 to 15 minutes. This method works best when preparing soft parts of a plant such as the leaf or flower petals.

Decocting is the other way to create medicinal tea. This method is reserved for the hard parts of a plant, like the root, rhizome, nuts, seeds, bark, and stem. After all, it takes more time and heat to extract the healing qualities from these woody sections. To make a decoction simply place water and allocated herb in a pot. Slowly bring it to a boil, cover and let simmer for 15 to 30 minutes.

For those too busy or impatient to watch a simmering pot, or when you need to prepare a combination of soft and hard herbal parts, use the thermos method of decocting. Begin by powdering your herbs (both hard and soft portions) in a blender or coffee grinder. Place powder in a thermos, add boiling water and cap. Leave the mixture for 40 minutes. Strain the tea before drinking.

HOW MUCH, HOW OFTEN   As with tinctures, how much tea you take can vary according to what herb or herbs you choose. Again, here I offer general guidelines. If you experience any adverse reaction after taking an herb, stop immediately or consult with a professional trained in this area.

As a general rule, add 1 tbsp. of herb to 1 cup of water to make medicinal herbal tea; most tea bags contain 2 tsp. of dried herb. If you're treating yourself for an acute, short-term illness like a cold, drink one cup of tea every one to three hours. Do this for five to 10 days. If you need to repeat this cycle, take two to three days off, and start again.

For more chronic conditions like arthritis, or as a preventive measure, drink one cup of tea three times per day. Continue this trend for eight weeks, then take a two-week rest.

Be imaginative with your teas. Many can also be used in other ways. After preparing your tea using the above guidelines, try the following: add tea to a bath (two cups to a tub of water or sitz bath); as a douche for a vaginal infection; as a mouthwash for a gum condition or gargle for a sore throat; as a wash for a skin problem. Remember to adjust the temperature of the tea accordingly and don't burn yourself.

Herbal Glossary

Listed below are all the herbs mentioned in this book. They are presented in alphabetical order by common name; the scientific name follows in parentheses. For your information, I describe how each herb works. As a safety precaution, I also list situations where specific herbs should *not* be used.

Aconite (*Aconitum napellus*). Painkiller, sedative, decreases fevers. NOTE: THIS IS A VERY POISONOUS HERB; DO NOT TAKE BY MOUTH EXCEPT UNDER THE GUIDANCE OF A TRAINED PROFESSIONAL. This herb is often in ear drop medication, and can be safely used by consumers.

Agrimony (*Agrimonia eupatoria*). Heals wounds, helps the liver, promotes bile flow, diuretic, astringent, tonic.

Alfalfa (*Medicago sativa*). Stops bleeding, diuretic, estrogen-like, nutritious. NOTE: Avoid during pregnancy.

Aloe (*Aloe vera*). Heals wounds (internally and externally), soothing (external), enhances menstrual flow, helps the liver, kills worms, cathartic. NOTE: Avoid during pregnancy and during breast feeding; do not give to children internally.

American Cranesbill (*Geranium maculatum*). Astringent, stops bleeding (internally and externally), anti-inflammatory, heals wounds.

Angelica (*Angelica archangelica*). Controls gas, stimulates appetite, expectorant for coughs, eases spasms, induces perspiration. NOTE: Do not take large amounts without professional guidance.

Astragalus (*Astragalus membranaceus*). Antiviral activity, enhances immunity.

Balmony (*chelone glabra*). Helps the liver, promotes bile flow, mild laxative, general tonic for digestion, controls nausea and vomiting.

Barberry (*Berberis vulgaris*). Helps the liver, promotes bile flow, laxative, controls nausea and vomiting, bitter. NOTE: Avoid during pregnancy.

Bayberry (*Myrica cerifera*). Astringent, induces perspiration. NOTE: Large amounts may cause gas or nausea and vomiting.

Bilberry (*Vaccinium myrtillus*). Astringent, antiseptic, blood sugar lowering action, may improve vision (cataracts, macular degeneration, glaucoma), strengthens blood vessels.

Bitter Melon (*Momordica charantia*). Blood sugar lowering action.

Black Catechu (*Acacia catechu*). Astringent, antiseptic.

Black Walnut (*Juglans nigra*). Cathartic.

Black Willow (*Salix nigra*). Painkiller, lowers fever, anti-inflammatory, heals wounds, astringent.

Blue Flag (*Iris versicolor*). Helps the liver, promotes bile flow, laxative, diuretic, anti-inflammatory, promotes salivation. NOTE: Large amounts might cause nausea, vomiting, or facial neuralgias. Picking this plant might cause a rash.

Boneset (*Eupatorium perfoliatum*). Induces perspiration, clears respiratory mucus, eases spasms, bitter, diuretic.

Borage (*Borago officinalis*). Revives adrenal glands, anti-inflammatory, diuretic, induces perspiration, expectorant for coughs, stimulates breast milk.

Burdock (*Arctium lappa*). Bitter, laxative, diuretic, restores general health, heals wounds.

Butcher's Broom (*Ruscus aculeatus*). Lowers fevers, diuretic, constricts blood vessels. NOTE: Avoid if you have high blood pressure.

Cabbage (*Brassica spp*). Heals intestinal ulcers.

Calendula (*Calendula officinalis*). Heals wounds (externally and internally), anti-inflammatory, kills germs, astringent, promotes bile flow, brings on menstruation.

Cascara (*Cascara sagrada*). Laxative, purgative, appetite stimulant.

Catnip (*Nepeta cataria*). Controls gas, sedative, eases spasms, induces perspiration, astringent.

Cayenne (*Capsicum annum*). Kills germs, controls gas, promotes salivation, reduces respiratory mucus, controls nausea and vomiting, induces perspiration, reduces cholesterol and triglycerides, painkiller (externally in creams). NOTE: Do not apply cayenne cream to irritated or broken skin.

Celery Seed (*Apium graveolens*). Diuretic, controls gas, sedative.

Chamomile (*Chamaemelum nobile or Matricaria recutita*). Eases spasms, controls gas, anti-inflammatory, painkiller, heals wounds, sedative, induces perspiration.

Chickweed (*Stellaria media*). Heals wounds; soothing (externally) for wounds, itching, irritation, and arthritic joints.

Cleavers (*Galium aparine*). Diuretic, astringent, anti-inflammatory, helps the liver, laxative, heals wounds.

Coltsfoot (*Tussilago farfara*). Expectorant, controls coughs, soothing, tones the lungs, reduces respiratory mucus, anti-inflammatory, diuretic.

Comfrey (*Symphytum officinale*). Heals wounds (externally), soothing, astringent, expectorant. NOTE: Don't apply comfrey to very deep wounds as this can cause wound to heal over too quickly.

Corn Silk (*Zea mays*). Diuretic, soothing, prevents kidney stones.

Couchgrass (*Agropyron repens*). Diuretic, kills germs, soothing, prevents kidney stones.

Daisy (*Bellis perennis*). Heals wounds, expectorant, astringent.

Dandelion (*Taraxacum officinale*). Helps the liver, promotes bile flow, diuretic, laxative.

Devil's Claw (*Harpogophytum procumbens*). Anti-inflammatory, painkiller

Echinacea (*Echinacea spp*). Enhances immunity, kills germs.

Elder (*Sambucus nigra*). Induces perspiration (flowers, berries), diuretic (whole plant), laxative (berries), expectorant (leaves), heals wounds and soothing (externally—leaves). NOTE: Actions depend on part of plant used.

Elecampane (*Inula helenium*). Controls coughs, expectorant, induces perspiration, kills germs, controls respiratory mucus, helps the liver, heals wounds, bitter.

Ephedra (*Ephedra sinica*). Fights allergies, stimulates blood circulation, increases blood pressure, promotes weight loss, stimulating. NOTE: Due to its stimulating qualities, ephedra can cause anxiety, insomnia, irritability in susceptible people. Avoid taking if you are pregnant, have high blood pressure, heart disease, diabetes, thyroid troubles, trouble urinating due to an enlarged prostate, or if you take antidepressant or blood pressure medication.

Eyebright (*Euphrasia officinalis*). Eye conditions, astringent, anti-inflammatory, controls respiratory mucus, heals wounds.

Fenugreek (*Trigonella foenum-graecum*). Heals wounds, soothing, controls gas, expectorant, promotes milk production, promotes menstruation.

Feverfew (*Tanacetum parthenium*). Dilates blood vessels, anti-inflammatory, relaxing, bitter, stimulates uterus. NOTE: Avoid during pregnancy.

Figwort (*Scrophularia nodosa*). Restores health, diuretic, heart stimulant, laxative, heals wounds, blood sugar-lowering action. NOTE: Use only under professional supervision.

Flax (*Linum usitatissimum*). Laxative, soothing, controls coughs, heals wounds. NOTE: Flax seed oil can cause gas.

Garlic (*Allium sativum*). Kills germs, enhances immunity, lowers blood pressure, protects heart and blood vessels, anti-inflammatory, diuretic, blood sugar-lowering action, expectorant, promotes menstruation, controls gas.

Gentian (*Gentiana lutea*). Bitter, promotes salivation, promotes bile flow, gastrointestinal tonic, kills germs, helps the liver, promotes menstruation.

Ginger (*Zingiber officinale*). Controls gas, promotes salivation, enhances perspiration, anti-inflammatory, controls nausea and vomiting, decreases cholesterol, kills germs, anti-ulcer, painkiller.

Ginkgo (*Ginkgo biloba*). Helps the brain, nervous system, and blood vessels.

Ginseng (*Panax ginseng* or *Eleutherococcus senticosus*). These are actually two different species. *Panax:* Fights fatigue, anti-stress, blood sugar-lowering action, enhances immunity, helps the liver. *Eleuthero:* Supports and enhances adrenal function and immunity. NOTE: Avoid during pregnancy. Can cause a stimulant effect in some people; avoid taking late in the day. Women do better with Eleuthero.

Goat's Rue (*Galega officinalis*). Blood sugar-lowering action, induces perspiration, diuretic, promotes milk production.

Golden Seal (*Hydrastis canadensis*). Enhances immunity, kills germs, lowers fevers, bitter, laxative, astringent, promotes bile flow, helps the liver, heals wounds, promotes menstruation, expectorant. NOTE: Avoid during pregnancy.

Gotu Kola (*Centella asiatica*). Heals wounds (externally and internally), aids hair and nail growth, reduces cellulite, helps the liver, increases mental abilities, improves vein health.

Greater Plantain (*Plantago major*). Heals wounds, soothing, astringent, diuretic, expectorant.

Grindelia (*Grindelia camporum*). Eases spasms, expectorant, lowers blood pressure.

Gymnema (*Gymnema sylvestre*). Blood sugar-lowering actions (in diabetics), reduces sweet taste (when applied directly to tongue).

Hawthorn (*Crataegus laevigata* or *Crataegus oxycantha*). Heart tonic, lowers blood pressure, diuretic.

Hops (*Humulus lupulus*). Sedative, bitter, painkiller, astringent. NOTE: Avoid in cases of chronic or severe depression.

Horse Chestnut (*Aesculus hippocastanum*). Tones blood vessels, astringent—externally or internally. NOTE: USE HERB EXTERNALLY ONLY; TAKE INTERNALLY ONLY UNDER PROFESSIONAL SUPERVISION AS SEED IS POTENTIALLY POISONOUS.

Horsetail (*Equisetum arvense*). Heals wounds (externally), astringent, diuretic.

Hyssop (*Hyssopus officinalis*). Expectorant, eases spasms, induces perspiration, sedative, controls gas, heals wounds, helps the liver, controls respiratory mucus.

Jamaican Dogwood (*Piscidia piscipula*). Painkiller, sedative. NOTE: Do not take large amounts.

Lady's Slipper (*Cypripedium calceolus*). Sedative, painkiller, eases spasms. NOTE: Large doses can cause hallucinations.

Licorice (*Glycyrrhiza glabra*). Anti-inflammatory, aids adrenal glands, stimulates immunity, kills germs, helps the liver, estrogen-like action, anti-allergy, soothing, mild laxative, eases spasms, expectorant. Often used as a flavoring with other herbs. NOTE: Do not take for more than six weeks unless under care of professional. Avoid if you have high blood pressure, kidney problems, or take digitalis.

Linden or Lime Blossom (*Tilia x vulgaris*). Sedative, eases spasms, aids circulation, induces perspiration, diuretic.

Marshmallow (*Althea officinalis*). Root: soothing, heals wounds, diuretic; use this part of the marshmallow plant for the gastrointestinal tract. Leaf: soothing, diuretic, expectorant, reduces respiratory mucus; use this part of the marshmallow plant for all other ailments.

Meadow Sweet (*Filipendula ulmaria*). Painkiller, lowers fevers, controls nausea and vomiting, anti-inflammatory, astringent, anti-rheumatic.

Milk Thistle (*Silybum marianum*). Helps/protects the liver, promotes bile flow, promotes milk production, soothing.

Mouse Ear (*Pilosella officinarum*). Heals wounds (externally), eases spasms, expectorant, reduces respiratory mucus, astringent.

Mullein (*Verbascum thapsus*). Expectorant, reduces respiratory mucus, soothing, tones the lungs, diuretic, sedative, heals wounds (externally).

Nettles or Stinging Nettles (*Urtica dioca*). Anti-allergy, astringent, diuretic, nutritious. NOTE: Touching the fresh plant can cause a rash.

Oats (*Avena sativa*). Supports the nervous system, soothing, heals wounds (external and internal), nutritious.

Oregon Grape (*Mahonia aquifolium*). Helps the liver, promotes bile flow, laxative, controls nausea and vomiting; used for skin conditions.

Osha root (*Ligusticum porteri*). Enhances immunity, kills germs.

Pasque Flower (*Pulsatilla vulgaris*). Sedative, painkiller, eases spasms, kills germs, promotes menstruation. NOTE: DO NOT USE THE FRESH PLANT.

Passion Flower (*Passiflora incarnata*). Sedative, sleeping aid, eases spasms, painkiller.

Pau D'Arco or Tahebo (*Tabebuia avellandae*). Anti-cancer (shrinks tumors and reduces pain).

Pennyroyal (*Mentha pulegium*). Promotes menstruation, controls gas, eases spasms. NOTE: Avoid during pregnancy or if you have kidney problems.

Peppermint (*Mentha piperita*). Controls gas, supports nervous system, eases spasms, controls nausea and vomiting, painkiller, kills germs. NOTE: Avoid peppermint oil internally during pregnancy or with children.

Pleurisy Root (*Asclepias tuberosa*). Expectorant, eases spasms, induces perspiration, controls gas. NOTE: Very large amounts can cause vomiting and diarrhea.

Psyllium (*Plantago psyllium*). Laxative, soothing.

Red Clover (*Trifolium pratense*). Skin conditions, expectorant, eases spasms, heals wounds, anti-cancer, sedative.

Rhubarb Root (*Rheum palmatum*). Laxative, bitter, astringent. NOTE: Taking this herb can make your urine appear yellow or red. Do not take if you have kidney stones.

Rosemary (*Rosmarinus officinalis*). Controls gas, eases spasms, anti-depressant, kills germs, astringent, supports nervous system, diuretic, promotes bile flow, repels insects (oil—externally). NOTE: Don't take oil internally. Avoid during pregnancy.

Rue (*Ruta graveolens*). Promotes menstruation, eases spasms, controls coughs, kills germs, bitter. NOTE: Avoid during pregnancy. Do not take oil internally. Do not take large amounts unless under professional supervision.

Sage (*Salvia officinalis*). Controls gas, anti-inflammatory, kills germs, astringent, promotes menstruation, reduces perspiration, decreases milk production. NOTE: Avoid during pregnancy.

Sarsaparilla (*Smilax sarsaparilla*). Promotes health, anti-gout, anti-rheumatic, "blood cleanser."

Senega (*Polygala senega*). Expectorant, induces perspiration, promotes salivation.

Senna (*Senna alexandrina*). Laxative.

Skullcap (*Scutellaria laterifolia*). Sedative, eases spasms, painkiller.

Slippery Elm (*Ulmus rubra*). Soothing, astringent, heals wounds (externally), nutritious.

St. John's Wort (*Hypericum perforatum*). Painkiller, antidepressant, sedative, anti-viral; externally—heals wounds, anti-inflammatory. NOTE: Makes susceptible people more sensitive to strong sunlight and tanning booths.

Stone Root (*Collinsonia canadensis*). Prevents kidney stones, diuretic, induces perspiration. Used for hemorrhoids in Europe where it's referred to as Pilewort.

Sumac (*Rhus aromatica*). Astringent.

Sundew (*Drosera rotundifolia*). Soothing, expectorant, eases spasms.

Tea Tree (*Melaleuca alternifolia*). Oil used externally: as a liniment, kills germs, repels insects. Tea taken internally: controls gas, eases spasms, expectorant. NOTE: Do not take the oil by mouth.

Thuja (*Thuja occidentalis*). Expectorant, astringent, diuretic, induces perspiration; kills worms, kills warts (externally). NOTE: Avoid during pregnancy. Do not take the oil by mouth.

Thyme (*Thymus vulgaris*). Controls gas, kills germs, astringent, controls respiratory mucus, induces perspiration; heals wounds (externally). NOTE: Do not take the oil by mouth.

Tormentil (*Potentilla erecta*). Astringent; heals wounds (externally). NOTE: THIS IS A STRONG HERB. USE CAUTIOUSLY BOTH INTERNALLY AND EXTERNALLY. DO NOT TAKE LARGE AMOUNTS FOR EXTENDED PERIODS OF TIME UNLESS UNDER PROFESSIONAL SUPERVISION.

Turmeric (*Curcuma longa*). Anti-inflammatory, helps the liver, kills germs, controls gas, supports the GI tract, lowers cholesterol. NOTE: At very high doses, can causes gastric ulcers.

Uva Ursi or Bearberry (*Arctostaphylos uva ursi*). Diuretic, astringent, soothing, prevents kidney stones, kills germs. NOTE: If used for extended periods, can cause constipation.

Valerian (*Valeriana officinalis*). Sedative, eases spasms, lowers blood pressure, controls gas, sleeping aid.

Vervain (*Verbena officinalis*). Sedative, eases spasms, painkiller, induces perspiration, expectorant, helps the liver; heals wounds (externally).

White Horehound (*Marrubium vulgare*). Expectorant, eases spasms, bitter, induces perspiration; heals wounds (externally).

Wild Indigo (*Baptisia tinctoria*). Kills germs, reduces fevers, reduces respiratory mucus, improves general health.

Witch Hazel (*Hamamelis virginiana*). Astringent, anti-inflammatory; heals wounds (externally).

Yarrow (*Achillea millefolium*). Induces perspiration, lowers blood pressure, diuretic, kills germs, astringent, stimulates digestion, supports blood vessels, helps the liver. NOTE: Large amounts can cause headaches and dizziness.

Yellow Dock (*Rumex crispus*). Laxative, helps the liver, promotes bile flow, astringent. NOTE: Large amounts can cause nausea.

Appendix B

Sixty Common Homeopathic Remedies and How to Use Them

This 200-year-old therapy has regained considerable popularity in the last 20 years due to its safety and effectiveness. Homeopathic remedies—of which there exist over 2000—are minute amounts of plant, mineral, or animal substances used to cure a wide variety of ailments. Remedies are diluted so few or no side effects occur. In fact, the more dilute a remedy, the more potent it is. It's believed that the vigorous shaking (called succussions) used to prepare these medicines help potentize them.

It's the principles of homeopathy that separate it from conventional medicine. One principle says "like cures like," meaning the compound used to treat a disease produces symptoms of that disease when given to a healthy person but cures that disease when given to an ill person. For example, *Coffea cruda* (homeopathic coffee) is ideal when used for restless insomnia.

In classical homeopathy, the law of the single remedy says medicines should be given one at a time based on current symptoms. Because the patient and the disease are each seen as ever-changing, the remedy is adjusted as symptoms change. Individual treatment requires careful documentation of physical symptoms, emotional and mental balance, food cravings and aversions, sleeping habits and other signs. These symptoms are then matched to one remedy at an appropriate dose.

Over-the-Counter Homeopathy

Most homeopathic remedies are used and sold for acute, short-term illnesses. Some practitioners call this acute homeopathic prescribing, versus constitutional homeopathy which requires an in-depth interview and expert diagnosis by a homeopathic practition-er. The second difference between acute and constitutional care is that acute remedies are typically used in lower potencies and are taken more frequently. Using the former is much simpler than the latter, and with a little practice, a homeopathic remedy kit or local health food store that carries these remedies, and a handy reference guide (see below), you'll be set.

Now that you're ready, be prepared to look at illness in a whole different way. With most over-the-counter medicines, you take the same pill for a particular illness, no matter what the quali-ty of the ailment. However, if you stop and think about it, no two colds, for example, are exactly the same. For instance, one time you might feel drowsy and dull and your eyelids droopy. Your nose is running with a watery discharge and you don't feel thirsty. Gelsemium would be a good choice here. Next cold might involve burning eyes, nose, and lips, along with profuse, searing, clear dis-charge, and thirst. Allium cepa is a better selection for this cold. So your job when picking a homeopathic remedy is to watch your symptoms: what do they feel like, when do they occur, where do they occur, how intense are they, what makes them better or worse, do they change with time of day, do your feelings or thinking abil-ity change, what is the quality of the symptom (is the pain stabbing or dull; is the discharge clear or green). As you become more famil-iar with homeopathy, you'll know what to look for. Ideally as symp-toms change, you'll pick a new and more appropriate remedy.

For an acute illness or injury, take three to five pills (or drops, if liquid) *under* your tongue. Let the substance dissolve for at least 30 seconds. You can take a remedy as often as every 15 minutes for an immediate problem, or three times a day for an ongoing condi-tion like a cold. Here are some other peculiarities of homeopathic remedies:

- Take 15 minutes away from food or drink.
- Do not take the remedy with anything else. For example, don't swallow pills with water or juice.
- *Avoid coffee and coffee products while taking a homeopathic remedy; they seem to erase the effects of this medicine. Black and herbal teas are fine.

- *Also steer clear of strong smells such as tea tree oil, eucalyptus, camphor (found in lip chaps, tiger balm, Vick's Vapor Rub™, liniments, cough drops, Noxema™, some cosmetics, some nail polish removers, some facial cleansers) Read labels. Also avoid mint products; read your toothpaste label. For alternatives to these products, visit the health food store.

- Avoid electric blankets. Water bed heaters are OK.

- Don't touch the remedy with your hands, mouth, or tongue. If you spill some, don't put it back in the bottle. (The best way to take a remedy is to pour a small amount on a clean spoon first.)

- Keep your open remedy container away from strong odors. Besides the above, this includes perfumes, cooking smells, and fresh paint.

- Store in a cool, dark place, but not the fridge.

* These steps are vital when taking constitutional remedies, but not as necessary for acute remedies. However, the more you follow these guidelines, the better your remedy will work.

For more detailed information on this fascinating field, refer to the following books:

Homeopathic Self-Care by Robert Ullman, ND & Judyth Reichenberg-Ullman, ND, Prima, 1997.

Everybody's Guide to Homeopathic Medicines by Stephen Cummings & Dana Ullman, Jeremy Tarcher, 1984.

Homeopathic Medicine at Home by Maesimund B Panos, MD & Jane Heimlich, JP Tacher, 1980.

Homeopathy: Medicine of the New Man by George Vithoulkas.

Homeopathic Glossary

Listed on the following pages are all the homeopathic remedies mentioned in this book. They are laid out in alphabetical order by name. Included by each are some of the keynote or peculiar symptoms that apply to that remedy; use these to make your selection.

Aconite or Aconitum napellus. This remedy is good for the first 24 hours of an illness. Symptoms come on suddenly. You might feel restless and anxious. Fear or shock might be the cause of your illness. Heat is key: hot feeling in the head, nasal discharge that's hot, fever, burning skin; thirst for cold beverages. Rest makes you better; cold makes you worse.

Aesculus hippocastanum. There's a feeling of fullness, especially in the lower bowel. The result can be hemorrhoids and backaches. Cool open air makes you better; walking makes you worse.

Allium cepa. This remedy is derived from the red onion, hence the profuse tearing, red burning eyes, clear, irritating nasal discharge, and frequent sneezing; also thirst. Not surprisingly you crave raw onions. Cool open air makes you better; worse in the evening and indoors.

Alumina. Skin and mucous membranes are dry. Bodily functions are sluggish and there's a general debility apparent. Spirits are low, though mood varies. Worse when you wake in the morning; better in the evening.

Antimonium tartaricum. Used often in lung conditions where mucous rattles, but not much comes up. You feel drowsy, irritable, dizzy, chilly, and run-down, and don't want to be touched. Muscles might hurt. Coughing phlegm or belching makes you better; lying down is worse.

Apis mellifica. This remedy from the honeybee is good for insect nips or bee stings. Also appropriate for any rash or allergic reaction that's red, hot, swollen, and stings. Your mind is "busy as a bee." Anything hot—room, bath, or drinks—makes you worse; coolness makes you better.

Argentum nitricum. The key characteristics for this remedy are nervous system complaints—uncoordinated, headaches, trembling, and a general feeling of being out of balance both physically and mentally—and inflammation of mucous membranes like the lungs and intestines; much gas and belching. Although you might crave sweets, eating them makes you feel worse. Cold makes you feel better.

Arnica. This is a key remedy for trauma—physical or mental (like shock). Anytime you bruise, bleed, bump, or turn black and blue, take Arnica. Can also be used before intentional trauma like surgery or dental work. As might be expected, you feel worse when overdoing it and better lying down.

Arsenicum album. Great anxiety and restlessness are key characteristics here, as well as searing pain, discharge, diarrhea, or other bodily afflictions. Regardless of this burning, you feel chilly. Thus cold food and beverages make you feel worse (even though you desire sips of cold drinks); heat and warm drinks make you better.

Belladonna. Think bright red, dry, and hot for Belladonna. This can mean a fever, headache, sore throat—often right-sided. Symptoms, as for Aconite, appear suddenly, and once there, make you very sensitive to movement, light, and sound. You feel better alone in a quiet and dark room.

Bellis perennis. This is homeopathic daisy. Yet this delicate flower is effective against deep tissue injuries, such as after surgery, or other trauma like bruises and sprains. Oddly enough, one old Materia Medica states that Bellis, or daisy, is good for gardeners. Not too much makes you feel better if you fit this remedy; however, hot and cold bathing and lying on your left side will surely make you worse.

Borax. This is a canker sore remedy especially when thrush (yeast in the mouth) is also present. It's most effective in children. As might be expected, spicy, salty or acid foods like fruit make these sores hurt.

Bryonia. Most important to look for here are symptoms—be it a cough, headache, or back pain—made worse with any movement. You'll find you yearn for cold beverages, and feel better pushing or lying on the hurting side.

Calcarea fluorica. Varicose veins are often helped with this remedy, as are any conditions where glands or veins are hard and stony, like a breast lump or goiter. Applying heat makes the lump feel better; rest makes it worse.

Calcarea sulphurica. Thick, yellow, pus-like discharges from the skin, eyes, nose, acne, or other body part best describe this remedy.

Cantharis. This is homeopathic Spanish fly, and is a key remedy for abruptly appearing bladder infections with a burning pain. Heightened libido can also be present. If you have this sort of urinary infection, urinating probably makes it worse, rest makes it better.

Carbo vegetabilis. This is homeopathy's version of charcoal, and is useful for abdominal complaints like gas, bloating, and indigestion. Even a small amount of food is not tolerated well. This remedy can also be used for fainting; the person often feels lethargic, yet irritable. Rich food and resting make things worse; moving air such as from a fan or draft makes you feel better.

Chamomilla. This is a great children's remedy for that whiny, restless baby or kid who wants to be held, yet is inconsolable. He might be fussy and crying because of great pain, like an ear infection, teething, colic, or general peevishness. Watch for green diarrhea, an intolerance to touch and a yen for cold beverages. His symptoms and behavior worsen at night (of course) and during teething; carrying the child makes him feel better.

Cinchona officinalis. After a long and debilitating illness, especially where vital fluids are lost, turn to Cinchona. You find that you feel apathetic and that gas and sour belches are a problem. When you eat, food just seems to sit there. Motion, a drafty room or touch makes you worse; pressing against the sore area makes it better.

Cocculus indicus. This is the motion sickness remedy where nausea, weakness, and dizziness reign. You don't want to eat anything. Women with morning sickness can also use this remedy. As might be expected, travel (and loss of sleep) make symptoms worse; sitting makes them better.

Coffea cruda. This is homeopathic coffee, and as such its symptoms are easy to remember. If you feel overstimulated, nervous and hyper, Coffea (not coffee) is the answer. Also think of insomnia and a racing heart for this remedy. Sleep makes you better; too much excitement, sound, or touch makes you worse.

Colchicum. This remedy is specific for gout, and also helps chronic afflictions of the muscles, joints, and related tissues. Watch for redness, heat and swelling and a tearing pain, as well as prostration. Evening and motion make symptoms worse.

Collinsonia canadensis. This remedy helps the rectal area, be it for constipation or hemorrhoids. Itching may be present as well as the "sensation of sharp sticks in (the) rectum." Heat makes it better, cold worse.

Drosera rotundifolia. This is a fine remedy for violent, dry and deep coughs that make you gag or even vomit. These annoying symptoms might make you angry though open air makes you feel better. Late at night, talking and lying down make things worse.

Echinacea. Like its herbal counterpart, homeopathic echinacea is helpful for acute infections. A general fatigue can be present, as well as chilliness and nausea. You can also apply homeopathic lotion or cream directly on infected areas.

Equisetum. This is a bladder remedy, good for both urinary or bladder infections and bedwetting. Watch for a full feeling, but once you urinate it only drips. At the close of urination, there is severe pain. The right side is often worse.

Eupatroium perfoliatum. This is homeopathic Boneset, and again, like the herb, it helps painful muscles and limbs, especially during fever. Symptoms seem to come and go.

Euphrasia. Bland nasal discharge, burning tears, grogginess, irritability, and sinus headache are what to observe; it's the opposite of Allium cepa (see above). This is an important remedy for hay fever. Open air relieves symptoms, though they turn worse as evening approaches.

Ferrum phosphoricum. Choose this remedy for the beginning of a fever or cold; the face can be pale or flushed. Also look for weakness and irritability. Lying down makes symptoms better, but they are worse at night.

Gelsemium. The four "Ds" describe this remedy—dull, droopy, drowsy, and dizzy. You don't feel like drinking anything, and your whole body feels stiff and maybe chilly. You want to hibernate in your bedroom and close the door on the world. Fright can bring your illness on or make it worse; lying down with your head propped feels good.

Graphites. This remedy works well for various skin conditions and constipation. Skin tends to be unhealthy-looking and can have a sticky ooze seeping from lesions. Those who fit this remedy startle easily, and often are fair-skinned and sometimes overweight.

Hamamelis virginica. This is homeopathic witch hazel and can also be used for varicose veins and hemorrhoids. This sign to note is a "bruised soreness of affected parts." Also, hemorrhoids tend to bleed profusely. Warmth makes these conditions feel worse.

Hepar sulphuris calcareum. This remedy works well for inflamed wounds that tend to form pus like abscesses. You might also find that you're very sensitive to pain and other annoyances, and feel chilly. Heat makes the sore feel better; touching it or covering the body makes it and you feel worse.

Ignatia. This is a classic remedy for grief. For those times when you're very sad, sigh a great deal, and can't stop crying, think of Ignatia. You feel like you have a lump in your throat; can also be used for hurt feelings after disappointment. Taking deep breaths eases your grief.

Ipecac. Ipecac syrup makes you vomit and is used in cases of poisoning. Homeopathic Ipecac works the opposite way and eases nausea and vomiting; bleeding may accompany this. Not surprisingly, irritability is part of this picture. You're not thirsty, though cold drinks may make you feel better. Vomiting makes you feel worse.

Kali bichromicum. Use this remedy for the later stages of a cold or for sinus infections where the mucus is thick and yellow-green, and there's pain under your eyes and around your nose. You can also use this for coughs associated with asthma and bronchitis that are hacking and rattle. Morning is worse, heat improves symptoms.

Kali muriaticum. This remedy is most suitable for chronic conditions of the middle ear. Often the glands around the ear are also swollen, and you might hear snapping noises. Eating fatty foods makes it worse.

Lachesis. This remedy—derived from the Bushmaster snake—has all the features associated with this animal: dislike of anything tight around the middle or neck (or a lump in the throat) and fear of snakes. Many of the symptoms are left-sided, or at the very least move from left to right. Bleeding disorders often fit this remedy, like nosebleeds and abnormal menstrual periods. Sleep or touch makes symptoms worse; expressing feelings makes things better.

Ledum. For puncture wounds, insect bites or stings, smashed digits, this is where you start. Also good for bruised sprains and sore feet. Cold makes the injuries feel better, and warmth and movement worse.

Lycopodium. Unlike Lachesis, this remedy's symptoms tend to be right-sided or move from right to left. You might find your sweet tooth is stronger than usual. People who fit this remedy often feel fearful inside, but hide it with bravado. Gas and bloating are predominant even after a small amount of food, including typical gaseous foods like cabbage and beans. You probably feel chilly though warmth makes you feel worse. You're better off with warm drinks, and in fact yearn for them.

Muriaticum acidum. This is a fine remedy for hemorrhoids that are swollen, itchy, dark blue, protruding and very sensitive; they're so sensitive, in fact, that even wiping yourself with toilet paper is agonizing. Women who get hemorrhoids during pregnancy are often helped by this remedy. One characteristic that separates Muriaticum from the others is that urination makes the itching and protrusion worse, and may even initiate involuntary stool evacuation. This remedy can also be used for conditions of the mouth like canker sores, ulcers on the tongue, and eczema on the back of the hands.

Natrum phosphoricum. In this book, I recommend Natrum phos for vaginal yeast that's characterized by a creamy or honey-colored, sour-smelling and sometimes watery discharge. This is a good remedy for yeast infections caused by antibiotic use. It can also be used for similar discharges from the eyes and mouth, greenish diarrhea, hives, and jaundice.

Nux vomica. This is the workaholic remedy. Your mind is obsessed with business, you're impatient and irritable, your muscles are tense, you have heartburn and constipation and insomnia. You're drawn to stimulants like coffee and tobacco as well as alcohol, and hot, fatty foods. Resting makes you feel better, and eating any of your desired foods makes you worse.

Petroleum. This is another good motion sickness remedy, but is distinguished by a drunk feeling that goes with it. Your stomach feels very empty, and is better when you eat. Also watch for very dry, cracking skin that bleeds because it's so chapped. Warm air makes both these situations better.

Phosphorus. A tendency to bleed bright red blood and bruise are featured here. This can mean nosebleeds, coughing up blood, or excessive periods. Cold drinks, especially pop or seltzer, go down easily. And you feel better with company. Spicy and warm foods make you worse.

Podophyllum. This is a fine diarrhea remedy, especially for the early morning explosive kind that comes with cramps and creates weakness. This diarrhea can stem from an intestinal infection like traveler's diarrhea, or overwork. Lying on your stomach feels good.

Pulsatilla. You feel like a little baby, happy one minute, crying the next. You want attention, but are indecisive. Any other symptoms you might have—infected eyes with yellow-green goop, cough, diarrhea, irregular periods—are also changeable. You crave creamy foods like ice cream, and are not thirsty. Being outside makes you feel better.

Rhus toxicodendron. Joints stiff after overexertion injuries like sprains, strains, and tendonitis, can be relieved with warmth and movement. You struggle to find a comfortable position. Warmth feels good; cold and wet feel bad.

Ruta graveolens or Ruta. This is another injury remedy. Here look for a bruised, sore, and achy feeling—especially of the ankles and wrists. Headaches caused by eye-strain can also be relieved with a dose of Ruta. An achy flu might be helped in cases where overdoing it makes you tired.

Sabadilla. This remedy targets the mucous membranes of the nose and eyes. Copious, watery nasal drainage, red runny eyes, itchiness inside the nose—somewhat like hay fever—are better outdoors in open air. Children's diarrhea with constant cutting pain can also be relieved with this remedy. Warm food and drinks make things better; cold makes them worse.

Sabina. This remedy offers help for a very specific type of trouble: paralytic pain in the small of the back. It feels worse with the smallest movement and heat, although cool fresh air brings some relief. Can also be applied to uterine problems (including hemorrhaging) and gout.

Sepia. This remedy is often used with women who are experiencing hormonal problems, though vaginal infections that discharge foul-smelling, white or yellow-green secretions are also indicated. Itching is also apparent. Irritability and crying can be present. Staying busy and exercising make symptoms better; skipping a meal makes them worse.

Silicea or Silica. Low stamina distinguishes this remedy, as well as infected lumps and bumps like boils, cysts, and abscesses. You can add swollen lymph glands to this list and conditions that go along with it like sore throats and ear infections. Constipation with "bashful" stools is also a part of this remedy. Warmth makes these conditions better.

Spongia. This is a good cough remedy, particularly for the dry, croupy, barking kind. Breathing can be difficult, and you might find yourself constantly clearing your throat. Hoarseness is also apparent. Warm drinks relieve these symptoms, while talking, singing, breathing (especially cold air) make them worse.

Sulphuricum acidum or Sulphur. When you have itchy, red, burning skin, turn to Sulphur. Burning, foul-smelling diarrhea and heartburn are also aided. Bathing and warmth make these symptoms worse; cool air makes them better.

Tabacum. If the smell of tobacco makes your travel sickness worse, think of Tabacum—homeopathic tobacco. This nausea is incessant, and moving makes you vomit. A terrible sinking feeling lies in the pit of your stomach, and your head aches horribly. Open your eyes, and the room (or car) spins. Fresh air makes you feel better.

Thuja occidentalis or Thuja. This is *the* wart remedy though it can be used for other bodily ailments, particularly of the skin and genitourinary system. Signs to look for when considering Thuja in vaginal yeast infections are a profuse, thick, white discharge (could be greenish too) and a very sensitive vagina. Symptoms increase at night while in bed and after drinking coffee or eating fatty foods.

Uranium nitricum. This unusual remedy is specific for both gastric and duodenal ulcers. Excessive thirst and a ravenous appetite set it apart from other ulcer remedies. Other distinguishing signs to take note of are nausea, vomiting, burning in the stomach, and a boring pain in a bloated abdomen.

Urtica urens. This is homeopathic stinging nettles (also called itch weed), so you should have no troubles remembering symptoms that match: stinging, itchy, painful, swollen sores. These can be skin rashes, bug bites, burns, herpes, hives, chicken pox, or others. Any cool application makes these symptoms worse.

Zincum metallicum or Zincum. Zincum is classic for depression that's not only mental but physical as well. Healing is slow; there might be anemia and profound fatigue. It also works well for large varicose veins of the legs that feel weak, tremble and twitch. You might find your soles are sensitive too. But most important, you're constantly moving your feet and legs. For women, menstruation makes it worse.

Appendix C
Resource List

There are many worthwhile books and magazines available on natural health. Below are a few to get you started. Also see Appendices A and B for herbal and homeopathic books to read. Some laboratories that specialize in tests that aid the natural health practitioner are listed below as well.

Books

Alternative Medicine: The Definitive Guide compiled by The Burton Goldberg Group, Future Medicine Publishing, 1993.

Total Wellness by Joseph Pizzorno, ND, Prima, 1996.

Dr. Wright's Guide to Healing with Nutrition by Jonathan Wright, MD, Keats, 1990.

Encyclopedia of Natural Medicine by Michael Murray, ND, and Joseph Pizzorno, ND, Prima, 1991.

Eat Right for Your Type by Peter D'Adamo, ND, G.P. Putnam's Sons, 1996.

Perfect Health by Deepak Chopra, MD, Harmony Books, 1991.

Encyclopedia of Nutritional Supplements by Michael T. Murray, ND, Prima, 1996.

Spontaneous Healing by Andrew Weil, MD, Alfred Knopf, 1995.

How to Eat Away Arthritis by Lauri M. Aesoph, ND, Prentice Hall, 1996.

Periodicals

Most of these magazines you'll find in your local bookstore, grocery store, or health food store. I've supplied addresses for ones you need to order.

Delicious!

Natural Health

Let's Live

Nutrition Insights

Vegetarian Times

Alive (Canada)

Humor and Health Letter
PO Box 16814
Jackson, MS 39236
(601) 957-0075

Bimonthly newsletter on the research and clinical use of humor.

Journal of Nursing Jocularity
PO Box 40416
Mesa, AZ 85274
(602) 835-6165

A quarterly journal about the funny side of nursing.

Laboratories

Great Smokies Diagnostic Laboratory
18A Regent Park Boulevard
Asheville, NC 28806
(800) 522-4762

Meridian Valley Clinical Laboratory
24030 132nd Avenue SE
Kent, WA 98042
(800) 234-6825

Appendix D

Natural Health Practitioners

While learning to care for your health is wonderful, there are times when you need the help of a skilled professional. Below I offer tips on how to assess natural health practitioners in your area; I also give you professional organizations that can refer you to trained natural health caregivers.

Twenty Questions to Ask Your Practitioner

1. Where were you trained?
2. Are you licensed to practice in this state (or province)? If your state doesn't license the practitioner you wish to see, ask if he or she is licensed in another state or, at the very least, is qualified to obtain a license in another state.
3. How long have you been in practice?
4. How many cases of my condition have you treated?
5. Do you practice full- or part-time? If part-time, how often?
6. Are you available 24 hours a day?
7. What kind of treatments do you use?
8. What do you do if your treatment doesn't work?
9. Do you perform physical exams?
10. Do you use laboratory tests? Which ones?
11. Do you believe in combining natural and conventional treatments? If so, how do you do this?

12. If I bring in new information, will you discuss it with me?

13. What do you do in case of emergencies?

14. Do you refer to other doctors or practitioners in the community?

15. Do you consult with other doctors in the community, or else-where?

16. Do you have privileges or a professional relationship with the local hospital?

17. Will you talk with my MD or family physician?

18. What do you charge?

19. Will my insurance cover your service, treatments and/or labo-ratory tests?

20. Do you carry malpractice insurance?

Professional Associations

Naturopathic Physicians

American Association of Naturopathic Physicians
601 Valley Street, Suite 105
Seattle, WA 98109
(206) 298-0125

Canadian Naturopathic Association
4174 Dundas Street, Suite 304
Etobicoke, Ontario
Canada M8X 1X3
(416) 233-1043

Holistic Doctors (MDs, osteopathic, naturopathic, chiropractic)

American Holistic Medical Association
4101 Lake Boone Trail, Suite 201
Raleigh, NC 27617
(919) 787-5181

Oriental Medical Doctors

American Association of Acupuncture and Oriental Medicine
433 Front Street
Capasauqua, PA 18032
(610) 433-2448

Herbalists

American Herbalists Guild
PO Box 746555
Arvada, CO 80006

Herb Research Foundation
1007 Pearl Street, Suite 200
Boulder, CO 80302
(303) 449-2265

Homeopaths

Homeopathic Academy of Naturopathic Physicians (HANP)
PO Box 69565
Portland, OR 97201
(503) 795-0579

International Foundation for Homeopathy (IFH)
PO Box 7
Edmonds, WA 98020
(206) 776-1499

National Center for Homeopathy
801 North Fairfax Street, Suite 306
Alexandria, VA 22314
(703) 548-7790

Humor Specialists

American Association of Therapeutic Humor
222 Meramec, Suite 303
St. Louis, MO 63105
(314) 863-6232

Appendix E

Feedback From Readers—Your Makeover Ideas!

A book like this develops with help from lots of people. If while completing *Your Natural Health Makeover*, you discovered some ideas, hints, or tricks of your own, let me know. I'd love to hear what worked for you, and with your permission, might include it in a future work.

Send *your* makeover ideas to:

Lauri M. Aesoph, ND
717 South Duluth Avenue
Sioux Falls, SD 57104

Or e-mail me at: aesoph@worldnet.att.net

For More Information

Lauri Aesoph, ND, delights in educating people about natural health care and responsible ways to begin incorporating these principles into their lives. She has also written *How to Eat Away Arthritis* (Prentice Hall, 1996), available in bookstores. If you're interested in reading more of her writings and what she does, look her up on the Internet (http://www.healthy.net/aesoph or http://www.naturopathic.org/nd.homepages/dr.aesoph).

If you'd like Dr. Aesoph to speak at your group meeting, association gathering, convention, or other get-together about *Your Natural Health Makeover* or related natural health topics, contact her at 605-339-3645 or write to her at 717 South Duluth Avenue, Sioux Falls, South Dakota 57104.

References

Part One

Chapter 1

1. Whelan J. Health care tradeoffs: comparing the Canadian single-payer and the American multipayer systems. Pacific Northwest Executive. October 1990:2.

2. US Dept of Health & Human Services (Public Health Service), *The Surgeon General's Report on Nutrition and Health*, 1988, Rocklin, CA: Prima Publishing.

3. Diamant M & B Diamant. Abuse and timing of use of antibiotics in acute otitis media. Archives of Otolaryngology 1974; 100: 226–232.

4. *Physician's Desk Reference 1996 (50th edition)*, Medical Economics Co., Montvale, NJ.

5. Caudell KA. Psychoneuroimmunology and innovative behavioral interventions in patients with leukemia. Oncology Nursing Forum 1996; 23(3):493–502.

6. Bryla CM. The relationship between stress and the development of breast cancer: a literature review. Oncology Nursing Forum 1996; 23(3):441–448.

7. Ginsburg IH. Psychological and psychophysiological aspects of psoriasis. Dermatologic Clinics 1995 Oct; 13(4):793–804.

8. Monteiro da Silva AM et al. Psychosocial factors in inflammatory periodontal diseases. A review. Journal of Clinical Periodontology 1995; 22:516–526.

9. Cohen S. Psychological stress and susceptibility to upper respiratory infections. American Journal of Respiratory & Critical Care Medicine 1995; 152:S53–S58.

10. Goddard NC. 'Spirituality as integrative energy': a philosophical analysis as requisite precursor to holistic nursing practice. Journal of Advanced Nursing 1995;22:808–815.

11. Miller MA. Culture, spirituality, and women's health. Journal of Obstetric, Gynecologic & Neonatal Nursing 1995; 24(3):257–263.

12. Turner JA et al. The importance of placebo effects in pain treatment and research. Journal of the American Medical Association. 1994; 271(20):1609–1614.

13. Rabinovitz M & DH Van Thiel. Hepatotoxicity of nonsteroidal anti-inflammatory drugs. The American Journal of Gastroenterology 1992; 87(12):1696–1704.

14. Graham NMH et al. Adverse effects of aspirin, acetaminophen, and ibuprofen on immune function, viral shedding, and clinical status in rhinovirus-infected volunteers. The Journal of Infectious Diseases 1990;162:1277–1282.

15. Trovato A et al. Drug-nutrient interactions. American Family Physician 1991; 44(5):1651–1658.

Chapter 3

1. Guyton AC. Textbook of Medical Physiology (6th ed). Philadelphia: WB Saunders, 1981.

2. Mozafar A. Enrichment of some B-vitamins in plants with application of organic fertilizers. Plant and Soil 1994;167: 305–311.

3. van de Laar MAFJ & JK van der Korst. Rheumatoid arthritis, food, and allergy. Seminars in Arthritis and Rheumatism 1991; 21(1): 12–23.

4. Egger J et al. Is migraine food allergy? The Lancet 1983, October 15: 865–869.

5. Burks AW et al. Atopic dermatitis: clinical relevance of food hypersensitivity reactions. The Journal of Pediatrics 1988; 113(3): 447–451.

6. Oehling A. Importance of food allergy in childhood asthma Allergol et Immonpathol. 1981; Supplementum IX:71–73.

7. Bogaards JJP et al. Consumption of Brussels sprouts results in elevated alpha-class glutathione S-transferase levels in human blood plasma. Carcinogenesis 1994;15(5): 1073–1075.

8. Kiso Y et al. Antihepatotoxic principles of Curcuma longa rhizomes. Planta Medica 1983;49:185–187.

9. Imai K & K Nakachi. Cross sectional study of effects of drinking green tea on cardiovascular and liver diseases.

10. Kirchchoff R et al. Increase in choleresis by means of artichoke extract. Phytomedicine 1994;1:107–115.

11. Hikino H et al. Antihepatotoxic actions of flavonolignans from Silybum marianum fruits. Planta Medica 1984; 50: 248–250.

12. Blanchet KD. Dandelion. Alternative & Complementary Therapies 1995 Jan/Feb: 115–117.

13. Kaptchuk T. The Web that has no Weaver. New York: Congdon & Weed, 1983, pp. 129–130.

14. Grady H. Immunomodulation through castor oil packs. The Journal of Naturopathic Medicine 1997; 7(10): 84–89.

Chapter 4

1. Thorburn AW et al. Slowly digested and absorbed carbohydrate in traditional bushfoods: a protective factor against diabetes? American Journal of Clinical Nutrition 1987; 45: 98–106.

2. Price WA. *Nutrition and Physical Degeneration* (50th anniversary edition). New Canaan: Keats Publishing, 1989.

3. Anon. Taco belles. Globe & Mail (Toronto). February 11, 1995, pg D8.

4. Block G. Dietary guidelines and the results of food consumption surveys. American Journal of Clinical Nutrition 1991; 53: 356S–357S.

5. Anon. Food timetables. Mother Earth News, Oct/Nov 1991; 128:26.

6. Greenberg ER et al. Mortality associated with low plasma concentration of beta carotene and the effect of oral supplementation. The Journal of the American Medical Association 1996; 275(9): 699–703.

7. Block G. Vitamin C and cancer prevention: the epidemiologic evidence. American Journal of Clinical Nutrition 1991; 53: 270S–282S.

8. Seddon JM et al. Dietary carotenoids, vitamins A, C, and E, and advanced age-related macular degeneration. Journal of the American Medical Association 1994; 272:1413–1420.

9. McNutt K. The individualized prescriptive foods era has dawned. Nutrition Today, May/June 1993: 43–47.

10. Johnston BT et al. Acid perception in gastro-oesophageal reflux disease is dependent on psychosocial factors. Scandinavian Journal of Gastroenterology 1995; 30(1): 1–5.

11. Herlofson BB & P Barkvoll. Oral mucosal desquamation of pre- and postmenopausal women. A comparison of response to sodium lauryl sulphate in toothpastes. Journal of Clinical Periodontology 1996; 23(6): 567–571.

Chapter 5

1. Covert C. New soft drinks surge into stores with a jolt. Star Tribune (Minneapolis), February 23, 1997: E1.

2. Robertson W et al. Prevalence of urinary stone disease in vegetarians. European Urology 1982; 8:334–339.

3. Avorn J et al. Reduction of bacteruria and pyuria after ingestion of cranberry juice. Journal of the American Medical Association 1994; 271:751–754.

4. Ringsdorf WM et al. Sucrose, neutrophilic phagocytosis and resistance to disease. Dental Survey 1976; 52:46–48.

5. Sanchez A et al. Role of sugars in human neutrophilic phagocytosis. The American Journal of Clinical Nutrition 1973; 26:1180–1184.

6. Kilbourne JP. Cranberry juice in urinary tract infection. Journal of Naturopathic Medicine 1991; 2:45–47.

7. Ofek I et al. Anit-escherichia adhesion activity of cranberry and blueberry juices. New England Journal of Medicine 1991;324: 1599

8. Katzung BG. *Basic and Clinical Pharmacology (2nd edition)*. Los Altos, CA: Lange Medical Publications, 1984, pg 180.

9. Adetumbi MA et al. *Allium sativum* (garlic)—a natural antibiotic. Medical Hypotheses 1983; 12:227–237.

10. Ghannoum MA. Studies on the anticandidal mode of action of *Allium sativum* (garlic). Journal of General Microbiology 1988;134: 2917–2924.

11. Davis LE et al. Antifungal activity on human cerebrospinal fluid and plasma after intravenous administration of *Allium sativum*. Antimicrobial Agents and Chemotherapy 1990; 34(4): 651–653.

12. Mirelman D et al. Inhibition of growth of *Entamoeba histolytica* by allicin, the active principal of garlic extract (*Allium sativum*). The Journal of Infectious Diseases 1987;156(1): 243–244 (Letter).

13. Tsai Y et al. Antiviral properties of garlic: in vitro effects on influenza B, herpes simplex and coxsackie viruses. Planta Medica 1985: 460–461.

14. Pantoja CV et al. Diuretic, natriuretic and hypotensive effects produced by *Allium sativum* (garlic) in anaesthetized dogs. Journal of Ethnopharmacology 1991; 31: 325–331.

15. Brenner BM (ed). *Brenner & Rector's: The Kidney* (5th ed), Volume II. Philadelphia: WB Saunders Co, 1996.

16. Scott R et al. The importance of cadmium as a factor in calcified upper urinary tract stone disease—a prospective 7-year study. British Journal of Urology 1982; 54: 584–589.

17. Rose G. The influence of calcium content of water, intake of vegetables and fruit and of other food factors upon the incidence of renal calculi. Urological Research 1975; 3: 61–66.

18. Shaw P et al. Idiopathic hypercalciuria: its control with unprocessed bran. British Journal of Urology 1980; 52:426–429.

19. Griffith H et al. A control study of dietary factors in renal stone formation. British Journal of Urology 1981; 53: 416–420.

20. Thom J et al. The influence of refined carbohydrate on urinary calcium excretion. British Journal of Urology 1978; 50: 459–464.

21. Lemann J et al. Possible role of carbohydrate-induced hypercalciuria in calcium oxalate kidney-stone formation. New England Journal of Medicine 1969; 280: 232–237.

22. Zechner O et al. Nutritional risk factors in urinary stone disease. Journal of Urology 1981; 125: 51–55.

23. Harvey JA et al. Calcium citrate: reduced propensity for the crystallization of calcium oxalatein urine resulting from induced hypercalciuria of calcium supplementation. Journal of Clinical Endocrinology and Metabolism 1985; 61(6): 1223.

24. Harvey JA et al. Dose dependency of calcium absorption: a comparison of calcium carbonate and calcium citrate. Journal of Bone and Mineral Research 1988; 3(3): 253.

25. Curhan GC et al. Comparison of dietary calcium with supplemental calcium and other nutrients as factors affecting the risk for kidney stones in women. Annals of Internal Medicine 1997; 126(7): 497–505. ("calcium"-abstract)

Chapter 6

1. Ringsdorf WM et al. Sucrose, neutrophilic phagocytosis and resistance to disease. Dental Survey 1976; 52: 46–48.

2. Covert C. New soft drinks surge into stores with a jolt. Star Tribune (Minneapolis), February 23, 1997:E1.

3. Sanchez A et al. Role of sugars in human neutrophilic phagocytosis. The American Journal of Clinical Nutrition 1973; 26: 1180–1184.

4. Dale DC & DD Federman (eds). *Scientific American Medicine.* NYC: Scientific American, Inc, 1978–1997; Chapter XXIV, "Pathophysiology of Fever and Fever of Undetermined Origin."

5. Horowith BJ et al. Sugar chromatography studies in recurrent candida vulvovaginitis. The Journal of Reproductive Medicine 1984; 29:441–443.

6. Lefkowith JB. Do dietary fatty acids affect the interactions among macrophages, endothelial lesions, and thrombosis? American Journal of Clinical Nutrition 1992; 56: 808S.

7. Nirgiotis JG et al. Low-fat, high-carbohydrate diets improve wound healing and increase protein levels in surgically stressed rats. Journal of Pediatric Surgery 1991; 26(8): 925–29.

8. Pollmacher T et al. Influence of host defense activation on sleep in humans. Advances in Neuroimmunology 1995; 5(2):155–169.

9. Moldofsky H. Central nervous system and peripheral immune functions and the sleep-wake system. Journal of Psychiatry & Neuroscience. 1994; 19(5): 368–374.

10. Chandra RK. Effect of vitamin and trace-element supplementation on immune responses and infection in elderly subjects. Lancet 1992; 340: 1124–1127.

11. Prinz W et al. The effect of ascorbic acid supplementation on some parameters of the human immunological defence system. International Journal of Vitamin and Nutritional Research 1977; 47: 248–257.

12. Semba RD et al. Abnormal T-cell subset proportions in vitamin-A-deficient children. The Lancet 1993; 341: 5–8.

13. Beisel WR et al. Single-nutrient effects on immunologic functions. Journal of the American Medical Association 1981; 245(1): 53–58.

14. Lakshman K et al. Monitoring nutritional status in the critically ill adult. Journal of Clinical Monit 1986; 2(2): 114–120.

15. Caudell KA. Psychoneuroimmunology and innovative behavioral interventions in patients with leukemia. Oncology Nursing Forum 1996; 23(3): 493–502.

16. Cohen S. Psychological stress and susceptibility to upper respiratory infections. American Journal of Respiratory Critical Care Medicine 1995;152: 553–558.

17. Monteiro da Silva AM et al. Psychological factors in inflammatory periodontal diseases. Journal of Clinical Periodontology 1995; 22: 516–526.

18. Ginsburg IH. Psychological and psychophysiological aspects of psoriasis. Dermatologic Clinics 1995;13(4): 793–804.

19. Kiecolt-Glaser JK et al. Slowing of wound healing by psychological stress. Lancet 1995; 346:1194–1196.

20. Cohen S et al. Psychological stress and susceptibility to the common cold. The New England Journal of Medicine 1991; 325:606–612.

21. Anon. State-specific estimates of smoking-attributable mortality and years of potential life lost-United States, 1985. Journal of the American Medical Association 1989; 261(1): 23–25.

22. Anon. Smoking and immunity. The Lancet 1990; 335: 1561–1563.

23. Lowinson JH et al (eds). *Substance Abuse, A Comprehensive Textbook (2nd ed)*. Baltimore: Williams & Wilkins, 1992.

24. Piyathilake CJ et al. Local and systemic effects of cigarette smoking on folate and vitamin B-12. American Journal of Clinical Nutrition 1994; 60: 559–566.

25. American Thoracic Society, Medical Section of American Lung Assoc. Cigarette smoking and health. American Review of Respiratory Disease 1985; 132(5): 1133–1136.

26. American Thoracic Society, Medical Section of American Lung Assoc. Health effects of smoking on children. American Review of Respiratory Disease 1985; 132(5): 1137–1138.

27. Dunnet B. Drugs that suppress immunity. American Health; Nov 1986: 43.

28. Bayer BM et al. Acute infusions of cocaine result in time-and-dose-dependent effects on lymphocyte responses and corticosterone secretion in rats. Immunopharmacology 1995; 29(1): 19–28.

29. Kreek MJ et al. Drugs of abuse and immunosuppression. NIDA Research Monograph 1994;140: 89–93.

30. Mohs ME et al. Nutritional effects of marijuana, heroin, cocaine, and nicotine. Journal of the American Dietetic Association 1990; 90: 1261–1267.

31. Brayton RG et al. Effect of alcohol and various diseases on leukocyte mobilization, phagocytosis and intracellular bacterial killing. The New England Journal of Medicine 1970; 282(3): 123–128.

32. Graham NMH et al. Adverse effects of aspirin, acetominophen, and ibuprofen on immune function, viral shedding, and clinical status in rhinovirus-infected volunteers. Journal of Infectious Disease 1990;162:1277–1282.

33. Fujii T et al. Inhibitory effect of erythromycin on interleukin 8 production by 1 alpha, 25-dihydroxyvitamin D3-stimulated THP-1 cells. Antimicrobial Agents & Chemotherapy 1996;40(6): 1548–1551.

34. Rosaschino F et al. Evaluation of the immune status of children never treated with chemoantibiotics (children 3 to 6 years old). Minerva Pediatrica 1994; 46(11): 481–500.

35. Vojdani A et al. Immune alterations associated with exposure to toxic chemicals. Toxicology and Industrial Health 1992; 8(5): 239–254.

36. Miyakoshi H, Aoki T. Acting mechanisms of lentinan in humans—I. Augmentation of DNA synthesis and immunoglobulin production of peripheral mononuclear cells. International Journal of Immunopharmacology 1984; 6(4): 365–371.

37. Srivastava KC, T Mustafa. Ginger (*Zingiber officinale*) in rheumatism and musculoskeletal disorders. Medical Hypotheses 1992; 39: 342–348.

38. Jeevan A, Kripke ML. Ozone depletion and the immune system. The Lancet 1993; 342:1159–1160.

Chapter 7

1. Associated Press. Fatty diet hurts ability to deal with stress. Argus Leader, October 31, 1992, pg 3a.

2. Bolton S et al. A pilot study of some physiological and psychological effects of caffeine. The Journal of Orthomolecular Psychiatry;13(1): 34–41.

3. Brown DJ. *Herbal Prescriptions for Better Health*. Rocklin: Prima Publishing, 1996

4. Cousins N. *Anatomy of an Illness*. New York: Bantam Books, 1979.

5. Wooten P. Humor: an antidote for stress. http://www.mother.com/JestHome/anti-stress.html.

6. Berk L. Neuroendocrine and stress hormone changes during mirthful laughter. American Journal of Medical Sciences. 1989; 298: 390–396.

7. Berk L. Eustress of mirthful laughter modifies natural killer cell activity. Clinical Research 1989; 37(115).

Chapter 8

1. Komatsu A & I Sakurai. A study of the development of atherosclerosis in childhood and young adults: risk factors and the prevention of progression in Japan and the USA. The Pathobiological Determinants of Atherosclerosis in Youth (PDAY) Research Group. Pathology International 1996; 46(8): 541–547.

2. Kottke BA et al. Apolipoproteins and coronary artery disease. Mayo Clinic Proceedings 1986; 61.

3. Blieden LC et al. Non-traditional risk factors for atherosclerosis in high risk children. Israel Journal of Medical Sciences 1996; 32(12): 1255–61.

4. Ornish D et al. Can lifestyle changes reverse coronary heart disease? The Lancet 1990; 336:129–133.

5. Sacks FM & WW Willett. More on chewing the fat. The good fat and the good cholesterol. The New England Journal of Medicine 1991; 325(24):1740–1742.

6. Steinberg D. et al. Lipoproteins and atherogenesis. Journal of the American Medical Association 1990; 264:3047–3052.

7. Lichenstein AH. Trans fatty acids and hydrogenated fat—what do we know? Nutrition Today 1995; 30(3):102–107.

8. Blair SN et al. Physical fitness and all-cause mortality. Journal of the American Medical Association 1989; 262(17): 2395–2401.

9. Davidson MH et al. The hypocholesterolemic effects of beta-glucan in oatmeal and oat bran. Journal of the American Medical Association 1991; 265(14):1833–1839.

10. Glore SR et al. Soluble fiber and serum lipids: a literature review. Journal of the American Dietetic Association 1994; 94(4):425–436.

11. Hertog MGL et al. Dietary antioxidant flavonoids and risk of coronary heart disease: the Zutphen Elderly Study. The Lancet 1993; 342:1007–1011.

12. Riemersma RA et al. Risk of angina pectoris and plasma concentrations of vitamins A, C, and E and carotene. The Lancet 1991; 337(8732):1–5.

13. Manson JE et al. A prospective study of vitamin C and incidence of coronary heart disease in women. Circulation 1992; 85: 865.

14. Whang R et al. Refractory potassium repletion: a consequence of magnesium deficiency. Archives of Internal Medicine 1992;152:40–45.

15. Woods KL et al. Intravenous magnesium sulphate in suspected acute myocardial infarction: results of the second Leicester Intravenous Magnesium Intervention Trial (LIMIT-2). The Lancet 1992; 339:1553–1558.

16. Clarke R et al. Hyperhomocysteinemia: an independent risk factor for vascular disease. The New England Journal of Medicine 1991; 324(17):1149–1155.

17. Ferrannini E et al. Insulin resistance in essential hypertension. The New England Journal of Medicine 1987; 317:350–357.

18. Hodges RE & T Rebello. Carbohydrates and blood pressure. Annals of Internal Medicine 1983; 98(part 2):838–841.

19. Hall JH et al. Long-term survival in coenzyme Q10 treated congestive heart failure patients. Circulation 1990; 82(4), supplement III: 675.

20. Ernst E et al. Garlic and blood lipids. British Medical Journal 1985; 291:139.

21. Gujral S et al. Effects of ginger (*Zingebar officinale roscoe*) oleoresin on serum and hepatic cholesterol levels in cholesterol fed rats. Nutrition Reports International 1978;17: 183–189.

22. Wang J-P et al. Antiplatelet effect of capsaicin. Thrombosis Research 1984;36:497–507.

23. Shoji N et al. Cardiotonic principles of ginger (Zingiber officinale roscoe). Journal of Pharm Science 1982;10:1174–75.

24. Kiuchi F et al. Inhibitors of prostaglandin biosynthesis from ginger. Chem Pharm Bull 1982; 30: 754–757.

25. Srivastava K. Effects of aqueous extracts of onion, garlic and ginger on the platelet aggregation and metabolism of arachidonic acid in the blood vascular system: In vitro study. Prost Leukotri Med 1984;13: 227–35.

26. Wahlqvist M. Fish intake and arterial wall characteristics in healthy people and diabetic patients. The Lancet 1989; 944: 946.

27. Sharp DS & NL Benowitz. Pharmacoepidemiology of the effect of caffeine on blood pressure. Clinical Pharmacol Ther 1990;47:57–60.

28. Urgert R et al. Effects of cafestol and kahweol from coffee grounds on serum lipids and serum liver enzymes in humans. American Journal of Clinical Nutrition 1995; 61:144–145.

29. Imai K, Nakachi K. Cross sectional study of effects of drinking green tea on cardiovascular and liver diseases. British Medical Journal 1995; 310: 693–96

30. Facchini FS et al. Insulin resistance and cigarette smoking. The Lancet 1992;339:1128–1130.

31. Zhu B & WW Parmley. Hemodynamic and vascular effects of active and passive smoking. American Heart Journal 1995;130:1270–1275.

32. Timmreck TC & JF Randolph. Smoking cessation: clinical steps to improve compliance. Geriatrics 1993; 48(4): 63–70.

33. Rimm EB et al. Prospective study of alcohol consumption and risk of coronary disease in men. The Lancet 1991; 338: 464–468.

34. Regan TJ. Alcohol and the cardiovascular system. Journal of the American Medical Association 1990; 264(3): 377–381.

35. Longnecker MP et al. A meta-analysis of alcohol consumption in relation to risk of breast cancer. Journal of the American Medical Association 1988; 260(5): 652–656.

36. Yeung AC et al. The effect of atherosclerosis on the vasomotor response of coronary arteries to mental stress. The New England Journal of Medicine 1991; 325: 1551–1556.

37. Anon. Essence of stress. The Lancet 1994; 344:1713–1714.

38. Raymond C. Distrust, rage may be "toxic core" that puts "Type A" person at risk. Journal of the American Medical Association 1989; 261(6): 813.

39. Chopra D. Longevity Magazine 1989.

Chapter 10

1. Anon. Chronobiology and chronotherapy in medicine. Disease-a-Month 1995;16(8):506–575.

2. Tjoa WS et al. Circannual rhythm in human sperm count revealed by serially independent sampling. Fertility and Sterility 1982; 38:454–459.

3. Lieber CS. The metabolism of alcohol. Scientific American 1976, March: 25–33.

4. Gavaler JS et al. Alcohol and estrogen levels in postmenopausal women: the spectrum of effect. Alcoholism: Clinical and Experimental Research 1993;17(4): 786–790.

5. Dawood MY, JL McGuire, LM Demers (ed). *Premenstrual Syndrome & Dysmenorrhea*. Baltimore-Munich: Urban & Schwarzenberg, 1985.

6. Feldman HA et al. Impotence and its medical and psychosocial correlates: results of the Massachusetts Male Aging Study 1994;151: 54–61.

7. Nielsen FH et al. Effect of dietary boron on mineral, estrogen, and testosterone metabolism in postmenopausal women. Federation of American Societies for Experimental Biology 1987;1:394–397.

8. Snively WD, RL Westerman. Minnesota Medicine, June 1965.

9. Gonzalez-Reimers E et al. Relative and combined effects of ethanol and protein deficiency on gonadal function and histology. Alcohol 1994;11(5):355–360.

10. Porikos KP, TB Van Itallie. Diet-induced changes in serum transaminase and triglyceride levels in healthy adult men. Role of sucrose and excess calories. American Journal of Medicine 1983; 75: 624.

11. Shils ME, VR Young. *Modern Nutrition in Health and Disease (7th ed)*. Philadelphia: Lea & Febiger, 1988.

12. Nielsen FH. Nutritional requirements for boron, silicon, vanadium, nickel, and arsenic: current knowledge and speculation. Federation of American Societies for Experimental Biology 1991;5:2661–2667.

13. Takihara H et al. Zinc sulfate therapy for infertile male with or without varicocelectomy. Urology 1987; 29(6): 638–641.

14. Dincer SL et al. Thalassemia, zinc deficiency, and sexual dysfunction in women. Hospital Practice 1992; 27(4A): 35.

15. Morales A et al. Oral and topical treatment of erectile dysfunction. Urologic Clinics of North America 1995; 22(4): 879–886.

Chapter 11

1. Wisneski LA. Clinical management of postmenopausal osteoporosis. Southern Medical Journal 1992; 85: 832–39.

2. Nelson ME et al. A 1-y walking program and increased dietary calcium in postmenopausal women: effects on bone. American Journal of Clinical Nutrition 1991; 53: 1304–1311.

3. Ott SM. Bone density in adolescents. New England Journal of Medicine 1991; 325: 1646–1647.

4. Licata AA. Therapies for symptomatic primary osteoporosis. Geriatrics 1991; 46: 62–67.

5. Slemenda CW et al. Long-term bone loss in men: effects of genetic and environmental factors. Annals of Internal Medicine 1992; 117: 286–291.

6. Hernandez-Avila M et al. Caffeine, moderate alcohol intake, and risk of fractures of the hip and forearm in middle-aged women. American Journal of Clinical Nutrition 1991;54:157–163.

7. Mickelsen O & AG Marsh. Calcium requirement and diet. Nutrition Today, Jan/Feb 1989:28–32.

8. Eaton SB et al. *The Paleolithic Prescription.* New York: Harper & Row, Publishers, 1988.

9. Johnson K & EW Kligman. Preventive nutrition: disease-specific dietary interventions for older adults. Geriatrics 1992;47: 39–40, 45–49.

10. Werbach MR. *Nutritional Influences on Illness.* Tarzana: Third Line Press, 1988.

11. Andon MB et al. Spinal bone density and calcium intake in healthy postmenopausal women. American Journal of Clinical Nutrition 1991;54: 927–929.

12. Stevenson JC et al. Dietary intake of calcium and postmenopausal bone loss. British Medical Journal 1988; 297:15–17.

13. Iseri LT & JH French. Magnesium: nature's physiologic calcium blocker. American Heart Journal 1984;108: 188–193.

14. Medalle R et al. Vitamin D resistance in magnesium deficiency. American Journal of Clinical Nutrition 1976; 29: 854–858.

15. Nielsen FH et al. Effect of dietary boron on mineral, estrogen, and testosterone metabolism in postmenopausal women. Federation of American Societies for Experimental Biology 1987;1:394–397.

16. Raloff J. Reasons for boning up on manganese. Science News 1986; 130: 199.

17. Gaby AR & JV Wright. Nutrients and bone health. Published by: Wright/Gaby Nutrition Institute (1988): PO Box 21535, Baltimore, MD 21208.

18. McCaslin FE Jr & JM Janes. The effect of strontium lactate in the treatment of osteoporosis. Proceedings of Staff Meetings Mayo Clinic 1959; 34: 329–334.

19. Nielsen FH. Nutritional requirements for boron, silicon, vanadium, nickel, and arsenic: current knowledge and speculation. FASEB 1991; 5: 2661–2667.

20. Fehily AM et al. Factors affecting bone density in young adults. American Journal of Clinical Nutrition 1992; 56: 570–586.

21. Hart JP et al. Circulating vitamin K1 levels in fracture neck of femur. The Lancet 1984; II: 283.

22. Turnlund JR et al. Vitamin B6 depletion followed by repletion with animal or plant source diets and calcium and magnesium metabolism in young women. American Journal of Clinical Nutrition 1992; 56.

23. Thom J et al. The influence of refined carbohydrate on urinary calcium excretion. British Journal of Urology 1978; 50: 459–464.

24. Lemann J et al. Possible role of carbohydrate-induced hypercalciuria in calcium oxalate kidney-stone formation. New England Journal of Medicine 1969; 280: 232–237.

25. Mazess RB & HS Barden. Bone density in premenopausal women: effects of age, dietary intake, physical activity, smoking and birth-control pills. American Journal of Clinical Nutrition 1991; 53: 132–142.

26. Rao C et al. Influence of bioflavonoids on the metabolism and crosslinking of collagen. Italian Journal of Biochemistry 1981; 30: 259–270.

27. Sutton PRN. Acute dental caries, mental stress, immunity and the active passage of ions through the teeth. Medical Hypotheses 1990; 31:17.

28. Herlofson BB & P Barkvoll. Oral mucosal desquamation caused by two toothpaste detergents in an experimental model. European Journal of Oral Sciences 1996; 104(1): 21–26.

29. Skaare A et al. The effect of toothpaste containing triclosan on oral mucosal desquamation. A model study. Journal of Clinical Periodontology 1996; 23(12):1100–1103.

30. Herlofson BB et al. Increased human gingival blood flow induced by sodium lauryl sulphate. Journal of Clinical Periodontology 1996; 23(11):1004–1007.

31. Herlofson BB & P Barkvoll. Oral mucosal desquamation of pre- and postmenopausal women. A comparison of response to sodium lauryl sulphate in toothpastes. Journal of Clinical Periodontology 1996; 23(6): 567–571.

32. Addy M et al. Dentine hypersensitivity—effects of some proprietary mouthwashes on the dentine smear layer: a SEM study. Journal of Dentistry 1991;19(3):148–152.

33. Subcommittee on Risk Management of the Committee to Coordinate Environmental Health and Related Programs. *Dental Amalgam: A scientific review and recommended public health service strategy for research, education and regulation.* January 1993. Department of Health and Human Services. Public Health Service.

34. Nylander M et al. Mercury concentrations in the human brain and kidneys in relation to exposure from dental amalgam fillings. Swedish Dental Journal 1987;11:179–187.

35. Bland JS. Can mercury in dental fillings make you sick? Delicious! April 1995: 64.

36. Siblerud RL. The relationship between mercury from dental amalgam and mental health. American Journal of Psychotherapy 1989;XLIII(4):575–587.

37. Newman NM & RSM Ling. Acetabular bone destruction related to non-steroidal anti-inflammatory drugs. The Lancet 1985; July 6: 11–14.

38. Hudson TS. Osteoporosis: an overview for clinical practice. Journal of Naturopathic Medicine 1997; 7(1): 27–33.

Chapter 12

1. Sindrup JH et al. Nocturnal temperature and subcutaneous blood flow in humans. Clinical Physiology 1995; 15(6): 611–622.

2. Marshall LA. How pure is your water? Delicious! April 1995, pg 38.

3. Krause MV & LK Mahan. *Food, Nutrition, and Diet Therapy (7th ed)*. Philadelphia: WB Saunders Co, 1984.

4. Trevithick JR et al. Topical tocopherol acetate reduces post UVB, sunburn associated erythema, edema, and skin sensitivity in mice. Archives of Biochemistry and Biophysiology 1992; 296: 575–582.

5. Garland CF et al. Could sunscreens increase melanoma risk? American Journal of Public Health 1992; 82(4): 614–615.

6. Roan S. Worship your skin. Argus Leader, July 30, 1996.

7. Perasalo J. Traditional use of the sauna for hygiene and health in Finland. Annals of Clinical Research 1988; 20: 220–223.

Chapter 13

1. Age-related Macular Degeneration Study Group. Multicenter ophthalmic and nutritional age-related macular degeneration study—part 1: design, subjects and procedures. Journal of the American Optometric Association 1996; 67(1): 12–29.

2. Christen WG et al. A prospective study of cigarette smoking and risk of age-related macular degeneration in men. Journal of the American Medical Association 1996; 276(14): 1147–1151.

3. Schectman G et al. The influence of smoking on vitamin C status in adults. American Journal of Public Health 1989; 79(2):158–162.

4. Klein R, BEK Klein. Smoke gets in your eyes too (editorial). Journal of the American Medical Association 1996; 276(14): 1178–1179.

5. Hankinson SE et al. Nutrient intake and cataract extraction in women: a prospective study. British Medical Journal 1992; 305: 335–339.

6. Ritter LL et al. Alcohol use and lens opacities in the Beaver Dam Eye Study. Archives of Ophthalmology 1993;111:113–117.

7. Forman MR et al. Effect of alcohol consumption on plasma carotenoid con-
    centrations in premenopausal women: a controlled dietary study. American
    Journal of Clinical Nutrition 1995; 62:131–135.

8. Munoz B et al. Alcohol use and risk of posterior subcapsular opacities.
    Archives of Ophthalmology 1993; 111:110–112.

9. Seddon JM et al. Dietary carotenoids, vitamins A, C, and E, and advanced age-
    related macular degeneration. Journal of the American Medical Association
    1994; 272:1413–1420.

10. Murray M. *The Healing Power of Herbs*. Rocklin, CA: Prima Publishing, 1995.

11. Shils ME, VR Young. *Modern Nutrition in Health and Disease (7th ed)*.
    Philadelphia: Lea & Febiger, 1988.

12. Berson EL et al. A randomized trial of vitamin A and vitamin E supplementa-
    tion for retinitis pigmentosa. Archives of Ophthalmology 1993;111:761–772.

13. Fishbein S & S Goodstein. The pressure lowering effect of ascorbic acid.
    Annals of Ophthalmology 1972;4:487–491.

14. Anon. Vitamin C may enhance healing of caustic corneal burns. Journal of the
    American Medical Association 1980; 243(7): 623.

15. Newsome DA et al. Oral zinc in macular degeneration. Archives of
    Ophthalmology 1988;106:192–198.

16. Swanson A, A Truesdale. Elemental analysis in normal and cataractous human
    lens tissue. Biochem. Biophys. Res. Comm 1971; 45:1, 488–496.

17. Albert DM, FA Jakobiec. *Principles and Practice of Ophthalmology (vol 1)*.
    Philadelphia: WB Saunders, 1994.

18. The Revolutionary Health Committee of Hunan Province. *A Barefoot Doctor's
    Manual* (revised and enlarged edition), Seattle: Madrona Publishers, 1977.

Chapter 14

1. Anderson GH. Diet, neurotransmitter and brain function. British Medical
    Bulletin 1981; 37(1): 95–100.

2. DeLong GR. Effects of nutrition on brain development in humans. American
    Journal of Clinical Nutrition Supplement 1993; 57: 286S–290S.

3. Benton D & JP Buts. Vitamin/mineral supplementation and intelligence. The
    Lancet 1990; 335:1158–1160.

4. LaRue A et al. Nutritional status and cognitive functioning in a normally aging
    sample: a 6-y reassessment. American Journal of Clinical Nutrition 1997;
    65: 20–29.

5. Pizzorno J. *Total Wellness*. Rocklin, CA: Prima Publishing, 1996.

6. Guyton AC. *Textbook of Medical Physiology* (6th ed). Philadelphia: WB
    Saunders, 1981.

Part Two

1. Psychiatry Research, 1992; 43: 253–62.

2. Das SK et al. Deglycyrrhizinated liquorice in apthous ulcers. Journal of the Association of Physicians of India (JAPI) 1989; 37: 647.

3. Jacobs J et al. Treatment of acute childhood diarrhea with homeopathic medicine: a randomized clinical trial in Nicaragua. Pediatrics 1994; 93(5): 719–725.

4. Diamant M, B Diamant. Abuse and timing of use of antibiotics in acute otitis media. Archives of Otolaryngology 1974;100: 226–232.

5. Dale DC & DD Federman (eds). *Scientific American Medicine*. NYC: Scientific American, Inc, 1978–1997; Chapter XXIV, "Pathophysiology of Fever and Fever of Undetermined Origin."

6. Ball GV & LB Sorensen. Pathogenesis of hyperuricemia in saturnine gout. New England Journal of Medicine 1969; 280: 1199–1202.

7. Stein HB. Ascorbic acid-induced uricosuria: a consequence of megavitamin therapy. Annals of Internal Medicine 1976; 84: 385–388.

8. Gershon SL & IH Fox. Pharmacological effects of nicotinic acid on human purine metabolism. Journal of Laboratory and Clinical Medicine 1974; 84: 179–186.

9. Grant ECG. Food allergies and migraine. The Lancet 1979, May 5: 966–969.

10. Egg J et al. Is migraine food allergy? A double-blind controlled trial of oligoantigenic diet treatment. The Lancet, 1983, October 15: 865–869.

11. Mauskop A. Intravenous magnesium sulfate relieves migraine attacks in patients with low serum ionized magnesium levels: A pilot study. Clinical Science 1995; 89: 633–636.

12. Scattner P & D Randerson. Tiger Balm as a treatment of tension headache: A clinical trial in general practice. Australian Family Physician 1996; 25:216–222.

13. Kraft JR. Detection of diabetes mellitus in situ (occult diabetes). Laboratory Medicine 1975; 6(2):10.

14. Macintosh A. Dysglycemia: a misunderstood functional illness. Journal of Naturopathic Medicine 1997; 7(1): 78–83.

15. Ferrannini E et al. Insulin resistance in essential hypertension. New England Journal of Medicine 1987; 317: 350.

16. Facchini FS et al. Insulin resistance and cigarette smoking. The Lancet 1992; 339: 1128–1130.

17. Eby GA et al. Reduction in duration of common colds by zinc gluconate lozenges in a double-blind study. Antimicrobial Agents and Chemotherapy 1984; 25(1): 20–24.

18. Anon. Bugged by an ulcer? You could have a bug. Discover 1987 (May); pg 10.

Index

KOMANTCIA

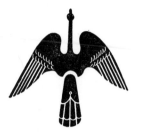

KOMANTCIA

BY HAROLD KEITH

THOMAS Y. CROWELL COMPANY

NEW YORK

J

9/66

Books by Harold Keith

SPORTS AND GAMES

RIFLES FOR WATIE

KOMANTCIA

for

JIM, JORENE, JAMIE, AND JERI FRAN

*who live in the Moobetahehoonoo country
of southwestern Oklahoma, scene
of much of this story*

CONTENTS

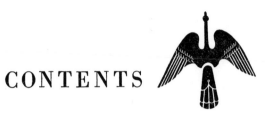

KOMANTCIA

1 · At the Rancho Pavón

The rain overtook them as they began the descent from the north Mexican highlands onto the plain of eastern Chihuahua. Slowly it crept eastward, pelting the shoulders, the backs, and sombreros of the travelers. Then it stopped. But its coming had wrought a miracle.

Flowers spangled the parched mesas with blossoms of pink, cream, and gold. The sodden soil smelled sweet in the icy air of late afternoon. Even the sinister thornbush looked friendly in its jacket of small green leaves with a scarlet blossom for a boutonniere. The desert had flared into color and life at the lash of the rain.

A long line of baggage mules laden with boxes and trunks serpentined in single file down the steep, cactus-studded trail. A bronco burro with a tinkling bell fastened to his neck led the way, a muleteer by his side.

Five travelers, superbly mounted on saddle horses, rode in the vanguard of the caravan. Pedro Pavón and his brother rode first. They looked so alike that any stranger could have told their blood relationship. Short in stature, they had long, thin necks and beautifully planed faces. Their dignified demeanor and the fashionable cut of their clothing indicated their high birth. Each wore tightly fitted gray trousers, frilled shirts banded at the waist with girdles of crimson silk, short coats, neat black boots, and Spanish capes.

1

Below, in a far-off oasis of sunshine, their uncle's rancho spread before them. The sprawl of its low adobe buildings, with their roof tiles of weathered red, their walls of glistening white and their crowns of pink almond blossoms soothed the harsh landscape. There were walled gardens of corn and beans, scores of neatly laid-out patios, and roads and courts freshly strewn with yellow gravel. The scene was such a faithful likeness of Pedro's native Andalusia that a wave of homesickness washed over him.

He stared at it with nostalgic pleasure as he lifted the bridle reins to slow the horse. He had deep, brooding eyes. Pride and aloofness showed in his brown face, and also a faint vestige of pain, as if some inner conflict were troubling him. He carried himself proudly in the saddle, as became a scion of a Spanish noble family.

"Look," he called in Spanish to Roberto, his twelve-year-old brother. "See how far it stretches." Pedro's voice was typically Andalusian, soft and musical.

Roberto squinted curiously through the thin mountain air. Unlike Pedro's, his skin was light, his lower lip was thick and protruding. His black, curly hair framed blue eyes. His boyish face held a fearless quality unusual for one of his years. As he spoke, he gestured vigorously. "Why shouldn't it stretch far? The guide says that the estate extends to hundreds of hectares. He says that in New Spain the ranchos are so enormous that one can ride for days without passing beyond the domain of a single man."

It had been a long, lonesome ride. Pedro was tired of the mountains of sandstone with the secate climbing to the summits of the flattopped semidomes and an occasional saguaro cactus thrusting itself out of the desert floor like a gigantic inverted tuning fork.

He stood in his stirrups to relax his legs and thighs and looked back over his shoulder. Behind him rode Doña Dolores, his mother, and Manuel, the tall *mozo,* or head servant. As a boy, Manuel's nose had been flattened by the kick of a horse and he wore a look of ineffable melancholy on his broken face as if he were continually in mourning over the displacement of his features. Actually, his sad look did not at all accord with his disposition. He knew horses and mules so well that his opinion about them was widely accepted in Seville. His family had been in the service of the Pavóns for five generations.

Doña Dolores was half Spanish, half gypsy. Her tiny shoes, adorned with buckles of silver, peeped out from beneath the folds of the great cape that protected her against the rain. A pink cameo pendant fastened to the lobe of one small ear was the only jewel visible. It was the gift of her husband Felipe, who had stayed behind in Seville to manage his tobacco factory. Over her brown hair she wore a lavender silk handkerchief tied so that one of the ends fell across her shoulder in the manner of a hood. Framed within the handkerchief was a strikingly beautiful face, gay and vivacious and perceptive.

Behind her and Manuel came Father Fita, the roundfaced padre who had loyally accompanied them all the way from Spain. Clad in black, he rode huddled forward in his saddle, his head bowed in meditation.

As they picked their way down the mountainside, Pedro noticed that the rancho buildings seemed more Moorish than they had from the summit. Colored tiles of black and green added decoration to the entrance portals. The upper windows were enhanced with graceful wrought-iron grates and were filled with potted flowers. Grass mats hung at the doors and windows to interrupt the fiery sun.

White walls, punctuated by semifortified entrances, encircled the entire establishment. The year was 1867 and the Rancho de Pavón lay just outside the raiding perimeter of the wild Comanche and Apache Indian tribes who lived across the Rio Grande.

In the entrance portal Don Luis Pavón, owner of the rancho, stood quietly waiting to greet the two long lines of animals approaching in separate trains down the mountainside. One train, he knew, bore his relatives from faraway Spain. The other train was strange to him. It arrived first, accompanied by a detachment of Mexican rurales clad in gray uniforms and leather leggings. Everybody in this caravan seemed eager to defer to the wishes of the fleshy señora in black who was helped from her horse by the captain of the rurales.

"Señora Ramiro, wife of the Spanish ambassador to Mexico," the captain murmured politely to Don Luis.

A girl dismounted behind the señora, gallantly assisted by two of the rurales. She looked like a pale, delicate fairy.

"Angelita, her daughter," the rurale leader added. "They are bound for Chihuahua to attend a *feria.*"

Don Luis bowed politely. "You and your daughter are most welcome here, señora. Your coming pleases us exceedingly." He spoke in slow, almost stately Spanish. He had the air of a man accustomed to authority and ease.

The señora turned her back on him and squinted with curious hostility at the approaching Pavón train.

"Isn't that the Pavón boy who was banished from Spain for attacking the governor?" she asked.

Don Luis' leathery cheeks reddened with surprise. Banished? Was that why his nephews were making such an unexpected trip to the New World? He had barely been notified of their coming by his brother Felipe.

"My nephew, señora. His mother and younger brother are with him. I am sure that the governor must have instigated the trouble by offending them first."

The señora snorted. "You are mistaken, señor. I know all about the case. I was in Seville when it happened. My sister has written me the latest details from Madrid." With an imperious swish of her skirts, she turned to her daughter. "Come, Angelita!"

Don Luis watched her flounce into a guesthouse. He had little time to think about the implications of her news. The second caravan had arrived.

Pedro, Roberto, and Doña Dolores, followed by their retinue, rode slowly up the pavement of black-and-white river pebbles to the entrance patio.

Don Luis stepped forward, extending his arms. His face was aglow with the happiness of a man who was seeing his brother's family for the first time.

"I am Luis Pavón, Felipe's brother. My home is yours."

The long ride apparently had not exhausted Doña Dolores. She took Don Luis' hand and dismounted easily, light as thistledown. As she stood beside him, she scarcely came to his shoulder, although he was a man of only medium height.

She smiled up at him. "Thank you. It is good to be here."

Don Luis inwardly congratulated his brother upon his choice of a wife. She had come of a wealthy family of Madrid gypsies whose wives and daughters were famous for their beauty and their love of fashion. They were all Spanish citizens, and in the clan was a gypsy lawyer and a famous gypsy bullfighter. Doña Dolores was influential in the Catholic Ladies' Aid, could quote the New Testament almost by heart, knew Cervantes and Shakespeare, and spoke Romany, Spanish, and French.

A cry of pleasure pealed from the doorway as the wife of Don Luis saw her guests. Doña Rita, small and blonde, hurried from the ranchhouse. Clasping both of Doña Dolores' small hands in hers, she kissed her warmly and embraced her. She embraced Pedro and Roberto and addressed them by their Christian names.

Pedro stood quietly at his mother's side, his dark face impassive. Then a driver from the Pavón train almost dropped a polished maple guitar case from a pack saddle. Pedro stepped quickly to the man's side and spoke to him in a low voice. Cringing from the boy's words, the driver shrank back against his mule. And Manuel, the *mozo* standing nearby, busied himself with his pack as if he did not want to be noticed.

"Come! Let us go inside where you can rest and be comfortable," Don Luis urged. "We'll have a glass of wine first, supper later. You must be weary from your long ride. After you've rested, I should like to hear about my brother. I'm sorry he could not come."

As they walked toward the ranchhouse, Don Luis studied Pedro, seeking to evaluate him. Don Luis had little affection for Spain, the decadent land of his birth. He knew what the average young Spanish aristocrat was like—proud, unintelligent, dreary, possessed of an exalted notion of his own personal dignity and preoccupied with dress, gossip, and love. But perhaps Pedro was different. Because of his love of music and the influence of his parents, this fifteen-year-old boy might not wholly fit the mold.

Don Luis paused at the doorway and struck his palms together sharply, twice. "Carlos! Put their belongings in the southwest downstairs rooms. And help with the unloading."

"Bueno!" Carlos, a fat little porter whose sombrero hung carelessly down his back, began to spout a torrent of Spanish, and rancho servants came running from all over the patio to obey him.

Manuel, of the Pavón train, quickly found himself the center of an excited group of porters who seemed to tumble over themselves helping him unload the luggage.

"Which is the guitar player?" Carlos asked.

"Is he the hawkfaced boy?"

"What's he like? We hear he has a fierce temper. We hear that in Monterrey he poured a plate of boiled fowl over the head of a waiter who accidentally spilled hot soup on his brother."

Manuel laughed as he wrestled with the network of rawhide ropes and wooden hooks that held the loads on the pack saddles. "He has spirit. Boils over like a pot of hot peppers occasionally. But what Spanish boy doesn't? Hand me that strap, will you please, *amigo*?" They scurried to assist him.

An old man wearing brown pantaloons and a short jacket ornamented with silver bullion stepped forward, holding his sombrero in his wrinkled hands. "Señor," he said respectfully, "the guide told us that his skill is so great that he can play a guitar that is not tuned." There was a touch of wonder in his creaking voice.

"They say that Roberto obeys his older brother like a child," added another.

Manuel grunted as he tugged at a rope. "Yes, the guitarist is very fond of his brother. Please be careful of that large bundle. It contains their bedding."

"Bedding? Señor, is it true that even on this trip, the brothers slept between silk sheets?"

"We hear that back in Spain they speak three languages and bathe each night in rosewater."

Manuel flashed a look of scorn on the interrogators. "The *guitarrista* speaks five languages in addition to Romany. Roberto speaks only three but he is learning a fourth. They live busy lives. Their mother takes them to visit the museum at Madrid twice a week. There they study the paintings under the personal direction of the curator. At their summer house in San Sebastián they attend the horseraces, the sailing regattas, and the bullfights."

"Don Luis says the younger has lung fever. What a pity!"

Manuel glared at him tolerantly. "It is Pedro, the guitar player, who has a touch of the lung fever. That's why his parents permit him to travel in the south of Spain each year with his mother's kinsmen, the gypsies. The doctor says the climate and the life in the open are good for him. And it's good for his playing, too. Each autumn, the best gypsy guitarists in the realm teach him all they know."

The old man in brown pantaloons again shoved himself forward. "Don Luis says he is the greatest young guitarist in the world."

Carlos corrected him. "He didn't say the greatest in the world, Pablo. Just the greatest in Spain."

Manuel looked pityingly at both of them. "It's all the same. The world's greatest guitarists have always come from Spain."

He unbuckled the pack saddle and peeled it off the mule's back. "*Arre, mula!*" he growled, and clouted it on the rump with his bare hand. Freed of its burden, the grateful beast broke into a shambling half trot, then laid down and rolled in the dust.

"Have patience," Manuel told them. "You will hear him soon. He never gets enough of his guitar. There has been little opportunity on this journey for him to enjoy it."

That very evening, Pedro Pavón gave his first concert in the New World. Don Luis had ordered a space cleared on a large patio of cobblestones and everyone on the rancho turned out. All around sat the men in clean white jackets and trousers and the women in brilliantly colored skirts and scarves. The children came, too. They knelt inside the circle of their fathers' arms or sat quietly in their mothers' laps. People were even clustered on the flattopped roofs of the adobe farm buildings.

As Don Luis and Pedro walked together to the patio, Don Luis said to his nephew, "Tell me, why did you choose to learn the guitar? When I think of the guitar, I think of an instrument used for playing accompaniments, or for having fun at parties."

A flush darkened Pedro's cheeks. He looked straight at his

uncle. "That is the only thing my father and I ever quarreled about. He wanted me to play the piano or the violin." Pedro patted the maple guitar case he was carrying. "Back in Andalusia I heard many instruments but all of them frightened me. When I listened to a violin I was conscious of its scratching tone and I said, '*Ai!* Not for me!' When I heard a piano I became terrified at its blurred thunder. It was the same with the violoncello. Although I loved music with all my heart and soul, I could not find an instrument I could love."

They had arrived at the patio. Carefully Pedro put down the maple case and leaned against the limestone wall. "Meanwhile, there was the guitar that I heard about me all the time. No matter how poorly or indifferently it was played, to me it sounded musical, beautiful. So I decided that I must have been waiting for the guitar from the time when I was born. And my mother supported me against my father. And he gave in."

Don Luis nodded thoughtfully and then excused himself. He turned to greet the ladies and escort them to the leather seats that were placed along the plaza wall.

Pedro, with his long tapering fingers, fashioned a brown paper *cigarrillo* as he watched the people gather. He had eagerly accepted Don Luis' invitation to play, rejecting the suggestion that he was tired. When he was playing, everything about him seemed vibrantly alive. In every kilometer of their long overland trek from Vera Cruz, he had been caught by some scene or sound or wayside scent. The melodies had come in a rush and he could hardly wait for the next camping spot so he could unleash his guitar and interpret them into music. But alas! The train could not always stop and many of the melodies escaped him forever, vanishing like the dewdrops glistening in the sunshine on the manzanillas growing along the trail. He lit his cigarette and inhaled deeply. As the blue smoke drifted aimlessly upward, he turned to listen to the local musicians Don Luis had brought in to lend variety to the occasion.

Two brothers with black, sleek heads played a mandolin duet. An itinerant troubadour sang several ballads, accompanying himself on a little Spanish harp. Finally, as the red moon climbed slowly over the flat adobe roofs, Don Luis turned to Pedro, smiled, and nodded.

Pedro rose and opened the guitar case. From its plush interior he lifted a blond instrument, age-browned and paper-thin. It was strung with gut and had ebony-pegged screws for tuning.

As soon as he touched it, Pedro felt a familiar tremor pass through him. His fingers tingled and his heart thumped with excitement. He marveled again at the overpowering effect the touch of the instrument always had upon him.

For a moment he held it lovingly. His mother had bought it for him after much searching and great expense. It was adorned with an inlay of rosewood, and its backs and sides were made of cherry. It was one of the best guitars old Kantun had made. What a Stradivarius was to a violinist, a Kantun was to a guitarist. They were very dear and very scarce.

Pedro sat in a chair and put the instrument across his right thigh. Like all Andalusians, he was a born exhibitionist. He had chosen his costume carefully: a lawn shirt with innumerable pleats, a short tight-fitting jacket of tan silk, a red silk sash wound tightly around his waist, and knee breeches of brown cloth. His feet were clad in morocco shoes ornamented with embroidery.

He wiped the strings with a satin handkerchief, then held his ear over the sounding hole. Gently twisting the pegs, he brushed the strings lightly with his thumb.

The sound climbed sweetly into the soft air and the audience grew quiet. Pedro noted with satisfaction that the tone was crisp and true. The guitar needed very little tuning in the dry mountain climate. He saw for the first time the proud Señora Ramiro and her daughter Angelita sitting in leather chairs along the plaza wall. He resolved to impress the girl with his music and to meet her later, if he could.

He began with a few quick exercises to limber his fingers, then the age-browned instrument began to sing. It had a full, rich resonance, a carrying power that reached into all the corners of the patio. At first Pedro played what was familiar to many of his listeners—Mozart, Scarlatti, Sor. He felt no tension of any kind. These people were friendly. Without pausing between numbers, he began a fugue by Bach. He saw his aunt lean forward with a little gasp of pleasure. Pedro knew that Bach was her favorite composer for both the organ and the clavichord. She had told him earlier that she had never heard the masters played on the guitar.

His left hand flashed three octaves up and down the ebony neck while his right hand whirred above the sounding hole. He played with a delicacy and sentiment that seemed to abhor all exaggeration. There was something in his music for everybody. He was listened to with religious silence.

Then he began to improvise. His black head was almost buried in the instrument's sounding hole as his brown fingers swept across the strings. He played with a constant sense of exploration. As he developed his theme, it became a gentle pastoral. The music sang along, softly and sweetly. He made the guitar echo the exact timbre of the bell worn by the little bronco burro that led their train down the steep mountain trail. In his imagination, Pedro introduced the rancho, a moorish-Spanish creation in the New World, and made his music express its activity, its hospitality, its peace, and finally his warm joy at being united with his father's kinsmen.

Then, yielding to his homesickness, he took his audience to a gypsy dance back in Granada, attacking the sounding board furiously, thwacking it to get the rhythmic effect of the dancers' heels and the click of their castanets. *Dzing! dzing!* rang the guitar. The rhythm was strong, the noise and speed electric. The rancho people began to tap their feet on the cobblestones. Their fingers snapped, their bodies swayed. They began to call out, *"Ole! Ole!"*

Abruptly, Pedro abandoned the dance and began a gypsy romance. His youthful tenor rang out upon the darkness clear and sweet as it slid mournfully from one note to another in a series of infinitesimal gradations: *"Enamoradita estoy, no me lo conoce nadie. . . ."*

> *I love, and no one knows I love you well.*
> *The deepest loves are those one doesn't tell.*

But mainly, he let his guitar tell the story. And all the time he played, Pedro kept stealing glances at Angelita. He knew that he had captivated her along with the rest of his audience. He could feel their approval in the darkness. He could hear their breathing quicken as their minds raced after the music, elated when it took a pleasant, familiar turn, displeased when it veered off at some unexpected tangent, yet so charmed and mesmerized by it that they could not have left it under any circumstances.

Afterward, Pedro came forward to meet the guests. Doña Rita, his aunt, had him by the arm. Before he could dispose of the half-smoked cigarette in his hand he was being introduced to the Señora Ramiro. And as he bowed, the ash dropped on Angelita's white gown. There was a tiny ruby smolder, a curl of smoke, the acrid smell of burning cloth. Señora Ramiro screamed. Pedro whipped off his silk jacket and flung it around Angelita to smother the tiny glow. He began to apologize. Señora Ramiro's facial muscles tightened into ugly knots and her fingernails became claws poised to scratch.

"You stupid gypsy lout!" she screeched.

Pedro stood still. He felt his insides gnarling and kinking. His mother and Father Fita moved quickly to his side.

Angelita looked appealingly at her mother, "No, *mamá!* I'm not burned. It was just an accident." She flashed one look at Pedro, then ran into her chamber. Her sobs echoed across the patio.

Pedro dimly heard his mother speak. There was scorn and pity in her lovely voice. "Señora, you have not the power to disparage my race. The origin of all mankind was the same. The man or woman of true quality is not one who decorates herself with genealogical tables but she whose actions and behavior cause her to be held in high repute. I am glad your daughter was not burned. I am sorry about her gown. I will be happy to replace it."

But Señora Ramiro merely sneered in answer and sailed from their presence like a proud sloop from a hostile harbor. Don Luis shook his head. "I always thought understanding came with age," he said. "Now I'm not so sure."

They dined that night in the Spanish manner, the men in one dining room, the ladies in another. The furniture was of mahogany, hand-carved a century earlier. Don Luis sat at the head of the men's table, straight and slender. Doña Rita presided at the women's. Her linen was very fine, and her silver bore the stamp of the royal arms of Spain.

The sight of the royal arms brought back afresh Pedro's recollection of his banishment. He wondered if he could ever erase the searing memory from his mind.

His debut at the Royal Theater in Madrid had been so successful that the foremost music critic of Spain had written, "After hearing the Pavón boy play, one has the voluptuous sense of passing the fingers through masses of richly colored jewels."

For nine wonderful days the name of Pedro Pavón rang through Spain like a deep-toned bell. He patronized the finest cafes, had his own box in the theater, and was saluted on the streets with a low bow by persons of taste and quality. Scores of people made congratulatory calls at his parents' home. It seemed that everybody in the realm wanted to hear him play.

A tour of Spain had been arranged for him and after it there was to be a tour of the Continent. He could hardly wait to play in all the distant and gorgeous theaters of the world, and to prove to the audiences of each that Spanish music had a charm all of its own and that the guitar was its finest medium.

Two days before his concert in Seville, he had practiced six hours so he would have time to visit his friends, the gypsies at the Granada, and enjoy one last musical spree with them. But that was not to be. Pedro shut his eyes. *Better not to think about it.*

He tried to concentrate on Doña Rita's excellent food—a savory cheese, lamb dressed with dried raisins, baked eggs and tamales, wine. But Pedro only picked at the food. Then came honeycakes and a delicious cinnamon-flavored chocolate that Doña Rita brewed in a small earthen pot. But Pedro scarcely touched it.

After dinner, his uncle led him into a small private room beside a fire of piñon knots. As Pedro entered, the sight of the coat of arms of the Pavón family leaped out at him from the wall over the fireplace. It had four quarterings: the first and fourth displayed a gold star of eight rays against a blue field, the second and third showed a black wolf walking fearlessly against a background of gold. Proudly, Pedro caught his breath. The antiquity and preeminence of the house of Pavón went so far back that historians had been unable to find its true beginning. And yet the ambassador's wife had had the insolence to identify him as a gypsy, ignoring his true blood!

As Pedro carefully formed a brown paper cigarette, his fingers trembled and he spilled tobacco on the black bearskin rug beneath his feet.

"Uncle, I'm in trouble," he blurted miserably.

Don Luis touched a lighted taper to Pedro's cigarette; then applied it to his own long cigar. "Your troubles are my troubles, nephew," he said, and settled back into his large leather chair.

Pedro was grateful for the opportunity to unburden himself. He told his uncle of his banishment and filled in the details Don Luis had not heard. Pedro's father was of noble birth, but because of his mother's gypsy ancestry the family was not always accepted at court functions. The marriage had cost Pedro's father the governorship: he had been the popular candidate but the appointment had gone instead to Carbonero Grimaldi, a pompous, arrogant noble who was the queen's favorite. All this infuriated Pedro.

He felt he had avenged his whole family on the night of his triumph in Madrid's Royal Theater. His guitar would get the approval he wanted for his family and for himself. He wanted the name Pavón to be known and respected the length and breadth of Spain. He had worked hard to develop the priceless gift of his music. And Spain had accepted it.

Pedro felt himself go tense as he tried to repress the recollection of that morning in Seville. He and Roberto were walking along the promenade just before dinner. It was the city's most prominent street and was most crowded at that time of day.

They heard the smooth roll of wheels and the *clop-clop-clop* of a fast-trotting horse. Sitting high in the royal chaise rode the new governor, Carbonero Grimaldi, bowing haughtily from right to left. People swept off their hats in obeisance.

Neither Pedro nor Roberto lifted his hat. As Grimaldi recognized them, his face flushed. He ordered his carriage stopped. Standing up, he struck Roberto, the nearest Pavón, across the shoulders with his riding whip.

"Gypsy dogs!"

Pedro leaped into the royal carriage. His long evenings of practice with the best knife fighters in the gypsy camps had not been wasted, especially the quickness he had learned when facing an enemy who was armed when he was not.

Grasping the governor's beefy wrist, Pedro jerked him out to the pavement and slapped him resoundingly half a dozen times across his fat, powdered cheeks. As a final gesture, he wrenched the whip away from the governor, broke it over his knee, and tossed its fragments into the street. Then the Pavón brothers turned their backs and resumed their promenade.

As they neared their home Roberto stopped and stared. "Brother, aren't those soldiers before our father's house?"

They were indeed. And before the affair was settled, the gypsy lawyer on their mother's side of the family had rushed by carriage from Madrid to aid their father in the defense. Although Pedro was the darling of the populace, the governor was the delegate of the queen. For his outrage upon the governor's dignity, it was finally agreed by a compromise that Pedro would be banished to New Spain to carry on his education at the university in Mexico City. But included in the compromise was permission to visit his uncle's ranch far to the north.

Don Luis looked at the tip of his cigar, then at Pedro. There was sympathy in the lean, understanding face.

"Forget Spain and live all your life in this fine, new country," Don Luis urged him warmly. "Why go back to the Old World? Every Spaniard who has a drop of daring in his soul comes to the new lands of America to drink the wine of freedom. Here he can intoxicate himself in adventure, make a quick fortune, and enjoy it where he made it. You, my nephew, can have such a fortune too. I will help you acquire it."

Pedro looked at his uncle respectfully.

"Music is my fortune, Uncle. And while I like what I have seen of your new country, there is no challenge in it for my music. I would seldom be heard."

Don Luis leaned forward. "Why not forget music until

later?" he entreated. "Here you can be a man! Here you will never be banished. Here you can rise! Here is glory, pleasure, wealth, a wonderful living. What's music compared to all this?"

Pedro realized that his uncle would never understand. . . .

Next morning, the party of the ambassador's wife departed shortly after sunup. From his bed, Pedro heard the creaking of their packsaddles and the jingle of their bridles. He had rested poorly and still felt a slight fatigue.

At his mother's insistence, he stayed in his room most of the day.

"My son, you must cultivate calmness," she said soothingly. "Life is too short to be spent nursing some furious passion. When you have made your place in the world with your music —and you shall—you will cease resenting these references to our Romany ancestry."

Pedro smiled wanly. "Thank you, dear Mother," he said, and patted her hand.

By midafternoon he felt so much better that when he asked his uncle about the extent of the rancho, Don Luis put the brothers on his personal saddlehorses and conducted them on a canter along the mesa to show them the range and scope of his holdings.

The ride made Pedro hungry. He ate heartily, and went early to the first-floor apartment where his aunt had established them. He was tired from the restlessness of the previous night and slept soundly.

Four hours after midnight, Pedro awakened. He was conscious of figures moving stealthily in the room. Blinking with drowsiness, he thought at first that Doña Rita's softly treading female servants were tidying up the chamber while the guests were still abed. Suddenly from the patio outside his window there burst a wild cry of horror. Pedro felt his scalp rise.

"Muchos indios! Muchos indios!"

He raised himself on his elbow. The terrible cry burst upon his ears again, louder, closer, more urgent. Running footsteps drummed on the cobblestones outside. Other yells of alarm rang out. A gun went off. Hoofbeats of running horses filled the courtyard.

Pedro's breath felt hot in his throat. He raised to his knees and looked around the large apartment. There was a stirring near his mother's bed on the other side of the wide room. In the gray light, he saw a figure rise and bend over her.

"No!" Pedro yelled. He ran across the apartment.

His mother somehow evaded the figure standing over her and ran lightly through the door onto the patio, but the man overtook her before she had gone half a dozen steps. Grasping her by one arm, he brought his cudgel down upon her head in a short, sideways arc.

As long as he lived, Pedro never forgot the sound of that blow. It reminded him of the squashing noise of a melon hurled against a stone wall.

Quickly, working with incredible swiftness, the attacker tore off the scalp with one powerful sweep. He was attaching the bloody trophy to his girdle when Pedro reached him.

With a strangled cry the boy slashed the murderer's cheek with his fingernails, scarifying it with four bloody furrows. He saw the face with its big nose that was hooked like the beak of an eagle. Evil and brutish, it looked ghastly in the light of the early dawn. Then a blow from behind felled Pedro.

2 · Terror at Dawn

When he opened his eyes, the cold gray of the eastern sky had become purple. He was sitting bareback on a horse. Groggily, he noticed that it was one of Don Luis' blooded animals, and he didn't understand. His head ached cruelly. He smelled smoke and saw long plumes of fire curling from a window down the court. Other naked figures emerged from the ranchhouse, carrying loot. The sickening knowledge struck Pedro that the ranch was being raided by Indians.

His mother's body, still and crumpled, lay in a small heap on the patio stones. He tried to go to her but he could not work his arms or legs. He had wit enough left to know what was going on but he couldn't move. The blow had partially paralyzed him. His head pained him sorely. He could feel blood from the wound on the back of his head oozing down inside his shirt.

The rancho bell clanged, tolling an alarm. Pedro shook his head, trying to clear it. If the bell was ringing, then the Indians must have possession of only a part of the ranch. The morning air was stinging cold. Pedro's senses began to return. Feeling came back into his limbs. He heard shouting. Gunfire echoed. He smelled powder.

The patio swarmed with strange, fierce-looking men mounted bareback on horses. They had weapons in their hands—lances, warclubs, knives. Most of them wore drooping yellow feathers in their straight, black hair. Pedro had never

19

seen anything like the looks on their faces, the cruelty and the bestiality. Nor had he ever seen such horses. There were browns, blacks, yellows, roans, pintos, buckskins, bays. They had thick, unruly manes and long tails that brushed the patio stones. Their feet were small, their limbs delicate, and their eyes mischievous and mean. They looked as wild as their riders, who controlled them with an easy expertness that seemed almost casual.

Again Pedro's eyes fell upon his mother's form. He stared at her, knowing she was dead yet unable to accept the fact. Weakly, he half slid, half fell off the horse and tried to crawl to her.

"Madre mia! Madrecita mia!" he breathed.

A quirt across his back stopped him. It burned like fire. He was jerked to his feet, picked up bodily, and flung astride the horse. Someone tied his feet underneath the horse's belly and his hands behind his back. Obviously, his captors intended to take him with them.

From a nearby doorway, Roberto ran out into the midst of the savages. His eyes were swollen with sleep and his curly black hair was mussed. He still wore his sleeping garments.

He made such a ludicrous figure that the mounted Indian nearest him broke into laughter. One urged his horse forward, hemming the boy against the wall. Roberto ran under the horse's neck. Another yelled at him and spurred his animal against him but Roberto dropped to hands and knees and dodged under the second horse's belly.

A third Indian flanked his horse forward and pointed his lance straight at Roberto's belly. On the Indian's chest and ribs were battle scars made obvious by green tattoo marks inscribed around them, as though the owner was proud of them.

Roberto looked him fearlessly in the eye. The Indian spoke in a strange tongue as he lifted his lance. Reaching down, he patted Roberto on the back.

"Bravo," he grunted.

Roberto seemed to decide that resistance was useless. He walked straight up to Green Tattoo Marks. The man reached down, took him by the hand, and extended his foot. Roberto stepped upon the moccasined foot and was hoisted onto the horse's back, in front of his captor. The man grunted an order and they all moved off.

As they trotted down the pavement of black-and-white river pebbles, the birds sang sweetly from the madrone trees along the way. The eastern horizon crimsoned prettily, dyeing the undersides of a nearby cloudbank lavender and gold. Heart-sick, Pedro wondered how there could be so much violence and suffering on such a beautiful July morning. He twisted, trying to look back. The effort agitated the welt across his back.

His lips moved. "O Virgin Mary, Mother of all Christians, living and dead. Behold me, dear Mary, supplicating thee to intercede for the soul of my dear departed mother . . ."

His horse shied as they passed the bodies of the dead rancho people lying along the roadside. Pedro saw his uncle lying face up in a sprawl, his head in a pool of blood. The brown beard pointed straight into the sky, and there was an expression of agony on his features. He had been lanced and scalped. The hilt of a broken sword was still clutched defiantly in his right hand. Pedro thought of his aunt, wondering what had been her fate.

Again he prayed. "Intercede also, Virgin Mary, for the soul of my dear departed uncle. Look with compassion upon us who are left to mourn . . ."

The horses began to gallop. Pedro threw one last look across his shoulder, searching for his mother's still form. Hot tears stung his eyes. He sobbed quietly.

An old gypsy song of mourning began taking form in his consciousness. In his stupefaction and grief he could not sing it. But the words and the tune kept running through his mind. . . .

Oh sweet Mother, thy mouth is closed and thy voice stilled.
  Thy feet go no more over the green heath,
Thy hands are dead and work no more!
  Oh Mother, thine eyes see not the greenwood,
Thy ears hear not the birds.
  Thou dost not kiss thy little flower.

All morning they traveled northward. The desert sun struck like a burning glass. In the growing heat, the deep cut across Pedro's back began to smart and swell. It pained him with each stride of his mount. He rode bareback until midday, then was changed to an Indian pony whose primitive wooden saddle had no stirrups. His bonds were removed and he had more freedom of movement. His bloody shirt was ripped from his crusted back and claimed by one of his captors. They started up again.

His mother's murderer rode just ahead and his sweetish, fetid smell kept coming back to Pedro. Like all the others, this man wore footwear of beaded buckskin and was naked except for a rude cloth contrivance about his crotch. This ingenious device was anchored by a buckskin string tied about the man's waist. A long length of dirty cloth that had once been white apparently had been drawn under the string at the waist and passed between the legs and brought back up under the string behind. The loose end in front hung nearly to his knees, the rear flap swung behind like a tail. The man constantly turned around and stared at Pedro malignantly, pointing significantly to the four red scars across his face as though plotting some terrible revenge.

The sun arched above them, then began to descend. Pedro felt his back blistering. The skin on the inside of his legs was rubbed raw by friction from the forked-stick saddle. Fierce pangs of hunger assailed him. He was worried about Roberto and kept looking ahead, trying in vain to identify his brother among the naked riders bobbing up and down on the horses. Dripping with sweat, he tried to smother the grunts of pain that escaped him.

When the sun set, the air became cooler and the riding somewhat easier. Pedro wondered when they would make camp, but still they loped silently across the miles. The sunset settled into darkness and the darkness into night, midnight, and early morning. Now it took all of Pedro's strength just to stay on the back of his horse. Dully, he fretted about how his brother was standing the cruel ride, for Roberto was only twelve.

It was when the sun arose on Pedro's right, showing they were still traveling north, that he saw Roberto for the first time since they had left the ranch. His brother had gone to sleep sitting up. The warrior with the green tattoo marks was holding the dozing boy in the saddle in front of him. Roberto's tousled black head was cradled against the man's chest. Pedro felt a great sense of relief.

Soon the sun's rays shone hotly again and Pedro felt his face blistering. He saw the skin peeling off his arms and breast and thighs. And where the sides of his legs rubbed against the crude saddle, his flesh was lacerated and torn. He rode with his chin sagging on his breast, and the pangs of his suffering came over him in dull waves.

Occasionally he raised his head and studied his captors. He had never seen such horsemen. Slovenly and ungraceful on the ground, they rode as though born on horseback and seemed to be part of the animals they straddled. Cautious and wary, they never manifested emotion or excitement. Many of them looked quite young. They all had hideous, repulsive faces.

Pedro felt sorry for Don Luis' blooded horses, accustomed only to regimented daily exercise, careful feeding, and affectionate treatment from the grooms. His captors had no regard for the physical welfare of the captured animals, running them at full speed over the stony ground and making no halts to breathe them.

Most heartless was Four Scars, his mother's murderer. He rode a small black that had been Doña Rita's favorite. Don Luis had told Pedro the animal was so gentle that it followed Doña Rita about the rancho like a dog. It had known no other rider but her. The Indian used his heavy Spanish spurs so viciously that the little horse's flanks were torn and bloody. The animal seemed terrified of its rider. Its eyes almost bulged out of its head, its mouth frothed, and a film of perspiration lathered its body. All day long the Indian pushed it cruelly in the desert heat.

Finally, in midafternoon of the second day, the gallant little beast began to flounder. Pedro saw blood on one hoof: it had cut its front fetlock on a rock. The Indian applied his quirt vigorously and for a few strides the animal accelerated its pace. Suddenly it lurched to its knees and fell on its side. The Indian leaped nimbly to the ground. Still holding the reins, he began to quirt the horse while it lay wheezing for breath. Then he began pounding it over the head with the butt of his quirt. The horse staggered to its feet. Instantly he leaped astride, whipping it with redoubled effort. The animal somehow broke into a slow, labored gallop and caught up with the others.

They camped that night in a copse of scrub pine. Bone-tired, Pedro felt himself pulled off his horse. At first he could not stand. The ground kept coming up to meet him. He was so accustomed to the motion of the horse that it seemed as if he were still astride. He got one foot under him and crawled to his feet. His body felt like one big scab.

Three fierce-looking warriors walked up, and without ceremony, pushed him down and began pulling off the rest of his clothing. Soon he was almost naked. Now one of them was wearing Pedro's red silk sleeping garments. Another wore the lace shirt and red broadcloth trousers that apparently had been taken from the sleeping room back at the rancho. Then they left him.

"Brother!" Roberto walked up, rubbing his numb limbs. He had been permitted to keep his clothing, probably because it was too small to fit his captors. He seemed unable to comprehend the events of the last two days and their own involvement in them.

"What do they intend doing with us?"

Pedro felt his brother's blind reliance on him. Desolation swept through him. He feared that the *indios* meant to kill them. He didn't understand why they waited.

"I don't know, Roberto. Perhaps we will be ransomed."

He told Roberto of the death of their mother, and of Don Luis. Incomprehension, then shock came into Roberto's boyish face. Pedro's heart went out to the boy. Moving closer, he smoothed Roberto's disheveled black hair and put his arms around his brother.

Roberto did not cry. A strange look came into his face. Roughly, he threw off Pedro's embrace and stared at him with hostility and disbelief.

"It's true, Roberto," Pedro insisted. As he repeated the story, and related details, certainty gradually came through to Roberto. But still he did not weep. He looked sullen and bewildered. He sat on the ground and stared absently at the rocks.

Pedro was concerned about his brother's hunger. He knew Roberto had not eaten a morsel of food for two days. Pedro himself was not hungry. His heart seemed swollen to an unnatural size within him and he felt he would never want food again.

But the raiders, he noticed, had their own way of solving the hunger problem: Quirt in hand, Four Scars walked up to Doña

Rita's suffering colt. Growling like a wild animal, he jumped threateningly, striking the ground with his quirt. As the colt lunged away, terror in its eyes, the Indian threw back his head and laughed, a laugh so cold and barbarous that Pedro felt tiny shivers of hate running up his spine. Four Scars reached behind him and drew from his wildcat quiver a short bow and a single stone-headed arrow. Fitting the arrow to the string, he drew it full length and released it into the colt's heaving flank. The animal dropped and kicked convulsively. Pedro saw with surprise that the shaft had penetrated so deeply that only the top of its feathered tuft showed in the animal's side.

Steaks were cut from the dead colt and quickly roasted over a fire. The Indians bolted down the half-cooked meat, wiping the grease from their mouths onto their leggings and breechclouts. The man with green tattoo marks indicated by pointing that Pedro and Roberto were welcome to eat some of the meat. Pedro refused. But Roberto nibbled tentatively at a fire-blackened rib.

Pedro resolved to escape that very night. After making the decision, he felt calmer. Any action was better than the agony that lay ahead. He would wait until his captors slept, then waken Roberto. They would take two horses and ride back to the ranch.

Because they had no blankets, the Indians lay closely together for warmth, like animals. Pedro was made to lie on the ground between two of them. They smelled so filthy that he shrank from their touch but they only snuggled closer. Revulsion surged through him but he had to bear it. Besides, it was warmer with them close to him.

In his drowsiness he wondered where the horses were tethered and which would carry them fastest. The moon was rising. His eyelids fluttered sleepily. The last thing he remembered was listening to the savage nearest him snore. The noise reminded him of something he once had seen in a zoo at

Granada, a bear sliding down a tree backward, noisily shredding bark with all four of its clawed feet.

He was roused by a kick before dawn. Awakening, he felt hungry and despondent. He had overslept. While the savages breakfasted on the cold horsemeat, Pedro sat with his back toward them, his thoughts alternately occupied by recollections of home and by contemplation of his present predicament. He thought again of escape, then rejected it. Escape would be far more difficult if he took Roberto and he would not think of leaving without his brother.

All morning he rode, staring stonily at the glistening brown back of Four Scars bobbing up and down in front of him. A *copla* suggested itself to him. He hummed the quatrain ever so lightly to take his mind off his wounds. *"Permita Dios de los cielos . . ."*

> *I hope to God I see you fall*
> *And die in frightful pain.*
> *I hope I live to hurl the stone*
> *That dashes out your brain.*

The sun grew hotter. Pedro rode in agony, his open welts smarting from the perspiration that ran down into them. Once they stopped at the river for a drink and Pedro saw Roberto briefly as side by side they bent over to gulp the brackish water.

"The leader made me sleep in his arms last night," Roberto reported. "He smelled horribly. I laid awake for three hours, waiting for him to go to sleep so I could escape. About midnight, just as I was about to try, he squeezed me real hard. It was as though he had read my thoughts in his dreams. It discouraged me. I went back to sleep and did not awaken until morning. If they're that alert I'm afraid we'll never get away."

The third night the Indians killed another horse for food. Although Pedro was weak with hunger, again he turned away with loathing when Four Scars handed him a hunk of the scorched horseflesh.

Rage burned suddenly in the Indian's face. Grasping his quirt, he dealt Pedro a blow that knocked him flat and raised a new red welt across his left shoulder.

Roberto, standing nearby, cried out hoarsely and leaped on Four Scars' back, fastening his teeth into the Indian's arm. With a howl of rage, Four Scars flung him to the ground and struck him twice with the quirt before the man with the green tattoo marks seized his arm, grunting a protest. It was plain he considered the younger Pavón his personal prize.

Four Scars turned to Pedro. Again he pointed to the scorched horseflesh. *"Tu kar roo!"* he grunted, commandingly, and raised his quirt.

Pedro bit into the burnt meat. Although it was stringy, it did not taste bad. As the juices went down his throat, his appetite was stimulated. He gulped the meat with relish, but when he reached for another roasted rib, Four Scars pushed him roughly away, refusing to let him have any more.

On the morning of the fourth day, they crossed a shallow river and passed several prairies of mesquite. Pedro noticed that the Indians veered to the east and sent out scouts ahead and to both sides. Once they intersected a rude cow trail and when Pedro saw in the soft sand the imprint of a man's shoe, he felt a thrill of hope. They must be nearing a settlement.

"Have courage," he called softly in Spanish to Roberto, riding nearby on a horse by himself. "I think we are passing near a white settlement."

To Pedro's consternation, Four Scars repeated the words in Spanish, then laughed tauntingly at Pedro's surprise. *"Somos comanches!* We are Comanches!" he boasted in Spanish, drumming his right fist on his chest. "We do not fear your white forts. We pass close to them to elude your warriors trying to intercept us farther out upon the prairie."

But Pedro felt encouraged anyhow, and resolved to talk to Roberto thereafter in German, a language his brother had just begun to study at the Royal Academy in Madrid.

Now the Comanches doubled their caution, moving slowly. Again they tied the wrists of each of their captives and bound their feet together beneath their horses' bellies with buckskin thongs. They stayed away from roads as much as possible, and whenever they had to cross one, sent three or four men back to erase their trail carefully with their hands. Pedro frowned in admiration. These barbarians were devilishly clever. When they finished their effacing, the road looked just as it had before they crossed it.

A peak arose to the north of them. It was covered with quartz outcroppings that blazed in the bright sunshine. It reminded Pedro of a large sugar loaf. They made a halt.

The man with green tattoo marks on his chest rode to the top of a nearby rise and carefully examined the horizon with a fieldglass. The hot wind ruffled the fringe of his leggings. He rode back and grunted an order. A hole was dug, a fire kindled in it, and a wet blanket placed over it. When the blanket was removed after a few minutes, a column of gray smoke climbed almost one hundred feet into the sky.

Soon Pedro saw a similar smoke spiral rising several miles to their left. An hour later, another band of Comanches rode up. Their horses were wet with sweat and obviously had been run hard. These Indians were well armed and heavily laden with loot—everything from calico dresses and blankets to pots and pans. There was blood on their lances and short war axes. One warrior had been shot through the shoulder. A rude poultice of prickly pear leaves was lashed to it, but there was no look of pain in his brutish face as he controlled his fractious mount with one hand.

"We shot the feathers out o' you, anyhow," chuckled an Irish voice nearby. The man was speaking in English.

Pedro saw him, a big fellow with a mop of red hair peppered with gray. He was barefoot, for his shoes had been taken from him as well as most of his clothing. He was standing with another prisoner, a black-haired man whose face was wild with fear. Both wore blue trousers with yellow braid down the sides.

"I'm Shamus and he's Frank. We're cavalrymen from Fort Concho," the Irishman told Pedro. "There's a company of cavalry trailin' us right now. But these brown devils will be hard to come up with."

Pedro stared at his blue trousers. His nostrils distended with suspicion. He did not trust soldiers. Some were friendly, others disloyal. All were blindly obedient to whatever master paid their wages. The queen's soldiers who had arrested him and Roberto had treated them roughly until his father secured their release. For whom were these men fighting? He had heard of the *americanos,* that virile young nation that had just concluded a bloody civil war. But he had never heard of Fort Concho.

"It's rare that these brown divils ever take grown men like us prisoners," Shamus went on. "Usually they want only white children whose minds and habits are pliable and who soon become as Comancheized as the Indians themselves. I'm surprised they haven't kilt Frank and me long ago. They must have something better in mind for us, eh Frank?" His deep, rolling tones sounded genial.

The other man made no answer. His hands were shaking with fright and it was apparent he saw no frivolity in their plight.

Speaking in English, Pedro told Shamus of their capture. When he related that they had been visiting in Mexico when taken, the soldier snorted and lost his geniality.

"Mexico!" he ejaculated bitterly. "That's a land of t'ieves. That's where they herd hogs and the flowers have no scent and the birds no song. That's where they dig for wood with a hoe, cut hay with an ax, and call my Blessed Redeemer Haysoos!" He was so vehement that Pedro fell silent.

Shamus was made to mount in front of a young brave, who was first disarmed so that the big soldier could not get at his weapons. Pedro, Roberto, and the other prisoners were similarly mounted and the party put in motion, heading northwest.

Now the land became more broken, with flattened-out limestone bluffs, deeply carved canyons, and small hills covered with scrub cedar and thorny mesquite. They will never find us in this desolate country, Pedro said to himself sadly.

The Comanches seemed concerned only for their rear, throwing out scouts behind and traveling along the high points where they had a commanding view of the surrounding country. Once they halted and quickly built another signal fire. As the queues of smoke lifted gracefully, Shamus turned grimly to Pedro.

"Telegraphin' their chums that they are bein' pursued," he surmised. "It's by this system that the various bands, separated from each other, keep in contact and maintain a spy system over the lands they raid and plunder. It bates the world, so it does." They resumed their flight, traveling hard.

In midafternoon Pedro heard the faint baying of bloodhounds behind them and his heart leaped hopefully. Green Tattoo Marks grunted an order. Two braves slid off their horses and set fire to the prairie grass behind them. The baying ceased.

Two hours later, Pedro heard the dogs baying again. Shamus pushed his red hair back out of his eyes. "Must be Rangers," he mused. "Probably took the dogs up in their saddles until they rode past the burned places."

Again Green Tattoo Marks grunted and motioned with his hand. He reminded Pedro of a skilled chess player three moves ahead of his opponent. This time another brave dismounted, a buckskin pouch in his hand, and began to pour its contents about the grass on the trail behind them.

Shamus sniffed, frowned, and looked glum. "Skunk musk. That'll knock the poor dogs out of time." Soon the baying behind them stopped again.

A halt was made and a hurried council held. Quickly the Indians separated, scattering in small groups. None of the four captives traveled together now. Each went in a different direction, accompanied by his own small guard. Pedro went with Four Scars. He saw Roberto, his frail shoulders rising and falling with the motion of his horse, turn and look at him beseechingly before riding off into a copse of mesquite with Green Tattoo Marks. An immense wave of loneliness washed over him.

"Don't fret, me dear," Shamus advised kindly, as he was hustled off with his group. "You'll see your brother again. These brown divils are separatin' now so the Rangers will have fifty maddenin' trails to follow 'stead a jist one. We'll all come togither some place up ahead."

The Comanches knew how to deal with pursuit. Riding hard, they deliberately moved westward into a desert area where there was no water and where their white pursuers could not follow them and live. The vegetation grew more scarce each mile they rode. The dry earth was covered with a whitish skim. The sun burned down mercilessly without a cloud or bush to relieve its awful glare. Although the Comanches punished themselves, they eliminated all pursuit. The white dust, stirred by the sultry south wind, tasted salty. It peppered Pedro's bare skin until he felt each pore was full. His eyes became inflamed and his skin began to crack. He could taste the blood from his bleeding lips and feel his tongue swelling.

The Indians ignored everybody's thirst until midafternoon

when a stop was made and a horse killed. With his brass-handled knife, Four Scars opened a vein in the dead animal's leg and the Indians drank the hot blood, forcing Pedro to drink some too. It tasted thick, salty, and warm but Pedro got some down. They resumed their flight at frenzied speed with the sun coming down so hot that the paint on the savages' faces began to melt and run down their cheeks in red-and-yellow smears.

Pedro was appalled by the Indians' inhuman treatment of their horses. There was nothing for the animals to drink, and galled animals were pushed most cruelly. Pedro saw blood flowing down the side of a pinto ridden by a buck. The skin and flesh on its back had been lacerated by a poorly fitting wooden saddle that Pedro judged was Comanche-made; yet the saddle stayed on, and the rider in it. Its plight reminded Pedro of something Shamus had said just before they separated. "When a horse breaks down and can't go a step further, a white man will abandon him. A Mexican will then mount him and ride him fifty miles more and leave him. Then one of these brown divils will mount him and ride him hard for a week."

They kept crossing ravines, the bottoms of which bore the marks of streams dried up. Once they came alongside a small rivulet where clear blue water ran fresh and abundant. However, to Pedro's sorrow, they passed it by and he realized it must be salty.

Weakness overcame him and he began to sway from side to side on his horse. In his delirium, his mind went groping back to his boyhood in Spain when the railroad train in which he and his father were riding through a drought-stricken area had finally arrived at a station in Castile. An ancient water seller, carrying well-filled canvas bags across his shoulders, passed beneath the train windows calling out in quavering Spanish, "Water! Fresh water! Water cooler than snow!"

On and on they traveled. The horizon was always a straight

line and nothing ever rose above it. The dismal sameness became maddening. There were no sounds save the horses'
muted hoofbeats in the hot sand. He was sure the Comanches
must be lost. It seemed to him that they had nothing by which
to calculate their progress.

I'll never escape back to the rancho through this awful desert, Pedro told himself wretchedly. I'll never see Roberto
again.

The next morning they came to an old wallow, or shallow
pond, with a few puddles of muddy water in it. The water was
fouled with green scum. Dead flies and bugs floated on its surface. It smelled bad. The Comanches dismounted. Pedro slid
off his horse and crawled weakly to the water.

Breaking off a handful of grass, he spread it on top of the
water, shut his eyes and began to suck the muddy fluid through
the grass, using it as a strainer. After his first long gulp, he became ill. Recovering, he drank deeply and this time felt better
and had less difficulty keeping the cloudy fluid down. When
they resumed traveling, they went more slowly as though the
danger of pursuit was past.

In the afternoon they emerged from the desert into a broken
country where veins of creamy gypsum showed amid low, rust-
red hills. Cactus grew tightly in the rocks and a few stemless
yuccas dotted the sand. Stunted oaks began to appear. After
what he had been riding through, it all looked wonderful to
Pedro.

An hour later, they rode along an incline and he saw below
a river rushing rapidly out of a rocky tableland. Its crystal
waters flashed in the sunlight. For half a mile the Comanches
rode along its stony heights, then descended to the almost perpendicular bank of the stream where scrub cedar and prickly
pear grew in the cliffs on both sides. Pedro doubted that they
could ever descend the steep cliff to the water. And even if

they could, he believed the stream impossible to cross, so deep was the cleft it rushed through. But an old Indian guided the party to a series of natural steps in the terraces of stone. Leading the horses carefully down these steps, they descended without trouble.

To Pedro's surprise, the river shoaled to a depth of only one foot and the water tasted warm. Men and beasts drank thirstily side by side and for a moment nothing could be heard save the sucking sounds of water going down hot throats and the relieved moans of the drinkers. Then they ascended the opposite bank along a similar series of carved steps which looked as if they had been fashioned centuries before. In late afternoon, they climbed onto a grassy tableland.

Cooler air refreshed them. Here the mesquite trees became instantly taller. Their green plumes, redolent with blossoms, nodded lazily in the breeze. The grass stretched into the distance like an immense grayish-green lawn. And when they camped that night and Pedro saw the heavy orange coloring in the evening sky accentuating the violet shadows of the bluffs, he felt uplifted. He thought his prayers to the Blessed Virgin had been answered and that she had persuaded God to paint the heavens purposely to hearten him.

They were riding through a small grove of gnarled oaks in midmorning of the following day when he heard a strange noise from afar. It sounded like the mewing of seagulls or the gabbling of wild geese. Pedro scanned the heavens but saw nothing. Again he heard the eerie noise. This time it came from upwind and he thought he could discern a human quality in it. Then the wind flawed it.

The Comanches were listening, too. Suddenly they broke into a warwhoop that rang through the woods. Digging their heels into the flanks of their tired horses, they urged them toward the noise. With a quirt, Four Scars struck Pedro's mount across the hind legs and the boy was almost unhorsed as his animal lunged forward with the others. As they swung helterskelter through the trees, Pedro had to dodge overhanging branches.

The mystery babble crystallized into a wind-borne blending of female voices singing a wild, savage song. It was the strangest singing he had ever heard. Although he did not understand the words, the theme of the discordance seemed a fierce, triumphant rejoicing, as though the singers were celebrating an event of barbaric importance.

As the running horses broke into a clearing, Pedro saw the approaching women. Some were mounted on ponies; others ran awkwardly on foot, holding to the legs of the mounted ones. They were coming at full speed.

Never had Pedro seen such hideous creatures. They were dressed in buff-colored deerskin with fringes along the sides of their short skirts and clusters of blue beads on their tunics. Their coarse, straight black hair was cropped and uncombed. The insides of their ears were painted red, and yellow lines were penciled under their eyes. They were dirty and sweaty. Judging from the looks of joy on their broad faces, they had run for miles in the heat to meet their men.

Pedro felt a powerful shove from behind and he fell to the ground on his arms and shoulders. Four Scars had pushed him off his horse. As he got to his feet, dizzy and shaken, he looked again at the approaching females. He realized that instead of pausing to greet their long absent menfolk, the Indian women were all running straight for him, screeching with rage.

Too weak to flee, he could only stare at them. They hurled themselves upon him like angry hens, striking him across the head and shoulders with blows that hurt like a man's. Fingernails tore through the skin on his bare chest, sending stabs of pain through him. He felt as if he were being scratched to death. As they beat him they screamed and shouted with maniacal fury. He buried his face in his arms for protection, and fell to the ground, their stinking bodies on top of him. His eyesight grew dim, his hearing faded, and consciousness mercifully slipped away.

The beating ended almost as speedily as it started and he found himself on hands and knees, his bruised body covered with scores of bloody scratches. To his surprise, the women now ignored him entirely as they turned to greet their husbands, fathers, and brothers. Later, he learned that the squaws were following a tribal custom: great honor went to the one who struck a captive the first blow and a gradually decreasing honor to the second, third, and fourth who did the same.

Pedro was jerked to his feet and thrown onto a horse. Surrounded by the howling mob, he was borne off in triumph to the band's permanent camp.

3 · The Bells of Death

The squaws walked, leading Pedro's horse and hurling shouts and jeers at him. He sat stolidly on the animal's back; his hands were tied, his shoulders drooped. His body felt as if it had been rubbed with a rasp. The scratches on his arms and stomach bled and stung. Twice he caught himself reeling; the beatings and hunger had made him weak.

They halted on an eminence and sent a young warrior ahead to inform the village that they were coming in. Despite the desperation of his plight, Pedro watched their preparations, fascinated by their vanity. The men smeared their faces and bodies with war paint. They rubbed down their horses with grass and polished their weapons. Wounds were circled with bright paint so they would be more noticeable.

Four Scars, adjudged to have most distinguished himself on the raid, won the honor of leading the party in. When he proudly held his lance aloft for all to see, Pedro tried not to look at the tiny tuft of chestnut hair that swung in the wind from its tip along with two other scalps. He rode behind Four Scars, followed by the other warriors who had taken scalps or participated in the raid. The women who had come to meet them had gone ahead, singing paeans of victory at the top of their voices. They ascended a small hill, and as he raised his eyes, Pedro saw the Comanche village in the distance.

Hundreds of small triangular shapes were banked closely to-

gether in a great horseshoe open at the north. In the light of
the morning sun they shone gray and reddish-yellow. They reminded Pedro of the hundreds of idle fishing boats with sails
drawn up like folded wings he had once seen in the great harbor of Cadiz. These must be the skin dwellings of his captors.
Curls of smoke twisted and coiled from their blackened tops,
forming a low cloud that overhung everything. Beyond the
camp, thousands of horses grazed in immense herds, speckling
the green prairie. Pedro forgot his doom and caught his breath
in wonder at the wild scene.

As they rode closer, he saw that the dwellings were conical
rather than triangular. Their walls of tanned hides seemed
sewn together and stretched, flesh side out, over a framework
of long poles, the ends of which stuck out the top. Crude circling stripes of red, blue, and green had been painted on some
of them. The smoke pall diffused a sour smell as though refuse
were being burned.

They were greeted at the village entrance by the savage
barking of scores of lean, ferocious-looking dogs whose long
pink tongues dangled over their white fangs. However, they
slunk away, howling in cowardice, when the party walked toward them and it occurred to Pedro that these dogs lived only
to devour carrion and refuse; they were not companions to
men. Throngs of squaws and naked children ran to greet them,
shouting and screaming with laughter. The bigger boys
scooped up dry horse droppings from the grass and pelted
Pedro. They clutched at him with their dirty hands.

Girls came running from all directions, little girls, big girls,
scraggly girls, smelly girls. Pedro did not understand their
screaming jargon, but when he felt the light, wet spatter of
their spittle on his bare skin, he had no doubt about their hostility. They fought and crowded and quarreled among themselves over who would touch or scratch him first.

A sense of remoteness such as he had never experienced before came over him. He rode proudly through their midst, pretending to ignore them. But he could not ignore their primitive fashions.

They had no conception of the modesty practiced by females of the world he had left. The youngest children ran around entirely naked, their brown skin glistening in the hot sunshine. One woman of the jeering horde carried her child wrapped in a blanket across her back. Without slackening pace or lessening her shouts of vituperation at Pedro, she pulled the infant down across her shoulder to give it the breast, and the child nursed hungrily while standing on its head, its bare heels sticking up in the air.

Many of the old women and nursing mothers in the procession had abandoned the jacket altogether, and exposed their bodies above the waist or covered it over with a loose piece of cloth.

The triumphant procession wound into the heart of the teeming tent city. Indians milled everywhere, thick as flies on the fruit of a mulberry tree. They swarmed in front of Pedro, behind him and on all sides, as far as his eyes could see. The odor of their unwashed bodies offended his nostrils. Those nearest him shouted taunts and shook weapons threateningly, striving to gain his eye. Although he ignored them, he was filled with apprehension. What did they intend to do with him? Pedro shuddered, remembering what had happened at the rancho. Then he looked upward at the clear blue sky. He thought, although I am in the midst of all these savages with no Christian soul near me, see how the Holy Mother hath preserved me in safety!

A busy domesticity existed everywhere. Women gossiped incessantly as they fetched wood or squatted along the ground, scraping flesh off hides pegged out upon the grass. Shrieking children overran the premises, wrestling, racing, or shooting at marks with small bows and arrows. Strips of meat were drying everywhere about the camp. Odors he had never smelled before came to Pedro; he could not classify them. Stacked on makeshift platforms of cut boughs near some of the lodges were lances, warclubs, and shields adorned with teeth and feathers. Old men sat quietly in the sunshine smoking pipes, oblivious to all the noisy activity about them.

They came at last to a large lodge in the center of the village. Two warriors dragged Pedro off his horse and pushed him roughly inside the tipi. It was dark and cool inside. Several old buffalo robes, reeking with ancient perspiration, served as a floor. Pedro sank gratefully onto one.

"Brother!"

Pedro's heart leaped joyfully as he heard that beloved voice. When his eyes became accustomed to the dark, he saw Roberto. Shamus and the trooper named Frank were with him. Each lay on his side with wrists and ankles bound securely. They looked tired and hungry and emaciated.

Despite their bonds, Pedro and Roberto crawled awkwardly together. Pedro raised his manacled wrists and dropped his arms around his brother's neck, embracing him. They leaned against each other, and exchanged accounts of what had happened to each since their separation on the desert.

"There are other white captives here, too, brother, mainly children," Roberto said. "I saw them as we rode up. I think this city must be a rendezvous for all the savages on these plains."

A guard entered and disdainfully tossed a quantity of dried buffalo meat onto the robes near the captives. They crawled to it and gulped it hungrily, paying no attention to its graininess.

Shamus, who lay on his side like a bull thrown and trussed by a vaquero, got to his knees and bolted his first bite hungrily. Then he grimaced and looked reproachfully at the Comanche sentinels who sat impassively all around them.

"Why didn't ye salt the meat more?" he demanded in English. Looking around at the other prisoners, he broke into an amused chuckle as though determined to have his fun no matter how serious their predicament.

He turned to Frank. "Well, old pal, I would rather be in Cork than starving here with these brown divils." Again his laughter rolled out in a pleasurable rumble.

But Frank seemed lost in another world. His black, whiskery chin was sunk on his chest, and he chewed his food with slow indifference, staring fixedly into space. "They are going to kill us," he told Pedro over and over, "although we have done nothing, nor have you."

In midafternoon, their guards forced them to their feet and led them outside the tipi. There the hundreds of Indians milling about greeted them with a hostile roar. Pedro, blinking in the bright sunlight, saw half a dozen other captives crouching in fear on the bank of the shallow river that ran in lazy whirls around the encampment. They were all children except for a young white woman, pale and disheveled, clad in the calico of the frontier. She clutched her child to her breast. The little blond girl looked only three years of age. The captive children were the dirtiest, loneliest, most forlorn children Pedro had ever seen.

Weak and terrified, they clung to each other desperately. Young as they were, they had grown up on the frontier and realized their plight and all its implications. Tears flowed down over the dust and sweat on their faces.

Shamus shook his great sorrel head and made clucking noises of sympathy in his throat. "Poor dears," he crooned, "they probably saw their folks murdered a few days ago down in Texas."

An Indian girl came out of the crowd of spectators and approached the cowering white children. Tall and supple, she walked with a smooth, easy grace; the bells on her moccasins jingled rhythmically and musically. Pedro knew she could not be more than thirteen or fourteen years of age. She dropped to her knees, paying no attention to the fact that her beaded buckskin skirt dragged in the wet river sand, but the children eyed her distrustfully, and shrank from her.

She held out her hands and looked sorrowfully into their faces, speaking kindly to them. Although they did not understand her speech, they did comprehend her kindness, and when one dirty little white boy conquered his fear and crept timidly into the shelter of her arms, the other children, hungry for affection, quickly followed. With a clump of clean grass, she wiped the tears and dirt from their faces and comforted them in low, compassionate tones.

Pedro watched incredulously. After encountering so much brutality, he knew he would never forget this interlude of kindness.

It ended all too soon. Some kind of bartering was in progress involving the young prisoners. As fast as an agreement was consummated, a band of Indians approached the white captives. The children recoiled, crying and whimpering with fear as they clutched their newfound Comanche friend about the neck. Although she did her best to console them, the savages roughly took the children away from her one by one and rode off with their screaming captives, splashing through the shallow stream and vanishing across the sage-dotted prairie. None of the feathered bands took more than one white captive.

A sardonic light came into Shamus' blue eyes. Cursing, he lifted his yoked wrists helplessly.

"Now I know what the brown divils are up to! 'Tis here they separate all kin—brother from sister, mother from child—so there'll be less chance for escape. They'll niver see each other agin. A white child who grows up with only Indians around him will soon be as much a Comanche as any Indian on the place!"

The white mother and her child were next torn apart. Pedro watched nervously. When the squaws came for her daughter, the young woman fought as fiercely as a wild animal mother protecting her young in the woods. Pedro felt intense admiration for her. She was the first white person he had seen stand up fearlessly to the Indians. Despite her heroism, her little girl was taken from her and borne off screaming in one direction while the mother was jerked away in another; she sobbed and entreated one minute, then tried to bite and scratch her captors the next.

" 'Tis the Valley of Tears this plaçe must be," intoned Shamus in hushed tones, "and that miserable little river yonder must be the Quitaque. And," he added devoutly, "the Lord be between her and all harm."

A group of warriors strode toward them, led by the Indian with the green tattoo marks on his chest. Pedro saw that he also had a green turtle rudely tattooed on his stomach.

He came up to Roberto and with one slash of the knife in his hand cut his bonds. Roberto stood, rubbing his wrists. He moved back against Pedro for protection. Pedro felt his own scalp rising and his heart pumping.

"Steady, lad!" Shamus counseled gently. "They've probably come to take your brother. 'Twill do no good to fight them as did the poor Texas lass. Perhaps they will treat him kindly."

Fury flamed through Pedro. Despite his leg bonds, he advanced on Green Turtle, hopping awkwardly.

"*No!*" he cried, hoarsely. But he stumbled and fell in the sand at the man's feet. A laugh of derision went up from hundreds of hostile throats.

Green Turtle looked down with contempt. Then he grunted a command, took Roberto by the arm, and moved off.

"Goodbye, dear Pedro," Roberto called, his young face stricken. "No matter where they take you, inquire about me and I will do the same about you."

Pedro could only lie in the sand, the unshed tears aching behind his eyes, wondering if he would ever see his brother again.

"*Adiós, caro* Pedro!" Roberto's voice kept pealing out, fainter and fainter, until finally it was lost in the answering shouts of the squaws who picked up the lad's words and mockingly relayed them back to Pedro.

Back in the center lodge, Shamus was talking. "Wurrah!" his deep voice came up from his chest in an annoyed rumble. "The United States governmint has no nature in thim. Hundreds of our people are captured or enslaved or killed each year by these brown divils. And what does the governmint do? Not'ing! If a fraction of the outrages these red heathen commit in the heart of our own kintry were committed by some foreign nation a t'ousand miles away—like England or Algeria or Mexico—our governmint would go to war tomorrow. Now that's the truth or I can't spake it."

The three of them had sat on the moldy robes all afternoon, surrounded by their implacable circle of guards. Frank lay flat on his stomach, his head in his arms and one knee drawn up under his chin. Pedro asked him how he could sleep in such an unnatural position.

"I'm not asleep," the trooper replied. "I am at prayer and lie this way so that our guards cannot observe what I am doing."

Night came, and with it, dread of what lay ahead. With every breath Pedro drew, the fact of Roberto's absence stabbed him afresh. He had to get his mind off it. He tried to imagine what lay ahead for Frank, for Shamus, for himself. He wondered what death at the hands of these barbarians was like. What means would they use?

Outside, a solitary drum began to beat, fast then slow. A far-off wailing of male and female voices accompanied it. Shamus strained against his bonds and raised his shaggy head so he could hear better.

Pedro listened too. His practiced ear caught the plural singing, the women in a high, reedy falsetto an octave above the men. Both sexes sang with all their strength, injuring the tone quality and clouding the melody but expressing the ardor of their emotion.

The lodge skins parted and several dark figures entered, cut the prisoners' bonds, and pushed them outside into the night. The singing was plainer as they walked toward it. Despite its excitement, the music seemed to possess a straining, pleading quality as though it were an entreaty to a heathen god. Pedro sensed that some type of ceremonial dance must be in progress, although the drum was beaten in a different measure from that of the song. He heard faintly the phrase "hah yah" over and over. The "yah" seemed more of a grunt than a musical note, as though the singers stamped their feet when they pronounced it.

The great village was very much awake. Every tipi was lighted by an inside fire that glowed redly through the skin walls, faintly tracing the conical shape of the dwelling. The lodges spread so interminably over knoll and dune that their illuminated shapes outlined the gentle contours of the land. The wind had slackened and the night air had a chill on it. The smoke from hundreds of campfires hung everywhere.

As the singing grew louder, Pedro felt his pulse pounding in his throat. He knew they would not have to wait long for whatever fate lay in store for them.

They walked until the lodges thinned out and came to a place where the ground slanted downward into a natural amphitheater. Here hundreds of spectators squatted along the gentle slope on all four sides. At the sight of the three prisoners, they set up a taunting roar. Pedro felt no fear until he looked down into the middle of the arena. There six posts of newly hewed cottonwood had been driven into the sand and ingeniously arranged in three crude gibbets of two puncheons

each. As he realized what they were, a feeling of stunned disbelief washed over him.

Several singers and a lone drummer sat in the arena's open
space. A fire of willow logs had been kindled nearby. Its light
glanced off the flashing eyes and bared teeth of the singers,
whose fervor increased as the shackled prisoners were brought
forward.

Several dried scalps swung from peeled wands implanted
in the sand, and these seemed to provide the theme of the
dance. One at a time, the warriors who had ravaged the rancho
danced forward and recited the details of their success in fierce
pantomine, acting out with startling realism each blow, each
knife thrust, each wound given and received. Pedro's mouth
tightened at the effrontery of their boasting, but the throng of
savage spectators applauded with fierce approval after each
performance, stamping their feet, clapping their hands, and
vigorously shaking their gourd rattles.

A new dancer burst upon the scene, his beaded ear pendants
and copper wire wristbands glinting in the firelight. With a
long, slow sweep of his hands through his hair, down his sides
and over his hips, he indicated that his enemy had been a
white woman. He spun, crouched and looked wildly about as
though his victim had eluded him. Then he bounded after her,
overtook her and with a grunt of rage, went through the action
of grasping her by an arm and swinging his war club downward.

Pedro's legs began to shake uncontrollably. The pantomim-
ist plucked his knife, stooped and pretended to tear off the
scalp. Then Four Scars abandoned his dumbshow performance
for reality, snatching up one of the scalp poles thrust into the
sand by the fire. The chestnut-brown hair on the small willow
hoop stirred in the wind. Flourishing it triumphantly, he
whirled around, arms spread, facing first one side of the as-

semblage, then the other, his evil face aflame with pride and passion. A roar of approbation arose, echoing off the distant bluffs. A wave of anguish overcame Pedro, and he closed his eyes, resolutely forcing his mind to shut out all of his surroundings.

Suddenly he felt his head jerked roughly upward. His eyes snapped open, and he saw that Four Scars was through; now it was time for the three captives to become participants.

They were prodded to their feet and led to the cottonwood posts. Quickly, rough hands stripped off all their remaining clothing. Their skin contrasted strangely. Frank's was white as marble. Shamus' body was covered with splotches of orange freckles and crests of curly red hair. Pedro looked down at himself. His skin was nearly as brown as that of the Indians. Shorter even than his captors, Pedro knew he must look like a callow boy. He was too shocked and terrified to be embarrassed at his nakedness. He had lost all hope.

Each captive was led to a gibbet. There were two posts for each of them. The hands of Shamus were lashed above his head, the right hand to one pole, the left to another. His ankles were similarly secured to the bottoms of the poles. He did not lose his aplomb. He turned his massive head so he could better face Frank.

"Well, old pal, when we get to the fort we'll have a divil of a story to tell the boys, won't we?" He tossed his red, curly hair out of his eyes and chuckled at the poor joke he had made.

When they came to tie Pedro, their fierce black eyes bored into his as though testing his nerve. Chin up, he walked resolutely to the stake, hoping he was hiding the terror he felt. As they fastened his ankles to the bottom of one pole, he looked coolly and defiantly from right to left at the hundreds of Indians clustered about. He was glad Roberto was not here to witness his doom.

And at the remembrance of Roberto a seed of fear suddenly germinated in the pit of Pedro's stomach. What would become of his young brother? How would his pliable young life be shaped if he grew up among these barbarians, amid their cruelty and violence? His brother had not yet learned the sweet solace available to him who turns to the Blessed Virgin for all needs of body and soul. Bitterly, Pedro shut his eyes, but Roberto would not be blotted out.

Legs spraddled and arms spread, he faced Frank and Shamus only five feet away. Everything had grown ominously quiet. Even the drums were hushed. All around him, the audience sat gravely still as if waiting for a new and more significant performance to begin.

Then Pedro heard the bells. Deadly as a rattlesnake's tail twitch, they jingled dryly from somewhere in the darkness. He swiveled his neck to right and left, searching for the sound and for sight of what was causing it, but he saw nothing. The noise persisted. With it came the measured beat of hundreds of feet stamping together somewhere on the sandy river soil. There was rhythm in the drumbeats, rhythm in the stamping, rhythm in the rustle of the bells.

Then he saw them. A long line of painted warriors emerged in single file from a lane in the crowd, led by one who wore a long flowing bonnet of white feathers. The men behind him had painted their faces black. A single yellow feather dangled from their braided scalplocks. Each carried a knife or tomahawk in one hand and a small flint stone, sharply pointed, in the other.

Pedro stared at them, entranced by the deliberateness and the regularity of their movements. They seemed in no hurry whatever, advancing at a slow, synchronized pace that was half shuffle, half walk. They glided forward, then backward, then right, then left, then forward again to tramp the ground so forcibly that the single slap of their moccasined feet echoing against the nearby bluff sounded as if hundreds of beavers had whacked their tails on the river bank with a mighty simultaneous wallop. The seated assemblage grew so hushed that Pedro could hear the crackling of the fire.

Shamus for the first time lost his sense of humor and looked grimly at the advancing line. Frank's whiskery face puckered. Eyes shut, he strained at his shackles and began to sob hysterically.

Pedro gaped at the leader. The man's stomach muscles twitched, his buttocks wagged, and the feathers in his headdress shook in the wind. Bowlegged and pigeontoed, he looked older than the others; his slit-black eyes bored hypnotically into Pedro's. The rattling of the bells grew louder and Pedro braced himself, determined not to reveal his fear, in order to triumph over them in at least one detail before he died.

As the long line glided past, weaving and pulsating like some gigantic serpent, two braves dashed from it. Seizing Frank and Shamus by the hair, with swift, dextrous strokes of their knives they scalped them, taking only a small segment of the skin and hair. Triumphantly, they lifted their trophies for all to see and the multitude responded with war whoops, gourd rattling, and clapping of hands.

Frank screamed as shrilly as a woman. A mad roar rumbled from the craggy chest of Shamus. Pedro closed his eyes. Quickly, one of the savages leaped to his side, clutched him by the hair and jerked his head back violently. Pedro realized they meant for him to see the suffering of his companions.

For a moment the bedlam ceased and the dancers retreated. They sat on the sandy ground, smoking their pipes, laughing, and ridiculing the prisoners. The respite didn't last long. Again the drums began to thud, accompanied by the jingling of bells and the rhythmic slapping of hundreds of moccasined feet as the warriors began a second approach.

This time they used their flints. As each warrior passed, he drew his stone point across the bare midriffs of the two troopers, being careful not to inflict a fatal wound.

Rage and revulsion shook Pedro. He wished he could do something for the two victims. He wished they'd come for him and get it over with.

Again there was a pause. Then the warriors rose, one by one, to form a third time their serpentining line. Shamus heaved his great head up and watched them dispassionately, his blue eyes glassy with the film of approaching death. Frank sagged unconscious on his scaffold.

Pedro's breath was hot in his throat. He prayed for his dying companions, then remembering his own ordeal that was yet to come, he licked his lips and murmured aloud, "Mother of God, help me!"

He prayed for calm, and by great effort got control of himself. He felt a strong need to express his Christian loyalty. Because he was an Andalusian, he took the Andalusian's most natural way to express himself. Lifting his gaze to the stars, he sucked in a long gulp of the night air and began to sing.

His mind had taken him back to Seville. It was the feast day of Corpus Christi. The figure of the Virgin was passing along the narrow street, which was thronged with people who had waited for hours.

His eyes fixed on Her face, Pedro sang the mournful *saeta* at the top of his boyish tenor:

> *With pikes and prongs and lances bright,*
> *They came for Jesus in the night. . . .*

Once more the torturers raised their war song and began their hideous dance of death, advancing, retreating, moving from right to left. But Pedro did not see them. His eyes were on the Virgin. He had mastery over himself now. His high, clear voice contrasting oddly with the barbaric uproar, he kept singing the *saeta* with all his strength. His voice pealed on, its sweet lamentation rising even above the savage war song and the hissing of the bells. . . .

When they cut him down, he almost fainted. The circulation of his legs was so deadened that he found it difficult to walk. He was too emotionally spent to rejoice over the miracle of his salvation.

4 · Bondage

It was smoky in Four Scars' tipi. A small blaze of buffalo chips smoldered from a fire hole in the center of the sandy floor but not all of the smoke escaped through the opening in the top. Buffalo skins spread in a circle around the inside perimeter of the lodge provided a place to sit in the daytime and to sleep at night.

Pedro lay in a stupor at the back of the lodge. His hair was matted with sand and sweat. He was filthy from not having bathed. His body prickled with scars, scabs, and half-healed blood clots; he was thirsty and feverish. Wearily he rolled his head and tried to focus his eyes on the people moving in the dim light of the fire.

Four Scars' Indian name was Belt Whip. He supported two wives. Caught While Mad, the elder, had hard black eyes and a tongue that made everybody quail. With the rib of an animal she stirred a sloppy stew bubbling in an iron pot over the fire. Apparently they ate at all hours of the day or night. Cedar, the younger wife, walked with a slight limp and stayed in the background.

Belt Whip and his surly son Two Hatchets sat on the buffalo skins, with their feet folded under them. Cedar placed short, flat pieces of wood on the floor before each. She moved awkwardly, for she was pregnant. Caught While Mad lifted the meat out of the kettle with her dirty fingers and placed it on the wooden platters.

Belt Whip broke off a morsel with his fingers. He lifted it to the sky as an offering to the Great Spirit, then buried it beneath the sandy floor; he wiped the soil from his hands on his breech-clout. He and Two Hatchets broke up the remaining meat with their fingers and swallowed it noisily. Pedro was offered none.

As he watched them he contrasted this dinner with the one regularly served in his mother's home in Seville. He could see her high-ceilinged dining chamber and the cloth of embroidered linen trimmed with lace. On the table would be strong wine, fresh fruit. There would be chickpeas, a fish salad, cutlets neatly baked, and a delicious cold soup. He could see his mother take off her drawing-room gloves and pull on the white table gloves that always lay beside her spotless napkin. Pedro's hate burned fiercely as he watched Belt Whip finish his meal.

When the men were done, Cedar offered them water in a terrapin shell. They sucked it into their mouths, spat it out upon their hands, and rubbed their faces. As the women ate, the father and son enjoyed a pipe together. Then the fire was banked and the family lay down to sleep on the spread-out robes.

Pedro turned over on the cast-off skin that was his bed and closed his eyes. He was accustomed to living in a tent during his summer wanderings with the gypsies but he always had his own tent; he loathed being confined in such proximity with four filthy savages.

He rested poorly. The hellish din of the scalp dance rang in his head. He lay in an agonized stupor, and thanked the Virgin Mary for his deliverance.

Finally he turned over on his stomach, the only part of his body he could lie upon with some degree of comfort, and forced himself to make an estimate of his situation. He doubted if he could long endure captivity. But he still lived. His glass was not yet run.

What should be his course? He had neither horse nor provisions. Even if he could steal a horse, he lacked the strength to ride it. Worst of all, he knew nothing of the country's geography. The only territory with which he was even slightly familiar was the one they had just passed over with such terrible hardship. Pedro knew that he could never again find it alone or exist if he tried to cross it. Besides, he would be watched closely, night and day. He locked his jaws to stifle his heartsickness. For the present, the only course open to him was to accept his hard lot and try to survive.

The smoked thinned out. Cool air drifted in. Finally he slept.

A kick awakened him. He cringed, blinking his eyes. The bearskin door had been rolled back and the warm sunshine filtered through. The family had breakfasted.

Belt Whip stood over Pedro, holding a single-shot musket. Then he walked to the rear of the lodge and sat down, facing the door. "Come here, my dog," he ordered in Spanish.

Pedro obeyed. Belt Whip signaled Pedro to drop to his knees.

When Pedro complied, Belt Whip cocked the gun and held it against Pedro's breast. He put his finger on the trigger.

Pedro looked at him coolly. If he must die, this way would be quick and he would be spared months of servitude. But he was sure that his enemy would not shoot.

Belt Whip lowered the weapon. He pulled the hammer back with his thumb and showed Pedro it was unloaded. With a bitter look, he began to load the gun. First he thrust in a paper cartridge and poured powder into the muzzle. With a ramrod, he forced more powder and a lead ball down the barrel. He stuck a percussion cap on the nipple. Then he drew the hammer back with his thumb, cocking the weapon, and put the gun to Pedro's forehead with a furious air. Again he fingered the trigger.

Again Pedro looked him in the eye. Although he tried not to

show fear, he felt the veins standing out on his forehead like small ropes. Belt Whip saw them, too. He threw back his head and deep, taunting laughter rumbled from his throat. He rolled on the ground in merriment.

Instantly, Pedro became vigilant, waiting for his enemy to lay down the gun. He determined to snatch it up and shoot Belt Whip. He would shoot him through the stomach to prolong his suffering. But the Indian seemed to read his thoughts. With no interruption of his laughter, he was careful to hold the weapon in Pedro's face. Pedro resolved to be a better actor the next time such an opportunity offered itself.

Later, Belt Whip and Two Hatchets thrust large quantities of arrows into their skin quivers, picked up their bows, and taking extra horses, rode off. They took the musket with them. Pedro decided that they had gone hunting and would be absent several days. Caught While Mad left the tipi and returned at once with three more squaws as ugly and dirty as herself.

They charged Pedro, knocking him off his feet. As he fell, he kicked out, feeling his bare foot drive into a face, then he rolled free. Screeching angrily, they rushed him again. They were strong as men and wrestled him to the ground.

He fought furiously against the odorous weight of them, but his strength quickly ebbed. They sat on him, holding him down with ease. With a pair of crude bone tweezers, one began to pull out every hair she found growing on his face. Pedro felt pain in his ears, as though something sharp was being thrust through the lobes. The pain was renewed again and again, despite his struggling. Jabbering with triumph, they oiled his hair and anointed his features with what felt like soft clay.

He cursed them weakly, but he had to submit. His earlobes stung painfully and bled freely. When they allowed him to feel his ears he discovered that several small sharp cactus spines had been thrust entirely through them.

They let him get up. He crouched on one knee, weak and off guard. Suddenly Caught While Mad knelt, scooped up a handful of dead ashes from the fire, and threw them in his eyes.

Blinded, he wallowed about, afraid he would never see again. He heard the women screeching with laughter. His eyes smarted, causing tears that washed out the sediment. When he could see, he discovered that they were all gone save Cedar, the lame squaw.

Pedro looked at his body. He had lost so much weight that his skin hung in loose folds. His scalp was matted with sores. He was prostrated by exhaustion, and the deep coughs of lung fever wracked his frail frame. For a moment he wished he were dead.

He saw Cedar watching him with compassion. Despite her broad, homely countenance her black eyes were not unkind. She picked up one of the unwashed wooden slabs and dipped her hand into the iron kettle. She brought bits of the unsavory-looking stew to him. It looked filthy. But Pedro was starving and it smelled wonderful.

He gulped it down and found it savory. She fed him two more helpings. While he slabbered down the food, she stood at the lodge door watching. Apparently she did not want anybody to know that she had fed him.

His ears still pained him. Why had they done him this cruelty? As she saw him finger his ears, she slipped a wire bracelet from her wrist and held it to his ear as an ornament to show him his ears had been punctured to admit the earrings worn by Comanche men.

She brought him some water in a skin pouch and watched as he gulped it down. She chewed some yucca roots, warmed the residue by the fire, and applied it to the lacerations festering on his body. Pedro felt better. His courage began to return.

A warm thread of thankfulness ran through him. Cedar was

the first Indian who had shown him any kindness. He thought of the many kindnesses that had been done him all his life by his mother, his father, teachers, servants, his nurse. It had never occurred to him to thank any of them. He had accepted their attentions as his due. For the first time he began to appreciate the measure of their devotion. He realized that the greatest kindness of all must be that for which the giver has no motive, and gets nothing in return.

With the men gone, Pedro learned to perform all the menial tasks of a slave, cutting and fetching wood, pounding corn, skinning game, dragging away dung, carrying water, and helping the women scrape flesh from pegged-out buffalo hides. Although some of his strength returned, he still felt depressed. In Spain, he had been waited on by several menials, including a body servant who even helped him dress. Now he was a domestic in the lodge of a savage who had slain his mother and reduced him to captivity. How quickly his lot had changed.

Cedar permitted him brief spells of rest when Caught While Mad was out of the lodge. During these periods of respite, he dozed uncomfortably in a sitting posture within the tipi. It was while he rested in this position that he discovered he was an object of great curiosity in the village. Every time he awakened, he saw eyes watching him from the lodge door or from underneath the tipi flap. Everywhere he went, he felt curious, hostile stares.

The Indian children seemed to fear him. They constantly avoided him. Once when he walked from the timber with an armload of wood, he surprised a group of them playing. They fled screaming at his approach. Then he remembered something Shamus had told him.

" 'Tis no wonder they hate all white men. The only ones they see are the whisky peddlers and the squaw men. It is from them that they get their ideas about our character and morality."

Next morning, Cedar handed Pedro a buffalo pouch and with explanatory gestures made him understand that he was to go to the nearby river and fetch water. Pedro welcomed the task; it would provide him his first opportunity to bathe. As he walked barefoot from the village, the hot river sand burned his feet. A gust of wind whipped dirt into his eyes and mouth. He spat it out, hating the unfriendly climate.

At the river bank, he paused to watch a group of Comanche boys about his own age practice riding feats. At home, Pedro had been the best rider in the royal stables.

He held his breath in admiration of their skill and daring. They all mounted from the right side. Most rode bareback but occasionally one used a crude wooden saddle with a bearskin for a pad. Their ponies were creams, buckskins, and piebalds.

As they ran them at full speed, they would lean low and snatch up objects from the prairie. Two of them, riding full tilt, converged on either side of a prostrate comrade, and stooping at the same instant, picked him up and swung his body across the horse of one of them.

"*Ai!*" Pedro told himself in wonder. "Their horsemanship begins where ours in Spain leaves off."

Obviously they were rehearsing procedures they might be expected to perform in battle. Pedro had never seen a people so devoted to fighting. At night he was kept awake by beating drums and martial singing. Almost every day he saw men wearing war paint riding about the village to enlist volunteers for raids. One day Pedro had counted six raiding parties parading through the camp at different times before leaving in separate directions.

Pedro continued to watch the youthful riders. One after another, they rode pellmell past a toppled cottonwood. Its uprooted base was their target. As they sped past it, they dropped their bodies upon the far side of their horses until nothing showed but a heel hooked over the racing animal's backbone.

Thus screened from the weapons of an imaginary enemy, each rider discharged arrow after arrow underneath his pony's neck into the cottonwood's roots.

One wiry young brave who wore a yellow feather in his black hair went even further. He threw himself up from a horizontal position on the right side of his flying mount and changed to a similar spot on the horse's opposite side, without dropping his bow, shield, or long lance. Pedro could hardly believe his eyes.

A white horse with a long strip of red calico streaming gaily from its tail galloped past at full speed. With arms outstretched for balance, its rider stood on the animal's withers, whooping in an exultant treble. The rider had thick, coarse lips and broad nostrils and wore a blouse brilliantly banded with beading. When Pedro saw that the raven-black hair was banged to the eyelids, he realized, incredulously, that the rider was a girl!

They practiced hard another five minutes, then the boys raced to the river for a cooling dip and the girl angled off toward the camp.

Pedro laid down his water paunch, stripped off his clothing, entered the stream, and began splashing warm water over himself. As he stepped dripping from the stream, he saw that the boy riders had finished their ablutions downstream and had joined him. Most of them wore blue breechclouts, wire earrings, and moccasins.

Their leader was the youth with the yellow feather. He was examining Pedro's torn trousers, holding them up to ridicule in Comanche. His remarks were greeted with laughter. Another young man picked up the water paunch.

Pedro reached for his trousers but was pushed roughly away. They closed in on him, hooting and jeering. The one who wore the yellow feather threw sand on him. Others pelted him with dry horse dung. A sandstone rock struck him in the head, dazing him. Other rocks thudded into his body.

Yellow Feather grasped Pedro about the middle and threw him heavily. With shrill cries, the others began to beat him with sticks. He fought as best he could but his feeble strength soon gave out. He was lapsing into unconsciousness when he heard a woman's voice scolding them. It was Cedar. Despite her pregnancy, she rained blows upon them with a stick, drove them off, and rescued Pedro's clothing.

Pedro was so sore and spent that he could hardly rise. His body was covered with fresh bruises and sores. His nose bled and the wound in his head hurt. He was embarrassed to have the lame squaw see him naked. She pointed to the water and Pedro waded in to take another bath. Then he drew on his torn trousers, filled the paunch, and followed her back to the tipi.

Then she did her crude doctoring job all over again, chewing yucca roots, warming them by the fire, and applying the crude lotion to his wounds. As he submitted, hate for his tormentors smothered him anew.

"Boys no good," she said with signs and a smattering of Spanish and Comanche. She made him understand, as best she could, that the young man with the yellow feather was Wolf Milk, the son of a chief. Many expensive gifts had been given away in his name and he had had his own religious articles from an early age.

When Pedro asked her about the girl rider, Cedar struggled again to explain as best she could that she was called To-a-nick-pe, "The Boy." Renowned as a rider and horse thief, she rarely let a horse-stealing expedition depart without her. Pedro marveled at this. He had never seen such an athletic people. Even their females rode like centaurs.

Encouraged by Cedar's friendliness, Pedro asked, with gestures, why Belt Whip had not killed him when the rancho was raided. Shamus had told him that the Comanches usually killed all their victims save children.

With fluent motions, she replied that because of the rich

clothing he wore at the time of his capture, Belt Whip had realized that he was wealthy and probably intended asking a ransom for him. Then, too, her husband liked to keep an occasional captive to torment and mistreat. It would satisfy his instinct for deviltry and it gave him prestige in the village. Pedro sat silent, dreading what lay ahead.

His depression worsened when Belt Whip and Two Hatchets returned next morning from their hunt. He had not known of their arrival until he heard Belt Whip call in Spanish from the outside of the tipi.

"Hola, my dog!"

Although Pedro went outside immediately, the lord of the lodge was not satisfied. Belt Whip gestured toward his pack pony some distance from the tipi. The pack pony bore a deer, freshly killed and dressed. Pedro obediently shouldered the deer and started to walk toward the lodge. The corpse was heavy and he had difficulty supporting it. He heard a swish and felt the bite of Belt Whip's hair bridle about his bare ankles. The pain was so blinding that he almost dropped the deer.

Each time Belt Whip swung his bridle, his laughter rang through the village; the crack of the bridle and the accompanying guffaw sounded almost as one.

Two Hatchets, in order to outdo his father, cut Pedro across the back with a long willow switch. Striving to avoid both lashings, Pedro stumbled into an awkward run. With loud yells of enjoyment, Belt Whip and Two Hatchets only increased the tempo of the punishment.

Running the gauntlet of the switch, the bridle, and the rope, Pedro dragged the deer inside the tipi. There he lay gasping for breath, too exhausted to curse his tormentors or to examine his welts.

Pedro did not always find the inside of the tipi a refuge. Not only was he living in a crowded space with people whom he hated, but the small living enclosure gave him a caged-bird feeling. His only relief came late at night when all the guests who visited almost constantly, chattering and feasting, had departed, and the snores of the lodge's occupants indicated that everyone was asleep. Then the cool night air began to seep underneath the raised tipi walls and Pedro would sink into slumber.

Belt Whip's family had no regular time for eating, although a morning and evening meal was generally served by the women. The dining procedure rarely varied. Belt Whip and Two Hatchets were served first. Then the women ate. Pedro was allowed to scavenge what was left. Later, Cedar explained that he was made to eat by himself so he would not disturb Belt Whip's medicine.

He was too starved to be fastidious about the food. Once Two Hatchets brought home several terrapins and threw them alive into the tipi cooking hole. As fast as they sought to escape, he kicked them back into the fire until they were roasted. Then the family rolled them out of the ashes, broke their shells with rocks, and ate with enjoyment. Much to his surprise, Pedro found the meat delicious.

August passed. The sun burned down, turning the buffalo grass the color of straw, but always the nights were cool. Life with the Comanches, Pedro discovered, moved with the urgencies of water, fuel, and sanitation. Because five people were living in one crowded tipi where all the cooking, eating, and sleeping were done, filth and nastiness were rampant. No furniture existed save the buffalo-robe bedding, a few cooking utensils, and several parfleche bags, skin containers filled with dried meat and clothing. Caught While Mad was such a poor housekeeper that no article was kept in its place but lay at random where it had last been dropped.

Hardest of all for Pedro to bear was what he considered their immodesty. Since there was no privacy in the lodge, there could be no decorum. The daily personal functions which Europeans performed in seclusion were discharged publicly by the Comanches. He remembered the cleanliness of the gypsies, who always washed their hands before eating, whose lives were spent protecting the virginity of their girls.

Always he thought of escape, yearning for it with every facet of his being. He could not bear to think of a long captivity amid all this degradation. He built in his mind a fierce determination to elude his captors somehow.

Cedar seemed to trust him completely. She would send him out at night into the moonlight to fetch buffalo chips for cooking. Nearly every tipi gleamed yellow and from inside came the cheerful murmur of many voices as the whole camp hummed with social living. Pedro heard the coarse, ribald voices of men as they gambled. Children cried and their mothers sang to them to quiet them. Old men jabbered and Pedro guessed that they were relating stories of their youth. Occasionally Pedro passed a pair of whispering lovers standing together inside a single blanket. Ponies nickered, dogs whined, and the rancid odor of burning buffalo chips was everywhere on the air.

One night he heard from somewhere out on the dark prairie a wolf's melancholy baying; it was a sharp bark that became a series of staccato yelps and ended in a long, quivering howl. Pedro looked at the sky and remembered nostalgically that the same blazing stars and serene moon riding over this savage village also swung over the tiled roofs of Andalusia. With a tug of affection, he wondered what his father was doing tonight.

He knew Felipe had not yet had time to be informed about the raid on the rancho in northern Chihuahua, for the mail was carried on a long slow ocean voyage. But he knew that when his father heard the news, he would hurry by boat to the rancho and start proceedings for the recovery of his sons. But ships and mule trains moved slowly, and even after his father arrived, how would he ever find Pedro and Roberto in this remote wilderness?

Escape was the only solution. But as the hot days passed, one after another, no way of escape suggested itself. It became one of his daily tasks to carry food to Cedar's aged grandmother in an adjoining tipi. Pedro was astonished at his first sight of the old crone as she lay on a robe at the back of the lodge. Withered and half naked, she smiled up at him, revealing pink, toothless gums. Her disordered gray hair fell down over her sunken shoulders, and her shriveled breasts hung like pendants.

Her eyes brightened with excitement when she saw the food. While Pedro propped her up, Cedar fed her soup from a buffalo horn. In a mixture of Spanish, Comanche, and sign language, Cedar explained to Pedro that ever since she had been a little girl, she and her *kaku,* her maternal grandmother, had been very close. Because of Cedar's lameness, her grandmother had indulged her in everything. She gave Cedar her first doll and had helped the girl dress it in deerskin. She made a toy cradle board so that Cedar could carry the doll on her back in the manner of her mother.

Their relationship had been much more intimate than that between Cedar and her own mother. And now that her beloved *kaku* was prostrated with the infirmities of age, Cedar returned the devotion she had received.

Pedro was surprised at how easily he could understand Cedar, especially in the medium of Spanish and "hand talk," or sign language. He noticed how gracefully she gestured when she spoke with her hands.

Soon Pedro was sent alone to feed the old woman. He would linger and listen as she sang before she ate her meal. She sang in a high, thin, quavering voice with her gums slightly separated and motionless. The melody descended steadily from the first note to the last, and ended on a fallen key. Pedro had never heard such eerie singing. It seemed a primitive keening, something he could not fathom. This is one way in which Comanches and Andalusians are the same, he thought: we both like to set our souls free in song.

Because he was starved for the guitar playing that was food and drink to his nature, he felt a strange comradeship for the old hag. He longed to cradle a guitar in his lap. His fingers ached to pluck its strings. He constantly moved the fingers of his left hand in the correct spacings as he associated them with the melodies that raced through his thoughts.

The old woman's tipi afforded him a privacy he had nowhere else. Keeping his voice low, he often sang to her, laments that expressed his own grief and sorrow. One day he sang the *copla* that began *"Cautivo y prisionero . . ."*

> *A captive in a prison cell*
> *I sing the woes I feel,*
> *And thus I file away my chains,*
> *My chains of heavy steel.*

She listened to him gravely, her watery eyes widening in surprise. Obviously she was as wonderstruck by his singing as he had been by hers. She nodded her scraggly head approvingly when he finished, as if she understood his emotion and sympathized with it.

Pedro enjoyed this phase of his labors. And the old woman liked it, too, so much so that when Cedar went alone to feed her the old grandmother would scold Cedar, upset the food, and ask in a shrill voice for Pedro.

Day followed day. Each was marked by a routine of skinning and dragging and carrying, while the hot wind blew and blew and blew. Gradually Pedro adjusted to his new life. He learned to eat whatever was offered him. His craving for the highly seasoned foods to which he was accustomed became unbearable at times, yet he soon discovered that the filthy victuals which earlier had turned his stomach now tasted good.

His thick black hair grew so fast that he was constantly raking it out of his eyes; the squaws had greased it with the oil from an animal and the sun's heat had burned the oil into his scalp. They had started to braid it in two thin twists that fell down each shoulder; after the punctures in his ears had healed they thrust circles of silver wire into his lobes. Cedar had given him an old pair of moccasins. Although the string of white beads sewn along their heel was worn halfway off, Pedro liked them. They enabled him to walk noiselessly.

But the hard life and the cruelty continued. In his relationship with Belt Whip Pedro's servitude became so complete that his arrogant master had only to give him a nod and Pedro would hurry to gratify his wish, filling his drinking horn at the river when he was thirsty, spreading his robe, lighting his pipe, or catching lice for him to eat. As he ran here and there, he laughed to himself. Juan, his body servant in Seville, would enjoy seeing him now. He had often been sharp and dictatorial with Juan. Now he was learning first hand a domestic's true position in the master-servant relationship.

Pedro's only pleasure was learning the speech of his captors, because knowledge of it might some day help him to escape. The Comanche tongue did not puzzle him long. It was definitive, each word describing its object precisely. Pedro had been a skillful linguistic student at the Royal Academy and he quickly began to master the rudiments of his sixth language.

Three months after his capture, he could understand many commands. As he progressed from day to day, he discovered that the Comanche way of speaking was sonorous and flowing. It contained many rolling *r*'s. The words usually ended in a whispered vowel that strengthened the preceding consonant and helped him enunciate more clearly.

The squaws helped him learn the language, too. When they told him to do something and he did not understand, they would grasp one of his sore ears, point toward what they wanted done, and repeat the Comanche phrase describing it.

Pedro was still the object of much cruelty in the village. When he went for water, the Comanche boys hazed him mercilessly. As fast as his old lacerations healed, new ones would be opened.

Belt Whip, too, enjoyed devising new ways of tormenting him. One afternoon, Belt Whip rode home from a hunt and called in a loud voice from outside the tipi, "Come here, my dog."

When Pedro appeared, Belt Whip seized him by the hair and one leg, picked him up, and thrust his face into a mess of rotting deer offal. Pedro struggled vainly. Belt Whip kept rubbing his face in the reeking refuse. As he did so, his deep laughter rolled out.

Later, when Cedar gave Pedro some water to wash with, his head ached cruelly and he staggered from weakness. He was so angry that his hands shook. He felt his resentment welling to the point of explosion and yet he knew that if he did retaliate, Belt Whip would not hesitate to kill him.

Death for Pedro was only a pulse beat away in any event. If Belt Whip did not slay him, he knew that he might die of starvation or illness. Shamus had told him that the Comanches' very existence was a fight for life that kept them at the peak of physical condition. None but the strongest could survive—and that was true of their captives. Pedro felt that in his own case the climax was near at hand.

After dark, he secretly fashioned a tiny likeness of the Holy Mother out of wet clay and smuggled it within the tipi, concealing it beneath the musty buffalo skin that comprised his bed. He was heartsick and desperate. In the event of death, he wanted to be prepared. "O most Holy Mary, Mother of goodness and mercy, when I consider my sins and think upon the moment of my death, I am filled with confusion and fear. O sweetest Mother, my only hope is in thy intercession. Do not forsake me. Do not fail to console me." After his prayer he felt calmer and again turned his thoughts to escape.

As he crouched in a corner of the lodge, he heard a camp crier ride past, calling an announcement. Apparently it was an important one, because the two wives, Caught While Mad and Cedar, exchanged looks of patient resignation in the dim light of the cooking fire.

The next morning they aroused Pedro before dawn. When he stepped outside into the cool air, the village looked as though a cyclone had whirled through it. The smoke-stained tipis were being torn down by the squaws and there was a great air of bustle. The camp was moving to a new location and the women were in a hurry to start; those who arrived first at the new site would get the choice locations.

Cedar showed Pedro how to stand on her shoulders and unfasten the wooden skewers, then pull down the tipi walls of buffalo hides. Quickly the hides and the poles that comprised the framework were packed on the horses and mules. They rolled up the buffalo-robe mattresses and loaded the parfleche bags and cooking utensils on the backs of the pack animals. Pedro was amazed at how speedily they finished their tasks. Obviously it was not the custom for the men of the band to help. While Pedro and the squaws lifted and grunted and strained, Belt Whip and Two Hatchets wandered aimlessly about, smoking their pipes. Moving was women's work.

Cedar turned next to the tipi of her grandmother. While she and Pedro dismantled it, the old woman lay outside on a robe. She had been dressed in her best beaded clothing; her face had been painted in her favorite way. Pedro had never seen the old woman so dressed up.

But the sparkle was gone from the old crone's eyes. Her cheeks had sunk, her lips were colorless. She was singing to herself in a weak monotone. Her voice was as hushed as the

final breath of a dying breeze; Pedro could not have heard her
had he not bent closely over her. As she kept mumbling over
and over one melancholy phrase in the same descending ca-
dence he recognized a line she had once sung when he fed her,
the words of which Cedar had later translated for him:

The stones are all that last long . . .

A tiny smile touched her lips when she saw him. Weakly she
raised one dirty, withered hand. Pedro took it, amazed at its
lightness. He tried to think of something to say.

Her fingers became limp and her eyes went blank as glass.
He thought for a moment that she was dead. Then he saw her
lips move silently, as if she were still trying to mouth the words
of the song.

Nearby stood a pony. The ends of two long tipi poles were
tied to each of its sides; the other ends dragged the ground,
forming a travois. Robes had been fastened between the poles
to make a bed. It would be a long, rough ride in the torrid
prairie sun. Pedro wondered if the old woman could survive
it.

Caught While Mad yelled at the mules. The caravan moved
off. Cedar took one last look at her grandmother lying on the
ground, a look in which poignancy and fear were strangely in-
termixed, then turned her back and limped off after the pack
animals.

Pedro overtook her, and pulling at her sleeve, pointed questioningly at the old woman back on the prairie.

Cedar shook her head vigorously. In a mixture of Spanish,
Comanche, and sign language, the lame squaw made him understand that her grandmother, too old and decrepit to travel,
was being "thrown away."

He pointed to the space on the travois where the old woman
could have ridden. Hostility came into Cedar's plain, broad
face. She shook her black head fiercely and tried to make

Pedro understand that while she still liked and respected her *kaku,* they were powerless to do anything but desert her because an evil spirit had taken possession of her body and they were afraid of it.

Pedro stared at her. The pack animals, their swaying backs concealed by piles of family belongings, walked steadily away from him. Belt Whip rode back, growling angrily, and struck Pedro with his bow. Pedro snatched up his burden, a heavy parfleche bag, and swung it over one shoulder. With his right hand he picked up a heavy iron pot. Its bail cut through his palm. Staggering under the weight of his load, he began to walk.

After Belt Whip had ridden past him, Pedro risked one look back over his shoulder. Behind him, not one tipi was left of what had been the vast Indian village. The entire town—homes, furniture, population—was moving off on the backs of the ponies and mules. All that was left were the darkly crimsoned buttes, the glint of the morning sun on the river water, and the hundreds of little curls of smoke rising from the abandoned fireholes in the flattened circles of grass where the tipis had stood.

One lone occupant remained. Pedro could see the pathetically small protuberance lying motionless amid the waving prairie grass.

Ahead, the long, multicolored cavalcade serpentined slowly through the sandhills. Everyone rode but Pedro and the squaws. He knew they would trudge all day in the hot wind, bowed down by their loads. Already his right hand ached from the heavy burden it hefted, although he had walked only two hundred yards.

From another travois on his right, he saw the sparkling black eyes of children peeping out at him. Dogs of all breeds ran everywhere, tails tucked between their legs, snapping and snarling at each other and howling hideously when some squaw caught them stealing food and aimed a blow at them. A frightened packhorse bolted, spilling its freight along the prairie. A squaw pursued it, yelling like a man. Soon she began arguing with another squaw over ownership of some of the scattered articles. They started to exchange blows.

Pedro took no amusement from the scene. His mind was busy with the heat, the ugliness of the land, and the weight of the burden he carried. Most of all, he could not understand the depravity of a people who would abandon an old woman to the wolves.

5 · The Buffalo Surround

The autumnal buffalo hunt came in early November when the coats of the great beasts were furring brownish-black. For Pedro this brought the hardest labor of his captivity. But he enjoyed it because it took him away from the village and out onto the open plains. And it gave him a look at the higher country to the west. There might be escape in that direction.

He had sensed that an important event was at hand when he saw the women erecting scaffolds upon which to dry the meat, when he heard the warriors singing in unison at the hunting dance, when he watched the old men cut dogwood shoots for extra arrows and fit turkey feathers in the grooves along the shafts.

The hunting party, Belt Whip and Two Hatchets among them, departed, festooned with weapons. Outside the tipis, the women and children stood admiringly, whooping and singing. The gaiety and anticipation infected even Pedro.

When he accompanied the squaws who followed the men on the two-day journey to the buffalo surround, he was permitted to ride one of the packhorses. At first, the land seemed sandy and worthless. Nothing much grew on it save yucca, cactus, and pepperwood. Even the mesquite grew stunted with dead limbs sticking abjectly out their tops, as if ashamed of the general desolation.

However, as they ascended a steep rise and came out upon a

73

high tableland, the ground flattened out and the short, curly buffalo grass afforded a beautiful sight. Its yellowish-gray blades grew only two or three inches above the ground but it turfed so thickly that it excluded everything else. Pedro knew that in Spain a rancher searching for pasture would have passed it by, but Cedar told him that the grass remained nutritious even after it had turned yellow in the fall. She said the buffalo thrived on it and the Comanche ponies ate it so greedily that they sated their appetites much more quickly than on other grasses.

The sight took Pedro back to his studies in Madrid. He had read with excitement the chronicles of the explorer Coronado and his helmet-crested Spanish horsemen who had found land similar to this as they ranged hundreds of leagues north of New Spain in the New World. Like every Spanish boy, Pedro had devoured the testimonies of the conquistadores and their feats. In the letters Coronado had written back to the king, he had told of wild cows and plains so flat and barren that whenever one looked at the cows one could see the sky between their legs.

Coronado and his chroniclers had also described the little field tents of the inhabitants, how they cooked their food with cow dung. They told of the grass so short that after it was trampled upon it stood up again as clean and straight as before. Pedro wondered if he was now riding over the prairies Coronado had seen three hundred years earlier.

He noticed hundreds of small mounds of fresh earth, the burrows of small barking animals. There were whole towns of them. The little brown creatures scurried into their holes when the skinning caravan passed. Owls perched solemnly on some of the mounds. Occasionally a packhorse would lunge quickly to one side to avoid a coiled rattlesnake.

A shout arose from the women ahead. Caught While Mad dismounted at once and put her ear on the ground. Curious,

Pedro did the same. To his surprise, he felt the earth tremble slightly and imagined he heard a barely perceptible rumble, like far-off thunder.

The women began to chatter excitedly, and whipped up their mounts. As Pedro followed, he noticed that portions of the prairie passing beneath them looked as if it had just been freshly plowed. The yucca had been trampled flat from the hooves of a great herd of running animals. He saw the fresh droppings, fetid and green. Ahead, a cloud of dust rose on the horizon and he heard an occasional far-off gunshot.

Soon they began to come upon evidences of the hunt. Bodies of great shaggy beasts dotted the prairie. They had tufted tails and black, bushy manes. Some had fallen so hard that the short, curved horns had broken off.

The corpses were still warm and bleeding. The feathered end of an arrow stuck out of the right flank of each, between the last rib and the hip bone, and Pedro marveled at how unerringly the light shafts had found the vital spot. For a moment, a feeling of envy came over him, a hollow realization that he had missed a thrilling adventure. It was the first time since his captivity that he had experienced an emotion even remotely friendly to this hostile country and his life in it.

As each corpse was encountered, the women would pause to examine the markings on the arrow. If it bore the imprint of her husband, she halted and her work began. If not, she would arise, leap nimbly astride her packhorse and continue until she found what she was looking for. Soon Pedro heard the whoop of Caught While Mad. While Cedar and Pedro stayed to skin the animal, Caught While Mad ran on in search of another buffalo corpse.

Cedar showed Pedro how to grasp the dead bull by the tail and the horns and heft him over on his belly with all four feet spread, ready for the butchering. In such a position, the bull looked like an immense dog, asleep with his head cradled between its forepaws. Then she tied the packhorses to one of the dead animal's upthrust horns and went to work. With a sharp stone knife she slashed across the neck, folding the brisket back so the forequarters could be detached at the joint. She cut down the spine, being careful not to damage the sinews, which were removed intact. Then she showed Pedro how to peel the hide down both sides and disjoint the hindquarters. She sliced the flank and removed it with the brisket in one thin roll of meat. Pedro watched carefully. This knowledge could be useful. When he made his dash for freedom, he might have to kill and butcher his own food as he traveled.

After taking out the entrails, she isolated the ribs with longitudinal slices and grasped their lower ends with both her hands. Then she wrenched them upward to break them off from the backbone. She was neat and expert. Soon all that remained of the beast was the head, rump, and connecting spine. Using the hide as a bag, they wrapped up the meat and bones, ready to load them on the packhorses.

Everywhere the women and older children feasted while they worked, ignoring the large, smelly piles of offal that were black with crawling flies. Pedro's eyes settled on a skinning crew nearby. He saw one sweaty squaw gash with a knife the udder of a dead cow and place her mouth over the rent. Then she sucked the mixture of warm blood and milk. Another, working on the other end of the animal, ripped open the skin between the prongs of the lower jawbone and pulled the severed tongue through the orifice; obviously it too was regarded as a delicacy. He sickened at what he saw next. A squaw was eating from one end of an entrail, stripping it of its contents by pulling it between two fingers, while a dog slunk up and seized the other end and began to gorge himself.

As fast as the skinners finished with a corpse and abandoned it, droves of Indian dogs worried the bones. Packs of wolves hovered boldly on the flanks, feasting hungrily on the more isolated carcasses. The women butchered and skinned most of the day until finally they had more meat and pelts than their pack animals could carry. They worked so fast that when they finished the sun still rode two hours above the western horizon.

Pedro was resting at the last carcass, when he noticed a mounted Indian herder about his own age smoking a cigarette as he watched over a nearby herd of horses. An overpowering yearning for tobacco assailed Pedro. He hadn't smoked since his capture five months before.

At a nod of permission from Cedar, he walked over to the boy, who wore earrings of long, thin shells. The loose flap of his blue breechclout whipped in the hot wind.

"Pah-mo," began Pedro, boldly, using the Comanche word for tobacco. With a mixture of sign language and Comanche words he knew, he endeavored to explain what he wanted.

The herdboy looked at Pedro queerly. Reaching leisurely inside his breechclout, he produced a catbrier leaf and a small quantity of what looked like tobacco. Deliberately, he fashioned a cigarette, his brown eyes warily studying every detail of Pedro's appearance.

He placed the new cigarette in his mouth and ignited it from his own. He presented it butt foremost to Pedro, who took it with fingers still bloody from the day's butchering. The herdboy's polite gesture of lighting the cigarette and his manner of proffering it seemed to belie his Comanche appearance.

"Thank you for tobacco," said Pedro in broken Comanche.

He took a long pull from the cigarette and nearly gagged. What he had drawn deeply into his lungs was not tobacco. It was only a crude substitute.

The herdboy said, *"Perdoneme,* señor. All I have is some crushed sumac leaves mixed with a little tobacco we get once a year from the Mexican traders. I do not even have a cornhusk to roll it in."

Pedro jerked his head up. The herdboy had spoken in purest New World Spanish.

The herdboy continued, "Are you not the one they spared that night they killed the two soldiers?"

Pedro nodded. He identified himself and briefly told his story. The herdboy threw away his cigarette and listened intently. As he listened, his smooth face changed from fascination to incredulity, as though Pedro's account were too extraordinary to believe.

"I, too, am a prisoner," he announced, finally. "I am Tito Gonzales. I was born at Elota in the state of Durango in Mexican Spain. When I was nine years old, the Comanches raided our country and took me away. They also took fourteen of our mules and the horse my father had given me. When they closed in on our *casa,* my father had only one bullet left. I saw him kiss my mama, then shoot her through the head. All our men shoot their women rather than let them be captured by the Indians. Then the Indians lanced my father through the stomach and rode off with me. I have lived with them five years."

Pedro stood frozen. Tito's tale was even more tragic than his own. Perhaps one who had suffered so greatly from Comanche cruelty would be willing to join him when he made his break for freedom. Two might have a better chance than one.

With the end of the jawrope in his hand, Tito leaned closer to slap a fly on his pony's neck. Pedro was horrified to see several holes in Tito's ears.

Tito explained. "Seven times I try to escape. Each time they recapture me and burn a hole in my ear as punishment." With steady fingers, he rolled himself another catbrier cigarette.

Pedro could scarcely believe his eyes. The young brave before him was bare from the waist up and his reddish-brown skin gleamed in the sunshine. His eyebrows had been plucked out by the roots. He wore breechclout and moccasins as authoritatively as any Indian in camp and he sat his pony with indolent ease. He looked and smelled like a Comanche, yet not a drop of Comanche blood flowed in his veins. What a rapid amalgamation these Indians could accomplish! With a tiny crawl of fear, he thought of Roberto. What progress had the Indians made in transforming his brother? Did Roberto still live?

Tito talked on, the cigarette drooping out of the corner of his mouth. "There are many Mexican captives and a few fair-haired, blue-eyed ones among these Comanches. Because of their warrior losses from their constant wars, they need the captured Mexican children to replenish the tribe. Some of the worst Indians of all are former captives whom the savages have Indianized. These Comanches know nothing of the virtues we Christians are taught in the church. They regard the stealing of horses and mules, the murder and scalping of settlers, and the capture of women and children as marks of valor. They have no sense of wrongdoing as we know it."

Tito looked curiously at Pedro. "What warrior captured you?"

"Belt Whip."

Tito's face froze with dread. He had trouble taking his cigarette out of his mouth. "He is one of the worst, señor. You must watch him carefully. I have heard that he sometimes disembowels his captives, cuts their bellies open, when he is drinking liquor. And if they try to escape, he sometimes does it even when he is not drinking."

Pedro felt his spine tense. If Tito had tried seven times to escape and always failed, what chance had he? But he had to do something. He doubted if he had strength enough for the knifeplay he had learned in the gypsy camps of Barcelona. Perhaps an escape attempt would be a better gamble. Provided he tried in some other direction than that over which he had been brought.

He asked, "What do you know of the lands north, west, and east of here?"

"West of here are the New Mexican settlements, but nobody

there would help you, señor. They are in league with the Indians and send their traders twice a year to traffic with them. To the north are more Indians—Utes and Cheyennes. They are almost as bad as the Comanches. I do not know what is east of here. More Indians, I think."

Pedro's eye explored the snuff-colored prairie in all four directions. They looked equally formidable. The orange light of late afternoon intensified the dark lavender shadows in the arroyos. The dry air had become sharper and a savage hunger began to pinch at his vitals. They hadn't eaten since morning, before the hunters went out.

Tito reached down and patted his pony's shoulder. "I am sorry for you, señor, but you cannot escape from these savages. They know this whole land, every path and waterhole in it as I knew my town plaza in Durango. They can trail you at a trot. They know how to survive while you are starving. By using smoke signals they enlist the aid of other bands ahead to intercept you. They would recapture you in two or three days at most, probably much sooner. And remember Belt Whip's knife." With an eloquent gesture of his right hand, Tito feigned a circling thrust across his middle.

Pedro took a final pull on his catbrier cigarette. He threw down the stub and stepped upon it, then looked up at Tito.

"One thing more." He told Tito about Roberto. "Have you seen or heard of him?"

Tito shook his head. "No, señor. If he's still alive, he's with another band. Probably the Nokonis, the Wanderers. The band you and I belong to here is called the Cuchaneo, the Buffalo Eaters. There are many Comanche bands. All of them are bad."

Pedro thanked him and turned to go. He had seen Caught While Mad approaching with several heavily laden pack ponies.

"Señor." Tito threw a look over his shoulder at the herd,

then rode closer. "I am held captive by Gray Eagle and live in his lodge. If you ever do decide to escape, after you are permitted more freedom and learn your way about"—he fingered one of his maimed ears reflectively—"I might go with you. Two of us would have a better chance than one. But it would not be a very good chance."

Pedro nodded. *"Adiós,"* he said gravely.

Pedro returned to help Cedar load the pack animals. Belt Whip and Two Hatchets had hunted so well that there was no room on the packhorses for all the meat. Pedro had to carry a large quantity on his shoulder. Although he was ravenously hungry, he dared not touch a morsel of it.

As he trudged along behind the pack animals toward the hunting camp, he thought of what Tito had said about Belt Whip sometimes disemboweling his captives. Pedro reviewed in retrospect the knife-fighting techniques he had learned in the gypsy camp. The training had been his father's idea.

"A man skilled in weapons will never be in a hurry to seek a quarrel because the knowledge that he can defend himself renders him oblivious to affronts that would wound his pride were he unable to avenge them," Felipe had said.

His father had hired Cavo, a gypsy-Andalusian knife fighter of fifty who was active as a chickadee. The gypsy or Andalusian fights his enemy hand to hand with a knife. Cavo not only taught Pedro all the thrusts, but also how an unarmed person can defeat a man who attacks with a knife in his hand.

Cavo traveled with Pedro. Every day on the grass or bare ground between the wagons, Pedro practiced as assiduously with knives as he did with his guitar. At first he thought he would never master the art. Cavo could take his knife away from him in a flash but Pedro could never disarm Cavo.

"You have the quickest hands I have ever encountered but you don't know how to take advantage of your enemy's loss of equilibrium," Cavo would say.

The old man worked with Pedro twice a day, an hour at a time, for two whole summers. Pedro finally became so proficient with the safe, thick-edged practice knives that he could beat most of the young gypsies in camp.

But that had been more than a year ago. And Pedro had no idea how his skill would work against a Comanche or whether he had strength enough in his present half-starved condition to overcome anybody.

That night, there was great feasting at the hunting camp. Caught While Mad made Pedro stay outside while Belt Whip and Two Hatchets ate beneath the makeshift shelter of old skins draped over a pole reclining on crossed stakes. The autumn night grew chilly. Pedro shivered in his breechclout and moccasins until he could stand it no longer; he dug himself a burrow in the sand of a nearby arroyo for warmth. He thought, When the snows come I will need leggings, an old robe, and something to wrap around my feet. And the snows might come at any time.

For an hour he lay in his sandy cocoon, smelling the roasting food and listening to the coyotes as they barked in the frost-sharpened weather. Just as he had resigned himself to going to sleep hungry, he heard a furtive noise behind the lodge. A dark form had stolen out and stood with outstretched hands.

"There you are." Pedro recognized the voice and his heart leaped. Cedar handed him some fresh buffalo liver, cooked on the coals and spread with fresh marrow.

"Thank you for food," Pedro whispered gratefully. Seared by fire, the meat resisted his first bite. Then his teeth broke through to juicy sweetness. It was good to be alive and hungry.

As he licked his lips afterward, it occurred to him that he owed a great deal to Cedar.

6 · The Comanchero's Guitar

After each day's hunting, the work of fleshing the hides began. All over the hunting camp, the women staked out the skins, and placed them, hairy side down, on level ground that was exposed all day to the sun's rays. They cut small slits in the edges of the skins all around their circumference, then pinned the hides to the ground with small pegs driven through the slits. They spread wood ashes over the greasy surface and as soon as the lye had neutralized the fat, the fleshing began.

With a bone scraper, Pedro helped the women scrape the hide until every particle of flesh was removed and it was clean and white. The skin was then left three or four days to dry in the sunshine. After this was repeated several times the skin was worked by hand. Finally it became soft and pliable.

As soon as all the robes were cured, another hunt was made, until finally there was enough meat and skins to last through the winter.

On the last day of the hide fleshing, Pedro and Caught While Mad were working together when a rain squall came up suddenly. As the first cold drops fell, raising tiny scuds of dust, the squaw began to screech in alarm. Shouting to Pedro for help, she jerked out the pegs and snatched up the skins. Rain would cause them to shrivel and they would then be useless as merchandise.

Pedro rescued as many of the hides as she but two perfect

robes were drenched before he could take them inside the tipi. His heart sank at the thought of the wasted labor—the killing, butchering, skinning, and fleshing.

Caught While Mad had to vent her rage on someone. She picked up a coil of horsehair rope and began to beat Pedro. She kept her back to the only door by which he might have escaped, and in his writhings to avoid the lashing, he upset the pot of stew that was bubbling on the fire. As his foot came down on the red coals, he could not help but cry out.

He saw the squaw's eyes gleam murderously. Not only were the robes ruined but the stew spilled, as well. Abandoning the rope, she darted outside the tipi and snatched up Belt Whip's loaded musket. Pedro ran past her but she thrust out her foot and tripped him. He scrambled to his feet and began to run in a zigzag. He heard the roar of the gun, and a rope of red fire belched past him. He felt the rush of the ball as it thudded into the ground a foot away from him. Then snatching up Belt Whip's war ax, she hurled it at him with all her might. Pedro dodged and a yell of anger bubbled out of his throat. He picked up the ax and he heaved it back at her with all his strength, cursing her in Spanish. She avoided it as adroitly as he. She looked at him strangely, then turned and walked into the tipi.

To his surprise, Pedro found he fared much better for having opposed her. The incident had happened in the center of the hunting camp. Many people saw it. They looked at him with new respect. One squaw even gave him a black salve that smelled like oil to put on his burned heel. The burn made him walk with a limp but Pedro felt wonderful. He had learned that the Indians admired him for fighting back against the tyranny of the squaw. He resolved to remember this.

The first winter of Pedro's captivity began with a long siege of mild weather. The tamarisks growing along the river had turned to pale gold. The cottonwood leaves had changed from buttery yellow to ivory but they still stayed on. Each day, the sun came up and went down in the straw-colored buffalo grass. There were no clouds. Everyone still slept under the light-weight buffalo robes that had had the hair removed. Nature had turned its face toward winter but winter had not come.

One afternoon during the mild weather Pedro and Cedar were walking toward the river for water. A pack of dogs was barking with noisy truculence at something in the brush. The baying had an odd quality; they howled as if death were approaching. Pedro looked down the path.

"What's that?" he asked Cedar.

A group of jeering children were running after an old man, terribly stiffened by age. The man walked with the aid of a crooked stick, his head and shoulders bent over so far that he looked more like a dog than a man. Occasionally the old one would turn slowly and scold them in a bull-like voice that belied his feebleness.

On he plodded, at a tortoise pace. Although the sun shone down warmly, he wore about his middle a mangy buffalo robe that looked as time-worn as he did. His bones, almost as big as those of a horse, jutted through his withered skin; his joints protruded from his shrunken flesh like sinewy knobs. His hair, white as wool, dropped thinly to his frail shoulders. He was the only white-haired Comanche Pedro had ever seen. Apparently he had long ago outlived his usefulness and had been neglected and abandoned by the tribe.

He stopped and tried to roll a cigarette on his hip, out of the breeze, but his trembling fingers, gnarled by age, kept spilling the mixture of sumac and tobacco in the sand at his feet. Cedar went on alone but Pedro lingered, feeling pity.

"Buenos dias, grandfather," he greeted him. "May I help you?"

The old man slowly straightened to his full height and Pedro was astonished to discover that the top of his own head reached only to the ancient's chest. The Indian patriarch stood nearly six and one-half feet tall in his ragged moccasins. His face was as wrinkled as a sun-dried plum. His teeth were much worn and he had lost an ear. His brown eyes regarded Pedro coldly and censoriously.

Pedro took the cigarette materials from the ancient one's shaking fingers, poured the mixture of tobacco and sumac into an oak leaf, rolled it carefully, licked it, sealed it, and handed it back to him. For a moment, the old man lost his look of scorn. He stared at Pedro as one who is reminded of the bright, golden days of his youth.

His voice, deep and quavering, sounded as if it were rolling from the bottom of a cavern. "You speak the Spanish tongue as purely as did Anza many moons ago. I remember Anza and the Spanish. I fought against them. Anza tried to make our people dig in the soil and live in wooden houses at San Carlos. But the eagle does not nest in the martin's house. The antelope will not thrive in a pen. Anza found that out."

Pedro said, in his halting Comanche, "I have heard much of Anza. He died many years ago. He lived in Spain, which is many leagues east of here, across the ocean. My home was in Spain, too." His mind thrust itself back to his history classes in the Royal Academy. Calculating dates, he estimated that this filthy-looking grandsire must be more than ninety.

The ancient peered sourly at Pedro. "I have seen many captives but you are not Mexican. You are Spanish and I have not seen your kind since I was a young man. Where did we capture you?"

Pedro told him.

The old man sneered. "Why did you let us capture you? You Spanish must have grown soft, much softer than in Anza's day. Anza's Spanish fought fiercely with firesticks and long knives. They wore leggings and shirts of iron. What was the matter with you? Were you afraid to fight us?"

Hate twisted in Pedro as he relived the attack on his uncle's rancho. He watched the old man move off, plunging his crooked stick into the sand and staggering a little with each step, as though it was the labor of his life to put one foot down ahead of the other. The dogs redoubled their yelping but kept their distance. The children ran after him, making faces and ridiculing him with shrill cries. But they were careful not to get close.

Pedro wondered what would happen to the ancient one when the cutting edge of the cold that Cedar had promised came down from the northwest mountains.

"When it comes, it will be hard on the poor people," she had explained. "They have few robes and no boots."

As he watched the old one disappear, Pedro thought about Roberto, and a wave of apprehension engulfed him. He wondered where his brother was and whether he would be warm enough. His heart was sore as he turned back to follow Cedar to the river.

The mild weather stayed and there were those who chose to take advantage of it. One afternoon a camp crier rode through the village. Pedro knew enough Comanche to understand the man's announcement. "Trading tonight . . . trading and feasting . . . bring your robes."

There was hustle and excitement in Belt Whip's tipi. Supper was served before the sun set. Everyone ate so fast and left so much on the wooden slabs that for once plenty remained for Pedro. Cedar and Caught While Mad unpiled the buffalo robes taken in the fall hunt and carefully swept them off with a brush made from a skunk's tail. Pedro helped the women put the hides on the packhorses, and standing back, watched them ride off into the dusk.

He had no appetite for the leftover buffalo meat. He felt discouraged and feverish. As he limped outside to see the stars, his burned heel throbbed painfully. Everywhere people were hurrying to the trading. He heard the squaws chattering as they led pack ponies burdened down with robes. Soon the tipis were deserted and quiet.

The night air had a chill in it. Pedro wondered if he would be alive to wear the winter boots Cedar was secretly making for him from the buffalo robe ruined by the rain. She was making them Comanche fashion, with the woolly hair of the buffalo inside.

A strange sound came to his ears, a strange, civilized sound that could not possibly exist in this wilderness of cacti and sage. It was the sound of a guitar being plucked. As it died in the wind, Pedro smiled sadly to himself. In his loneliness, his ears were playing him tricks.

He heard it again, a soft strumming, muted by the wind. The thin, high notes carried clearly above the babble of the distant trading. His ears were not playing him tricks. If there was a guitar in the camp, then there must be a white man playing it. Yet Cedar had told him the Comanches would never permit a white man to come into their homeland.

The breeze lulled and the far-off music became so distinct that he could hear the melody. Although the playing was listless and unimpressive, to Pedro it sounded beautiful. A thrill of hope flamed through him.

He sprang to his feet, oblivious to the pain of his crippled heel. He began to walk toward the music. Forgotten was Cedar's warning that under pain of death he must never go farther from the lodge than the river.

As Pedro passed the empty tipis, one by one, the guitar gradually became louder and clearer. He broke into a jerky trot. Stumbling along, he prayed that the music was not a figment of his imagination. He joined a few stragglers going to the trading. In the semidarkness no one recognized him. He came to an open spot on the prairie, illuminated by huge fires, and his jaw slacked with surprise.

Half a dozen swarthy-faced white men, dressed almost wholly in greasy leather, stood behind crude tables set before a row of skin tents. They wore sombreros on their tously black heads and big-roweled Spanish spurs on their booted feet. They were bartering with the Indians, taking the choicest robes and giving in return ammunition, knives, calico, beads, and steel for arrow points. Behind them, looking strange and ghost-like in the shadows, loomed the great wooden-wheeled carts in which they hauled their merchandise. Pedro remembered the mysterious wheel tracks that scored the prairie when he was brought to the village as a captive.

Hubbub and confusion reigned. The braves stalked gravely from tent to tent, boldly fingering the articles on display and demanding to be waited on first. The squaws, loaded down with robes, pressed behind their husbands, jabbering excitedly and admiring the goods with the zest for shopping typical of women of all races.

A warm wave of hope ran through Pedro. I'll bolt into the midst of these swarthy tradesmen and ask asylum from the Comanches. Surely, they'll protect an unfortunate from the mother country and assist his return to civilization.

He looked warily about, his eyes measuring the distance past the Indians to the nearest group of traders. But as he edged closer, something in the faces of the leather-clad visitors restrained him, something hard and knavish and shrewdly acquisitive. He sensed that these were not honest merchants or they would not be trafficking with the Comanches, swapping them powder and cartridges and Minié balls with which to wage their bloody raids on the southern frontiers. Besides, none of the traders carried weapons and the Indians outnumbered them forty to one.

Pedro saw harnessed mules night-grazing on the nearby prairie. He knew they had drawn the huge carts. Obviously they belonged to the more well-to-do tradesmen.

Apparently the poorer merchants were off to one side, out of the mainstream of traffic. They had ragged little stalls and smaller clusters of wares—lead, paint, tobacco, cloth, trinkets, and a few bags of meal. Behind them the small burros that had carried their merchandise nibbled patiently on the buffalo grass.

It was here that Pedro found the guitarist, a young Mexican teamster who seemed to have no connection with the trading. By the light of the fire in front of the player, Pedro saw that he was about eighteen years of age. He had soft brown eyes and a wide, ugly mouth.

He sat idly on the ground, his back against a packsaddle, lazily pulling at the strings of a guitar as he watched the milling Indians. A rotting ring of buckskin whang was attached to the instrument so he could slip it about his neck and play while standing, if he wished. The whang looked as if it might snap at any moment.

He played indifferently but Pedro paid no attention to the playing. His eyes were glued upon the instrument itself. In the bright light of the fires, it looked old and cheap and shoddy and its flat back of warped ash had been varnished a yellowish brown. But Pedro eyed it lovingly.

He crowded close to the player, all the yearning of six long, pent-up months pushing on his heart. As he watched the player indolently manipulate the strings, his own fingers moved in rapport and he felt the blood pounding at his temples.

"Señor, may I try the instrument a moment? I would be most careful of it."

The Mexican youth's head jerked upward. His brown eyes widened in astonishment. Apparently his first inclination was to refuse. A scowl twisted his mouth. Hugging the instrument more closely to him, he ignored Pedro and continued playing.

But the proprietor of the stall, an older man, interceded. He was a villainous-looking fellow whose black mustache curled sardonically over his thick lips. He had the player's beautiful eyes and ugly mouth. Pedro thought they must be brothers.

"Permit him to hold it a moment, Ricardo. It will attract attention and be good for our enterprise. He will not injure it. Since he speaks our tongue so fluently he must be a captive." Smoke from his dark paper cigarette drifted maddeningly into Pedro's nostrils but his attention was riveted on the guitar.

Ricardo handed over the instrument. As Pedro held it, his throat thickened. With his hands, much roughened by weeks of flesh scraping, he reverently turned the instrument over and over, weighing it, feeling the scratches along its plain ash sides. Pedro feasted his eyes on the sounding hole, noted the worn ebony bridge and the frayed metal frets. Hot tears prickled his eyelids. At that moment he could have thrown himself into a mountain torrent to save a child or given the shirt off his back to a poor peasant. He felt capable of any sacrifice, so rich was he.

He looped the buckskin whang around his neck, and sat on the buffalo grass beside Ricardo. At first his fingers were stiff and cold and the touch of the instrument was strange. He held his ear over the sounding hole, and twisted the pegs with his left hand, then he brushed the strings with the thumb and fingers of his right, tuning with impatient speed.

He began a few quick exercises to supple his wrists and limber his fingers. Annoyed at his lost dexterity, he twisted his buttocks to better his seating position and licked his lips.

He increased his concentration on the warmup drill, his hands flashing and darting and blurring as though he had a dozen fingers on each. He ran the scales rapidly in single notes up and down through three octaves, listening keenly for the instrument's defects, adjusting his technique to compensate for them. The tones cleared and suddenly he began to embellish his exercise with clusters of chords. He plucked them first in crashing crescendos, then gradually softened them to melodious whispers until finally he was satisfied that his skill had begun to return, his wrists to loosen, and his fingertips to feel alive.

Oblivious to all else, Pedro started to play. Because of his elation, he began with a gypsy dance, clawing the strings madly and striking the sounding board like a drum. The music rose and fell in strong, exciting rhythms, sending wave after wave of sound over the sage-dotted terrain. Pedro sensed that Ricardo had shed his apathy and was staring in disbelief at his guitar as if he expected it to explode and the Devil to come striding out of the wreckage.

Then Pedro's long fingers with their dirty nails felt their way into Sor's beautiful "Preludio." The melancholy music sang along softly and sweetly, the melody borne by the silvery high strings, the bass simple and unadorned, yet every brief stab of it tuneful and harmonious. Ricardo's older brother stood transfixed, a tin cup of sugar clutched in one hand, his mustached mouth agape as he listened.

Others were listening too. Pedro was aware of them as he played. A young Comanche girl, attracted by the music, came toward him with a graceful motion; the gorgeous fringes on her buckskin sleeves swayed with every movement of her supple body and the narrow beading on her skirt glittered in the light of the fires. Pedro gave her a look of inquiry. Something about her seemed familiar.

Her long black hair was loose over her shoulders and there was a smell of fresh-scented cottonwood leaves about her. When Pedro looked directly at her he recognized the girl as the one who had befriended and comforted the white captive children on the Quitaque the afternoon before Frank and Shamus were tortured.

He was surprised to see how his music had transformed her. Her lips had parted and she looked as if she were about to burst into tears. Then she gained control of herself and stood listening, her hands clutching the mesquite post that supported the stall. Finally a small, dark woman came up, started to scold her, then herself became so attracted by the music that she stayed to hear it to the end.

Pedro finished the melody and paused, looking wryly at his fingers, bruised from their contact with the strings. He turned to the proprietor of the stand and spoke swiftly in Spanish. "I am Pedro Pavón. My home is in Andalusia, in southern Spain. My father is wealthy. If you can get information to him at some Spanish embassy, telling him where my brother and I are being held, he will reward you."

A shadow suddenly passed between Pedro and the white man. Pedro felt the buckskin whang around his back tighten and snap asunder as the guitar was jerked out of his hands. He turned in anger.

Belt Whip, grasping the instrument by the neck, swung it down powerfully on Pedro's head and shoulders. With a splintering crash of delicately built panels and a moaning of broken strings, the instrument burst in all directions. Pedro scrambled to his feet. The two Mexicans shrank back. They were three hundred miles from Las Vegas with armed Comanches all around them.

Murder blazed in Belt Whip's brutish face. Using the instrument as a club, he rained blows on Pedro.

But Pedro felt wonderful. He took the blows well. His body had become used to beatings. No matter how hard Belt Whip struck him, his brief restoration with his beloved music had lifted his spirit and sent it soaring. Like a soothing balm, the music had taken the pain out of all his hurts.

But the whipping wasn't the only forfeit Pedro paid. Early the next morning, Belt Whip summoned two evil-looking companions. One wore pieces of broken glass tied in his sidelocks for decorations. The other's cheeks were painted with horizontal black lines. Even outdoors, their bodies smelled rancid and greasy.

They grabbed Pedro and threw him on his back on the sand, staking his arms out, then his legs. Wild fear gushed through Pedro as he remembered the warning of Tito, the herdboy. He knew they were going to disembowel him. He looked desperately about and strained against his bonds but they held strongly.

Belt Whip drew his brass-handled knife out of one buckskin legging and stood staring down at Pedro, his eyes glittering mercilessly.

The Indian wiped his knife once across his breechclout and motioned to his two assistants. Obediently they crouched, one grasping Pedro's right leg firmly by the ankle, the other lying heavily across his stomach to pin him securely to the ground and block his view of the proceedings. The morning sun was just topping the nearby ridge, throwing off hues of pale orange, pink, and silvery green. It gave more light. Belt Whip, knife in hand, stepped between Pedro's outstretched legs and squatted. In an agony of despair Pedro mumbled, "Holy Mary, Mother of God, pray for me. . . ."

Coolly, Belt Whip went to work. Pedro felt an excruciating pain but not from the area of his stomach. Instead, the knife's razorlike edge cut across the tendon just below his right kneecap.

It was over in half a minute. Belt Whip knew what he was doing. He did not fully sever the tendon and thereby permanently cripple and reduce the value of his chattel. He wanted only to disable Pedro so that he could not walk long distances from the tipi.

For a full week, Pedro was kept tied down by day but freed at night. Every morning after staking him down anew, Belt Whip would bend the knee back and forth enough to tear the healing tissue and open the wound afresh. As the agonizing pains shot up his leg, Pedro cursed Belt Whip roundly, and his oaths blended with the Indian's resonant, delighted laughter.

The day finally came when Belt Whip freed his victim and Pedro dragged himself stiffly about the premises to do his chores, aided by a rude crutch he contrived from a stick of green cottonwood. So clever was Belt Whip's knowledge of the human anatomy and so skillful his surgery that Pedro was able to walk only a few steps before his knee cramped, compelling him to stop and sit on the ground. His plans for escape had been set back. But he had not been disemboweled, and for this he thanked the Holy Virgin over and over for answering his prayer.

That night, he had another reason for thanking the Holy Mother. As he sat in the sand outside the lodge, Cedar came up to him and gave him news, news that made happiness flash through him like a flame.

"Your brother is camped nearby with Green Turtle's band," she said softly. "They are on their way south to winter. Your brother asked Green Turtle if he might see you. Green Turtle talked this afternoon to Belt Whip. You will be permitted to see your brother in the morning."

7 · The Persimmon Hunt

Outside Belt Whip's tipi, Pedro and Roberto looked each other over after the first joyous embrace. Distress clouded Roberto's face when he saw in the many scabbed-over welts on Pedro's body evidence of the beatings he had suffered.

"What have they done to you, brother? You can hardly walk. Your head is swollen on one side. I feel scars on your back—scars from a flogging. There are fresh lacerations on your arms and shoulders."

Pedro explained briefly, minimizing his wounds. Like a distraught mother, he examined his younger brother from head to foot. Their separation of half a year had been the longest of their lives.

Roberto looked like a Comanche brave in miniature. His thick black hair, flourishing like a weed patch, was parted from the center of the forehead back to the crown, with a braid on each side. Feathers from a small bird were tied to his sidelocks. A streak of red had been painted down the part. The hair from his eyebrows had been plucked clean. Circles of brass dangled from his ears.

"They've treated me better lately," Roberto acknowledged. "At first they made me fight Indian boys my size. As fast as I'd vanquish one they'd bring another. Fighting is the passion of their lives. I fought so hard and so often that I got used to it. Worst of all is their food. Most of it isn't as good as our garbage in Seville. I had to force myself to eat it. I'm beginning to learn their language, too. I've missed you terribly, brother. I'm going to ask Green Turtle's squaw to trade for you so we can live together. Then you won't have to suffer these awful beatings."

Roberto boldly led the way to Green Turtle's camp nearby. Pedro limped after him. It was the most slovenly camp Pedro had ever seen. The flimsy lodges had only a few skins draped carelessly about the poles. Terrapin-shell utensils lay carelessly strewn about the ground. Roberto started at once to do extra chores for Green Turtle's squaw, a fleshy, motherly looking woman. Pedro knew she was Green Turtle's favorite wife because she wore a fringed appendage down the back of her dress upon which was painted a green turtle. Roberto fetched her a load of wood and two paunches of water. All the time he worked, he talked to her, pointing in Pedro's direction.

The squaw looked once at Pedro and shook her head. Roberto kept talking but Pedro knew it was useless. The Comanches did not allow captive brothers to grow up together in the same band. That was why Roberto had been torn from him at the Valley of Tears, near the Quitaque. Cedar had told him this months ago.

Finally Roberto walked over to Pedro, defeat in his face. "Don't give up hope. I'll ask my Indian father when he gets back from the trading."

Soon Green Turtle came striding back and sat down on the grass, examining a trinket he had just swapped for. Roberto hurried to get his red clay pipe, filled it for him, lit it at the cooking fire. Then he put his arm familiarly about the Indian's shoulders and put the question to him. But Green Turtle shook his head.

A qualm of uneasiness came over Pedro. It was not because of the refusal, either. A bond was forming between Roberto and Green Turtle. The Nokoni war chief obviously liked

Roberto and his winning ways. The quicker they both escaped from these savages, the better.

They were given a final moment together. It passed far too quickly. Pedro clasped Roberto in his arms.

"*Adiós,* Roberto!" he whispered. "Be cautious and alert. Be eternally vigilant for an opportunity to escape but don't take foolish risks. If you ever do get away, head for Chihuahua and our uncle's rancho. No matter where your band takes you, keep inquiring about me and I will ask about you. We must try to stay in communication with each other."

Roberto nodded obediently, his boyish face wretched and forlorn. When he looked again at the many abrasions on Pedro's body, his mouth trembled and tears welled into his eyes.

"*Adiós, caro* Pedro."

Pedro watched Roberto manfully square his shoulders and walk away. Soon his straight young back disappeared from view around the side of a lodge. Pedro gulped in a deep breath to fight off the wave of loneliness that engulfed him.

He knew that his brother was young and sweet and malleable. Because Roberto had not yet learned to love the Virgin, he was likely to absorb savage customs.

Pedro prayed hard: "Gently draw him, my Mother, into the fold of Christ. If thou dost not come to his assistance, he will go from good to bad. Let not his faith grow cold in need and danger."

Pedro limped back toward the light, his crude cottonwood crutch screaking dolefully each time he swung his weight upon it.

It was hard to get through the rest of the day. Discouragement weighed heavily upon him. If I ever get back to Spain, he told himself, I shall lie for hours in a soapy hot bath, washing this Comanche stench forever from my pores. I shall gorge myself on clean Spanish food. As he hobbled about the camp, doing the irksome chores assigned by the squaws, he tried to shut out the odors and the nastiness all about him. He tried to pretend he was back in Seville.

It was evening and he would be drawing deeply from a hot cigarette, savoring the good Moorish tobacco in it as Juan, his body servant, helped him dress for a night at the theater. On a nearby commode lay the genteel suit of crimson broadcloth with gold lace to cover it. As Juan helped him into the richly embroidered white silk shirt, Pedro could feel its soft cleanliness sliding over his bare skin and smell its delicate lavender perfume. He thought, Will my body always smell like an Indian's, even after I get back? Will my sores ever heal and my skin grow smoothly over them again?

The flint scraper shook in his hand. How could he go on day after day living a life he so detested? He resolved just to concentrate on getting past the days one at a time, living only for each day as it came.

The next day brought an unexpected event and Pedro was quick to credit his prayers for the good fortune it brought him. He had gone with Caught While Mad and the other squaws to gather ripe persimmons at the border of the camp. A young squaw from a neighborhood tipi, who traced the part line of her hair in vermilion, explained about the persimmons. They were good when eaten fresh, but it was important now to dry and store them for winter eating. The squaws put the ripe fruit into their mouths and sucked out the seeds with their tongue and teeth. Then they spat the residue into their hands and beat it into a pulp with small flat rocks. After drying it in the sunshine, they packed it away in cakes. Months later, the dehydrated fruit would be soaked in water and eaten.

Pedro had little difficulty in understanding the squaw's Comanche speech. His proficiency was fast improving. As he helped the squaws gather the fruit, he talked to them, practicing his speech and perfecting his inflections.

The shrill yelps of racing horsemen arose from the plain before them as the Comanche youths practiced their equestrian feats. Pedro saw Wolf Milk and his companions ride off into the woods. Soon they returned. Wolf Milk had something in his hands, something alive.

A small animal screamed in agony. Pedro felt his insides curdle.

"It's probably a rabbit," said the young squaw with the vermilion part line. "They will pull it apart while it is still alive. They will do it so you will go over there and try to make them stop. They want to torture you too."

Caught While Mad scowled at the young squaw. "Why don't you stop trying to advise everybody? You're too young to give advice. Besides, he's not anybody you should want to help anyhow. He's only a captive."

Pedro ignored Wolf Milk and the young riders. Bruises and welts from Belt Whip's latest whipping still mottled his body. He was scabbed all over. He wanted no more trouble.

He continued to shake the limbs of the persimmon trees, watching the ginger-colored fruit plop into the grass with a soft thud. He thought, what cold unfeeling devils these Comanche boys are. He knew that all human beings had cruel streaks in them but the Comanche's cruelty seemed inborn. As a boy, the Comanche delighted in torturing animals or birds; as a man he took pleasure in wrestling a cry of pain from an adult who was his captive or his torture victim.

Again the helpless rabbit shrieked in pain. This time the sound was prolonged and high-pitched. The guttural laughter of the young torturers drowned out the sound. Pedro felt the hackles rising on the back of his neck.

He dropped the paunch he had half filled with persimmons and began to walk toward Wolf Milk. He knew he was going to be flogged badly again but his anger outweighed his fear.

Wolf Milk and his companions watched him approach. Now they had the victim they really wanted.

Out of the corner of his eye Pedro noticed a movement in the sage. A man with bowed legs came out of a sand-plum thicket, a gray wolfskin robe wrapped closely about him. His presence was commanding. His weatherbeaten face was cunning and his slit-black eyes fierce as an eagle's. He dropped the jaw rope of the pinto he was leading and the animal stood as still as though it were cross-hobbled.

Pedro continued to advance on Wolf Milk and the arrogant young braves standing with him. He knew that whatever punishment he inflicted upon Wolf Milk he would have to deal out speedily, before the rest of the pack closed in. He walked straight up to Wolf Milk. Wolf Milk dropped the rabbit. As it lay upon the grass, its paws twitched convulsively. Wolf Milk seemed surprised at Pedro's boldness but his eyes danced wickedly. He seemed ready for anything but obviously he expected conversation first.

Pedro wasted no time exchanging taunts. Outrage had sharpened his reflexes. He moved quickly. He slapped Wolf Milk across the jaws with a blow that shook the young Indian's teeth. The blow cracked like a whip, and the sound of it carried to the busy squaws on the nearby hill and to the bow-legged man who had emerged from the sage.

Anger flared in Wolf Milk's face. He rushed, trying to get his hands on his smaller antagonist, but Pedro, using some of the knife-play tactics he had learned in the Gypsy camps, withdrew his body while keeping his balance. Just as Wolf Milk stumbled forward, reaching for him, Pedro grabbed him by his long, greased braids and jerked his head downward on his own upraised knee, breaking his nose.

The knee lift was accidental. Pedro's leg came up instinctively as he yanked downward. Still grasping his enemy's hair, he wrenched the Indian violently to the ground upon his back and pounded his head up and down against the hard earth. Blood gushed from Wolf Milk's broken nose.

Wolf Milk's face registered surprise, then truculence and determination. He seemed stolidly indifferent to the blood and the pain. He got his hands on Pedro's, finally succeeded in loosening them from his hair and with a single movement, rose from the flat of his back to his feet.

Suddenly Pedro felt himself pushed violently from behind into the path of his enemy. Wolf Milk closed with him, wrestling him to the grass. With the other young Comanches hovering over them shouting encouragement, Wolf Milk got hold of Pedro's hair and pressed his face so flat into the ground that Pedro's mouth filled with dirt. Pedro fought furiously but he felt the strength go out of him in a rush. He was weak from months of hunger. With a final effort he got to his knees. The other young savages joined the battle with cries of rage and he went down under the weight of a dozen bodies.

"A knife!" he heard the panting Wolf Milk implore in muffled Comanche. "Somebody give me a knife."

Howls of pain sounded dimly above Pedro. The weight on him quickly lightened. He turned over weakly on his side, spitting dirt out of his mouth. A man's deep voice was scolding Wolf Milk and his friends. They slunk off to the river to wash the blood from Wolf Milk's broken nose.

Pedro lay exhausted at the feet of his benefactor. He looked up and saw a pair of bowed legs clad in leggings, a gray wolf-skin robe, and the same cunning, weatherbeaten face that had come out of the sage while he was advancing on Wolf Milk. The man stood looking down upon him, his slit-black eyes thoughtful and impassive. He still held the quirt with which he had routed Pedro's tormentors.

He glanced at the watching squaws in the persimmon thicket.

"Whose captive is he?" he asked. His manner of asking was proud and disdainful.

"Belt Whip's," replied Caught While Mad. "He's worthless carrion," she added scornfully.

The bowlegged man looked around at the pinto gelding and whistled softly. Lifting its head, the animal began walking toward him. The man mounted the pinto and rode off toward the village without looking back.

At the tipi that night, Pedro's body was sore all over. Again Cedar gave him yucca roots which she had chewed and warmed by the fire for his fresh wounds. But Pedro felt good for having fought and hurt Wolf Milk. It pleased and strengthened him. He had suffered a beating, as usual, but this one was worth the suffering.

And he had learned a truism from it. An Indian off his horse was not a powerful man physically. His wrestling was just scuffling. Without weapons, he had little physical skill. It was another bit of knowledge to store away in his mind, something that might be useful when he made his break for freedom.

Cedar told him the man who had rescued him was Creek Water, the most noted Comanche chief in the band. Pedro understood now why Wolf Milk and his cronies had slunk off so fast. Besides, Cedar told him, they had violated the law regarding captives and they knew it. "Captives have the right of life, food, and protection."

Pedro drew himself taut. Life, food, and protection! What a mockery! He had nearly lost his life. The food he was given was abominable. And what did Comanche protection include? Protection from torture, from maiming, from disembowelment?

The next morning a cloud bank began slowly to form across the northwest sky. The wind arose. In the afternoon it changed to the north and before night settled in Pedro heard the camp crier announcing that the village would move.

He was up before dawn helping the squaws tear down the tipis. It was colder. A few flecks of snow fell, slanted in flight by the wind. The band was heading south to get away from it. The pack horses were fetched and loaded and the travois filled. The long procession started. This time Pedro carried a parfleche trunk containing buffalo meat.

He had walked only a quarter of a league when he saw something lying in the grass. He turned it over with his toe and his heart thumped with excitement. It was a small stone knife. When he picked it up he discovered that it was chipped so cleverly that its edges were sharp as a stiletto. In the confusion of moving, someone had probably dropped it.

Its horn handle fitted Pedro's hand snugly. He thrust it in his breechclout. At last he had a weapon to aid his escape. He was making progress toward freedom.

At the edge of camp, he heard a pack of dogs barking queerly. The object of their displeasure seemed to be a bundle of rags lying in a small depression. Their howling became so persistent that Pedro investigated and found the old white-headed man with one ear he had met walking near the river.

Clearly, time had caught up with the ancient one at last. He had been abandoned or "thrown away" and he seemed not to care. As he lay on his side on the cold ground, he looked as though he might be dreaming of the past when he sat his horse as a king and fought Anza's brightly armored Spanish hordes.

His gruff old voice mumbled a song. As he listened, Pedro could translate portions of it: "Old age is hard to bear . . . it hurts to use a cane . . . it hurts to pick it up . . . it hurts to walk with it . . . old age is hard to bear . . . but it comes."

Pedro paused in pity, hating the barbarous custom of deserting the hopelessly aged on moving day. He looked cautiously around him and saw that his group had gone ahead. Putting

down his load, he opened the parfleche trunk, took out a generous quantity of the dried buffalo meat and placed it in the
old man's wrinkled hands. He adjusted the ancient's robe so
that it was under him as well as over him, protecting him from
the cold.

Someone had obviously prepared the old man for death. He
had been bathed, his face daubed with vermilion, and his eyes
sealed with red clay. His small store of personal belongings had
been placed inside his robe. Suddenly the red clay parted and
cracked and the old man's eyes opened, fierce and rebuking.
He peered up at Pedro, scowling and blinking weakly as
though displeased at being awakened from his long sleep into
the spirit world.

A young squaw came past with two packhorses heavily
laden. She saw Pedro looking down at the old man. She
stopped and looked down at him, too.

"His name is Old Sore. He was a famous warrior of the old
times. He was born so long ago that only a few people are still
living who remember his feats. They say as a young man he
took so many scalps that his wives made a robe of them for
him. They say he could run down an elk on the smooth
prairie."

She shook her head sadly. "He asked to be prepared for
death and left alone. His grandniece is Hummingbird Woman
but her husband won't let him live with them. I helped her
bathe him and paint him and dress him for death. Hummingbird Woman and I will mourn him all the way to the new
camping place."

Pedro shouldered the parfleche trunk and set off in pursuit
of the caravan. The north wind blew at his back. The snow
sifted down, carpeting the grass and silvering the black
branches of the sand plum bushes along the route.

At the new camp he helped Cedar erect the tipi. She told
him that she had important news for him.

"You are going to live with Creek Water as soon as he returns from a scout. You belong to him now. He liked the way you fought Wolf Milk and his friends. If you are quick to learn the ways of a warrior, Creek Water may adopt you as his son. Belt Whip sold you for two issue blankets and six measures of corn."

Pedro stared at her. He could hardly believe his good fortune. Now he would be free of Belt Whip's tyranny. But he could not help feeling mortified, too. Although he was Pedro Herraro Vicente de la Pavón, the finest young guitarist in the world, a direct descendant of Ferdinand, the Catholic king, his Indian master thought so little of him that he had been sold for two dirty blankets and an armful of moldy corn.

Pedro resumed his labors. Using a digging stick, he planted the butt ends of the tipi poles two feet into the red soil so that the lodge would withstand the strongest winds. It really didn't matter that he had been sold so cheaply. He was not going to stay forever with these barbarians.

The next evening Pedro again heard the dogs howling weirdly. Their howling carried a strange intensity, as though death were approaching. And indeed it was.

A cracked voice bellowed irritably, "I want food and water." Pedro sat up, listening. The deep, discordant tones and the air of authority seemed familiar. The voice demanded again, "Get me food and water."

Pedro went outside and found Old Sore, the one-eared ancient, advancing up the trail at a snail's pace. Strengthened by the food Pedro had left for him, the old man had walked the fifteen miles from the former camping location and was just arriving, leaning on a crooked stick. He still had on all his burial clothing and carried in his hands the precious personal articles they had left with him in the burial robe.

Hummingbird Woman, who lived on the trail, heard him too and came outside. She whooped with pleasure and brought the old man into her tipi and warmed him by the fire. She hurried to get him food and drink before her husband returned from hunting.

Pedro was mystified. When Cedar's grandmother had been abandoned there had been no lamentation. And had she rejoined the camp, he doubted if there would have been whoops of joy. As he helped Cedar stake down the bottom tipi skins to keep out the cold night wind, he asked her about it.

Cedar replied in a matter-of-fact tone, "She was a woman. Her death was of no account."

8 · Old Sore

Creek Water summoned Pedro to his lodge and beckoned him to sit in front of him. As Pedro looked into the shrewd black eyes with no lashes above them and two crescents of dark blue painted under them, a growing caution filled him.

He thought that never in the Old World or the New World had he encountered such a commanding presence. Creek Water's coarse black hair, faintly powdered with the red dust of the land, hung in a tangle almost to his shoulders. He wore no decoration in it save a single eagle feather in his braided scalplock. He sat erect, motionless. Nothing about him moved but his glittering eyes, slightly slanted and black as obsidian, which now bored straight into Pedro's. For a moment Pedro had the chilling fear that this man could look into his heart and read his thoughts and intentions as easily as he could read his pinto's tracks on the prairie.

"This is what I want to say," Creek Water began gravely. "A boy growing into manhood is not taught by his father. His grandfather shows him how to ride, shoot, hunt, and trail. His grandfather teaches him what he needs to know about tribal legends and religious matters. A boy is allowed much liberty. He will not do any work about the camp such as you have been doing. A boy is respected and looked up to because he is going to be a warrior and his life may be short. He may die young in battle."

He described to Pedro the status in which he had been placed and promised he would formally adopt him if Pedro learned to be a good Comanche.

"But first, you will have to work hard to catch up with the other young men. You have no grandfather, so Old Sore will teach you. Old Sore knows more about war and hunting than any grandfather in camp. He was a famous warrior of the olden times. He lived in a day when our warriors took a knife and slit their horses' noses up to the gristle so that they could breathe in more air and run a long time without growing tired. Old Sore has lots of idle time and wants to be your teacher. I have given my consent."

Pedro listened and remained silent. He had been told by Cedar that Comanche parents leave most of the teaching and all the physical disciplining to some close relative while the child is growing up because too much parental regulation breeds animosity. He had been impressed by the wisdom of this. These Indians were far ahead of the Old World in much of their thinking. Apparently this theory was followed through adolescence, with the grandfather taking over as pedagogue when it came time to school the boy in the arts of war and the chase.

"While Old Sore trains you for war and the hunt, I will instruct you in the vision quest," Creek Water went on. "Selection of a man's medicine is the most sacred thing of his life. Power comes from visions. All your life you will need lots of power. You must also think of marriage. You will need horses and plunder to get a wife."

Pedro's pulse began to pound. The last indignity he would submit to in this primordial hellhole would be to take one of the unclean Comanche girls to wife.

Creek Water continued. "Old Sore was a great warrior before most of us were children. He is the best teacher you could have. He will teach you the old ways but you must learn the new ways, too. When he was a young man we hunted everything with bows and arrows. Now we have guns, and flint and steel to start our fires with. We don't slit our horses' noses anymore. After Old Sore teaches you the old way, I'd better teach you some of the new ways. Then you will know both. That will be good."

Pedro listened impassively, but he had no intention of learning either way. If his plan worked, he would soon be in northern Mexico and on his way to Spain.

Pedro sawed the jaw rope, halting the mule. The March sun, two hours high, warmed his bare back. He smelled the faint perfume of the wild plum blossoms blooming like white lace from the stunted clumps growing along a sandy knoll. The south wind blew so boisterously that it ruffled the feathers of a small brown owl perched on a nearby prairie-dog burrow, making the bird look puffy and disfigured.

For a month he had been taking his meals in the tipi of Porcupine Woman, Creek Water's oldest wife. Now he felt lean and fit. He had been treated with a respect he could scarcely become accustomed to. Porcupine Woman, fat-legged and friendly, and Creek Water's other two wives waited on him hand and foot. Once when Pedro had started to unsaddle his little mule, the youngest wife pushed him aside and did it herself. Offended at first, Pedro saw it was the custom all over the village. Older boys were persons of distinction here. At meals, the women served Creek Water first, then Pedro.

The month in camp had not been wasted. When Pedro's facial hair started to grow, the women had showed him how to pull it out with bone tweezers. As he looked at himself in the river one morning, he was surprised to discover that he looked as much like a Comanche as any boy in the band. His brows and cheeks were plucked clean. His black hair dangled in short braids down each shoulder. Porcupine Woman had shown him how to paint himself with pigment from berry juices. He learned that a warrior always carried paint and was expected to ornament himself with it upon special occasions or when strangers came. Pedro had tolerated all this because it gave him something to do, but in his heart he lived only for the day he could leave it all.

He watched Old Sore ride up on the old buckskin pony Creek Water had given him. On the ground, Old Sore seemed slow and slovenly. On a horse, the old man was exalted and graceful. He rode as if he had lived half his life in the saddle, controlling the animal with an authority so absolute that the shabby beast gave him instant obedience.

Pedro had never seen anybody sit a horse as peculiarly as did this gangling grandsire. Old Sore leaned so far forward that the upper part of his legs clutched the buckskin's bony body in an almost perpendicular position. But from the knee down, his legs were thrown back and his heels were thrust into the animal's flanks for a hold. His left hand held the jaw rope and in his right he carried a short stick with a rawhide thong on the end of it. A light flick of this against the animal's side punctuated every step of his mount, constantly reminding the pony of its complete subservience to him. He sat the animal strongly, with his weight borne by the crotch and thigh muscles. How he could ride thus and escape injury from the high pommel of his elm and rawhide saddle was something Pedro could not understand.

Pedro rode ahead, scanning the horizon warily, always weighing his chances for escape. Now that he was freed from the loathsome labor and despotism imposed by Belt Whip, he thought constantly of making a dash for freedom. He knew the peril that attended it. Creek Water would move like mechanical doom. Once Pedro left the village, a party would start instantly on his trail and messengers would be sent to bands far and near, warning the whole Comanche country to keep a sharp lookout for him.

They would light so many signal fires that the sky would be hazy with their smoke and he would have as much to fear from his front as from his rear. But he was resolved to make the effort. He doubted if Old Sore would constitute much of an obstacle despite his physical rejuvenation after a month of stuffing himself with the buffalo meat and pemmican provided by Creek Water. Old Sore's face, which had looked like a skull, was filling out. There was meat on his cheekbones now and the hollows around his eyes were disappearing. Even the dogs had stopped barking at him and the children jeered him no more.

Pedro slapped the end of the jaw rope impatiently against his legging. He would like to start off this very morning. He had food enough for three days. On moving day he had appropriated several strips of dried buffalo meat from the parfleche trunk he was carrying and cached it after dark in a hollow chinaberry tree near the river. All he needed was a good horse, but Creek Water had been careful not to give either of them a mount that would carry an escaping captive far. Until Pedro could find or steal such a horse he was as much a prisoner as if he still belonged to Belt Whip.

He was tired of having the old man constantly underfoot. Like all older boys, Pedro had been given a neighboring tipi to live in. Old Sore had moved in with him and his main purpose in living seemed to be to teach his young benefactor the things every Comanche learns early—how to hunt, use weapons, throw the lasso, ride and handle horses, and follow a trail—skills in which Pedro was almost totally lacking.

Now Pedro scowled at the grass bending before the breeze and listened to its steady, ceaseless whispering. He wanted no part of the tedious course of instruction Creek Water had planned for him. But something warned him not to underestimate this chief who was his new master.

He followed Old Sore through a hackberry grove and came out into sunlight that shone golden off a coppery slope of grass. Old Sore signaled him to dismount. They both slid off. The old man showed Pedro how to hopple his mule, wrapping a buckskin strip above the fetlock joints of the front and rear leg on the same side. However, he only staked his own mount.

"Don't ever stake a mule," Old Sore warned. "It will pull up the stake and run off. Then you have to walk back to camp."

Pedro himself had found the mule. One night he and Old Sore were sleeping outside Creek Water's hunting lodge. Suddenly Pedro was awakened by the roar of a wild animal almost in his face. As he opened his eyes, he beheld the mule standing over him, heehawing, its long ears wagging against the moon. Short-legged and big-bellied, the animal was so tame that when Old Sore's grass lasso, thrown with a swish from the adjacent bed, settled softly around its neck, it did not struggle. Old Sore fitted a noose around its underjaw and hoppled it. Next day it was quite docile, permitting Pedro to ride it at will. Since it was obviously a stray, Old Sore told Pedro the mule was his.

They walked fifty paces away from their mounts. Old Sore halted. All about them the tall grass rippled slowly in the wind. Pedro had never seen land like this. When he sat down in the grass, the country looked like a bowl and the horizon seemed to surround him on all sides. Half a league in the distance, he saw the haze of tipi smoke drifting above the village. An occasional bush of yucca or cholla was all that relieved the flat monotony of grass and wind.

Old Sore retreated behind a yucca, a mischievous glint in his irascible face. "Turn your back and wait until I tell you to turn around."

Pedro hesitated. He doubted the wisdom of turning his back on any Comanche, let alone one whose bloodstained hands had dispatched so many people into the spirit world. But he pulled a deep breath and turning his back, began to walk forward on the prairie.

He had gone only eight steps when Old Sore called challengingly, "Find me, *español*."

Pedro wheeled. The tall prairie grass leaned and doubled before the long wind flurries, its surface rapidly changing and blending in browns and yellows and greens in the early morning sunshine. Beyond it, the horse and the mule grazed quietly in the background. But where was Oid Sore?

Pedro examined the yucca bush behind which the tall old man had stood. He explored the terrain all around it. He searched the area where the horse and mule grazed. There was no break in the terrain, no secret shelter in which Old Sore might have hidden. It was as though some gigantic bird had swooped down to swallow him, then streaked away, faster than sound.

Pedro was still searching when he heard a taunting laugh behind him. "You almost trod on me twice, *español*. If I had been a snake, I could have bitten you."

Pedro spun around to see the old man arise, laughing and triumphant, within a pace of him.

Old Sore showed Pedro how to cover himself so cleverly with grass that he looked like a segment of the landscape; how to lie among the yuccas and so faithfully copy the structure of a bush that he appeared a part of it. He taught Pedro how to drape a skinned robe about him, and by partly covering himself with dirt, pass for a pink boulder when they were hunting or raiding in stony country.

Then he made Pedro do the hiding, and patiently corrected his many mistakes. As the afternoon passed, Pedro became very hungry. He complained about doing the same things over and over.

"Our children learn this game at an early age, *español*," the old man chided. "You are many years behind them. But I will teach you to catch up."

Pedro sighed. He had begun learning to be a Comanche by playing the game of children. There was so much to learn about concealment that Pedro was aghast at what he did not know. But he learned steadily, never forgetting a thing once he understood its purpose and was shown its method. He found that by applying himself, he forgot much of his boredom and time passed much faster.

His next instruction was in shooting. Pedro hoped that Old Sore would follow the new way and use the one-shot musket he had seen Creek Water carry on occasion. It was Pedro's plan to learn to load and shoot it, then eventually to steal the musket. A gun and ammunition would aid his escape effort tremendously.

But the old man would have none of it. "I have something to say about that," he told Pedro sternly. "This is something everybody ought to know, even Creek Water. Muskets are no good. You cannot load one on a horse. You cannot always get powder and bullets for one. They shoot too slowly. Creek Water likes them now because they are new. But when the newness wears off, he will be glad to go back to the bow and arrow."

He straightened and looked with affection at the plain bow in his hand. It was made of smooth wood from the Osage Orange, sinew-wrapped and tightly glued. Its taut string was contrived from horsetail hair twisted to form a strong cord.

"Now I will tell you about bows and arrows, *español*. They are noiseless. When you attack at night an arrow kills the enemy sentinel without awakening his friends. When you are on the chase or the hunt, you can kill two and sometimes three animals with the bow and arrow before the others in the herd are aware of you. Arrows are so light that you can wear them in a skin case over your right shoulder and never know they are there. You can use them at close quarters. You can shoot them so fast that before your first arrow has struck, your second is leaping off the bowstring. We should never give up the weapons of our ancestors."

He took Pedro out to the edge of the camp. Fitting an arrow to his bow, he drew it back strongly with his long right arm and discharged it almost three hundred paces into a distant sandbank. He twice split a last year's crow's nest in the fork of a cottonwood tree at a distance of forty paces.

He showed Pedro how to hold the bow, fit the arrow, and draw it back. They worked most of an afternoon, until Pedro's shoulders ached and his arms grew weary, before Old Sore seemed satisfied and promised Pedro he could start shooting by himself.

Always the old man was derisive of the new ways and loyal to the old. He liked horsetail bowstrings rather than those made of sinew because they did not break as readily and exposure to moisture did not affect them. When he grooved his war arrows, he scorned the common method of using straight furrows and rutted them in circular channels from the end of the feathers to the head of the point so that "more enemy's blood can leak out the grooves and weaken him." He winged his arrows with wild turkey-wing feathers, because those of the hawk and eagle were worthless when wetted by blood. He disliked the metal his tribesmen purchased from the New Mexican traders for their arrowheads; he preferred the old-style flint points because they were sharper and more apt to be fatal.

He taught Pedro how to select and cut wood that was free from knots for his bow, how to work it down to size while it was still green, how to season it, scrape it, and scour it with buffalo brains to make it pliable. Soon their tipi was filled with bow wood and arrow wood in various phases of seasoning. It reeked with odd odors, the most ill-smelling of which came from paunches partly filled with glue made from the rawhide chippings taken from the neck of a buffalo bull. Scores of arrow shafts were stacked near the fire for seasoning.

Every day, Old Sore showed Pedro how to take up the arrows, grease and warm the crooked sections in them, then bend them into shape with his hands and teeth. On cloudy days the tipi's interior was so dark that it was difficult for Pedro to walk about without treading on some implement of war. This would draw a bellow of annoyance from Old Sore, who seemed to have in the back of his hoary head a map of where he had placed everything. He never stepped on anything.

One night after a particularly tedious day of arrow making, Pedro was awakened from his deep sleep by a slight noise outside the tipi. He lay still, watching and listening. On the other side of the lodge Old Sore was snoring like a grandfather bullfrog bellowing in a swale.

The bottom of the tipi wall near Pedro began to raise slowly. He could barely see it in the half-light. Who sought to enter and why? He knew it was not a thief. Theft among the Comanches was so unusual that it was regarded as an abnormal act. Did someone wish to kill him? He reached stealthily into his breechclout and closed his fingers over the handle of the little stone knife. He silently gathered his body into a coil and waited.

The lodge skin lifted higher and higher. A black head and shoulders, cloaked in shadow, came thrusting through. Pedro's heart pounded. He got to his hands and knees and crept backwards a few inches.

A muffled titter of laughter, unmistakably feminine, came from the opening. Pedro sniffed with displeasure. The intruder was a girl. She smelled like most Comanche women, filthy and nasty.

Her fingers touched his bare leg, a brief touch that sent a shiver of disgust crawling up his spine. He sprang backward.

"Why are you here? What do you want?" he asked. She said nothing but kept coming. Now her hips and buttocks were underneath the flap.

Pedro leaped across the dark lodge floor where Old Sore was asleep and shook him. The old man awakened instantly.

"Somebody just crept into the lodge," Pedro whispered. "I think it's a girl." He looked over his shoulder for the intruder and saw her body disappear beneath the tipi flap.

The old man grunted once, an amused grunt, as though the matter had no importance.

"*Español,* you are advancing socially. Your visitor was a sleep-crawler."

He explained that sometimes bolder, unmarried girls crept into a boy's tipi at night to initiate him in lovemaking. They always kept their identity secret, for the sake of their reputations.

"Some maiden has noticed you and desires you. Why did you waken me, *español?* Why are you Spanish so strange? A well-mannered boy doesn't act like that. It's the girl's place to come to you and she did."

Pedro snorted disdainfully. "She smelled horrible, like the guts of a rotting deer."

"Why is that important?" the old man muttered sleepily. "After this, pinch your nose with your fingers so you can't smell her. Then try to be more friendly." He turned over on his side.

Pedro drew himself up angrily. He wanted no part of these dirty Comanche girls. He had no need for female companionship. He flopped down on his robe and stared into the darkness. The quicker he could steal a horse and be gone from this place the better he would like it.

March passed, full of wild winds and the dust they generated. When the buffalo grass began to green, Pedro knew that spring was coming. He welcomed his next field of instruction, how to ride and handle horses. In Andalusia, Manuel had taught him to ride with balance and control. Pedro had especially enjoyed the morning canter at his father's mountain stable with the son of the stablekeeper. After ascending the small mountain they could look down to the quiet little hamlet below and see roofs of weathered red glistening in the sunshine and hear the clucking of its chickens and the cries of playing children.

But there were no mountains here and no smooth-gaited horses with comfortable Spanish saddles. Old Sore galloped up on his old pony with five half-tamed *pookes,* or mustangs, on leash. The old man had brought along Arrow Bush, a herd boy about Pedro's age, to help him handle the fractious animals. They lost no time introducing Pedro to his new assignment.

Pedro discovered that the riding he had learned at the Royal Academy helped him very little here. Old Sore would have none of his upright stance, not even on the mule. Nor would he permit Pedro to ride like Arrow Bush and the other Comanche boys, whose short stirrups compelled them to sit almost on their tailbones with their heads carried forward. Old Sore made Pedro ride his way.

But first he told his pupil why the horse was important to the Comanches, a telling that was enriched with the old man's anecdotes about his boyhood, when the tribes still used dogs to draw their travois and the horse had not yet been acquired in large numbers.

"The horse made the Comanches great," the old man said. "Before the Great Spirit helped us take him from you Spaniards, we were just foot Indians. We didn't have much fun. There was little in life worth stealing except the women and you couldn't take them very far. But the horse changed everything. We found we could ride him on hunts and get more food, carry it farther, bring more of it back to camp. We could have the fun of stealing him from other tribes and from the

Mexicans and from the Spaniards. He was no trouble to feed because he ate grass and the bark of trees. We made saddles, robes, and rawhide thongs from his skin. We made ropes and bridles from his mane and tail. When food was scarce, we ate him. Horses are property. We make presents of them to get our wives and settle our quarrels. They made us better warriors, too."

He paused and began laboriously to roll one of his catbrier cigarettes on his hip, out of the wind. "When we got horses, we rode south and beat you Spaniards. We beat the Apaches and took their lands. We raided against Mexico, taking much plunder and many captives. We raided the Texas settlers, and punished them for using our domain. Because of the horse our lives became exciting and worth living. You must learn to love the horse, *español*. You must learn to steal him and ride him and we'll start right now on this blue mustang here. Come! We will find out what you can learn."

Pedro learned first how to stay on a bucking horse. Old Sore and Arrow Bush rode to one of the small prairie lakes for this instruction. Arrow Bush lassoed the blue, and threw it to the ground. He grasped its head and blew his breath into its nostrils to calm it while Old Sore looped a rope around its under jaw and fastened an elm saddle about its middle. When the horse was permitted to sit up, Pedro mounted and Old Sore handed him the rope end. Arrow Bush led the animal into the shallows of the lake, and yelling suddenly into its ear, freed it.

Instantly the mustang exploded, splashing water like a geyser. Pedro fought to stay on its back. Old Sore, a robe about his loins, loped along the bank on the old buckskin shouting advice.

"You will fall many times while learning," the old man bellowed. "But you cannot fall so hard in the water. And a horse cannot buck so hard in the water." He neglected to add that the water was as icy as a mountain freshet.

Even in the lake the ride was so rough that Pedro felt as if his guts were jumping up into his throat. He swallowed much of the water that gushed into his nose and mouth each time he was unhorsed. He almost wished himself back in Belt Whip's custody. Furious, he took his anger out on each horse he straddled, resolving with grim determination to master it so that he could start on another trial that would hasten his time of escape. Day after day he practiced until finally he learned to stick on the backs of the mustangs to Old Sore's satisfaction, first in the lake shallows and then on the nearby prairie.

And then came the time when Pedro was to attempt the difficult feat he had seen Wolf Milk and his friends perform of throwing himself on the side of his mount, leaving the enemy only a heel and one eye to shoot at. For this training Old Sore took him to the opposite side of the village to the deep river sand. There the horses could not run so fast, no matter how hard they tried. There the falling was softer. And Pedro Pavón fell many times.

He learned that Wolf Milk supported himself on the side of his horse by passing a short loop of rawhide attached to the pommel of the saddle over his head and under his arms. But this method was scorned by Old Sore.

The old man used a short hair halter which he looped under the horse's neck with both ends tightly braided into the mane on the withers, leaving a loop hanging beneath the neck and against the breast. Pedro had to grasp this with his left hand while sliding off the right side of his horse and fall into it with his elbow, bearing the weight of his body on his upper arm.

Pedro liked this method better. After several jolting spills, he learned to drop fearlessly into the sling, dragging his heel over the horse's back to steady himself. He then used the sling as a lever to return to his original seat in the saddle.

Next he learned to discharge his arrows from under the speeding pony's belly as well as from beneath its neck. And since the horse might be shot out from under him, he was thoroughly indoctrinated in the art of disengaging himself from the loop and jumping clear. He usually hit the sand on his feet but Old Sore taught him that whatever his landing fate, he must rise quickly, hold his shield in front of him and shoot his arrows from underneath it. He worked for hours at this rough feat. The old man galloped alongside on the mule, roaring advice as he corrected every detail.

Pedro almost hated Old Sore for his insistence on perfection. Driven to the point of rebellion, he sometimes swore that he would not submit to the old man's tyranny another day and would try to escape that very night. But at night he was too tired to even think about escape. And after a good sleep, he was always ready to go out again with the ancient one.

All through the rainy spring and the torrid summer they worked. The old man made Pedro constantly review all the skills he had been introduced to: concealment, shooting, riding, and arrow making, so his proficiency in each would not dull. When Creek Water, who was often absent on raids or council meetings, would return home, Old Sore would report to him on Pedro's progress.

Pedro was permitted to keep his knife and roam at will about the village, but for this he seldom had time because Old Sore kept him so busy. His relationship with Creek Water was briefer even than that of the average Comanche father and his son. Pedro thought it might be because he was still lacking in so many of the skills other sons learned from boyhood. But he knew that the chief was carefully following his improvement.

He sensed that Creek Water must know how hard the learning was because once the chief summoned him and said, "This is what I want to say. It is not the man who stays in the lodge who will be great. It is the man who works, sweats, and is always tired from going on the warpath. You are not ready to go on the warpath. But when you do go, do not turn around when you have gone part way. Go as far as you were going in the first place, then come back. The same thing is true of what Old Sore is teaching you now. Do not go part way. You must learn all the way. You must work and sweat. You must be a man."

So Pedro kept working and sweating even though his thoughts were always on escape. By the time Yuh-pah-ne, the fall, came and the buffalo grass turned gray and the winds howled mournfully through the tops of the tipi poles, Pedro was attaining such proficiency that the other youths resented it.

It was on such a day that Pedro went with Old Sore to take a bow to Big Crow, the father of Wolf Milk, whom he had over-thrown in the wrestling match. Big Crow, knowing Old Sore's skill, had asked him to make the bow for his son. It was mid-afternoon when they arrived at Big Crow's tipi to deliver the bow and accept the customary present, a horse. In accordance with Comanche custom, Big Crow's wife set food before them: a generous quantity of cold buffalo meat and mashed corn obtained from the Wichitas.

Wolf Milk had already received his spirit vision and was ready to take the warpath. He sat silently in a corner sharpening a metal arrowhead. Pedro saw with satisfaction that although Wolf Milk's broken nose had healed, it was still crooked.

The woman was civil enough when she first served the food. Then Pedro saw Wolf Milk whispering to her. When they finished eating and she started to clean up, she saved every morsel Old Sore had not eaten and stored it in a paunch hanging from a tipi pole. But everything Pedro had left she threw away. She even went to great pains to scrub with sand the wooden slab upon which he had dined.

When they rose to go, Wolf Milk turned to Old Sore. "Thank you, grandfather, for the bow." But he only stared at Pedro and did not speak. Pedro knew from that look that his enemies would like to destroy him. He resolved to be very alert. The sooner he could escape, the quicker he would be rid of this menace too.

He brooded on Wolf Milk's hatred during the night, and decided to find Tito Gonzales, the Mexican herdboy with the holes burned in his ears. Perhaps Tito would join him in an escape. Since Tito's post of duty was near the herd, he would be able to steal the horses they would need; moreover, he could steal good ones. They would need animals of stamina and speed.

The next afternoon, he rode past the herding grounds and looked about cautiously for Tito. Tito was not there. Pedro asked one of the herdboys where he could find Gray Eagle's captive.

Hate showed plainly in the herdboy's face as he recognized Pedro. "His flesh is rotting in the sunshine, if the wolves haven't already eaten it," he spat out. "He tried to run away again. This time he got as far as Pahseehoono, the Red River. When they brought him back, Gray Eagle thrust his lance clear through him and left his body lying on the prairie. They did not even bury it."

Shaken, Pedro rode slowly back to camp. He was saddened by the news of Tito's death. He had liked the young Mexican and pitied him for the tragic manner in which he had been orphaned. Now he was dead, his young life cruelly and painfully expunged. Surely one so unfortunate on earth would be well received in heaven.

As Pedro rode, he began to pray. "O Virgin Mary, Mother of all Christians, living and dead. Behold me, dear Mother, supplicating thee to intercede for the soul of dear departed Tito before the throne of Infinite Justice. . . ."

The first cold spell of winter struck that night and as Pedro lay in the dark listening to the winter wind drive sand particles against the tipi wall he planned the first step in his escape. With a surge of excitement he perfected it in all its details. It was a much better plan than any other because it would give him a long start on his pursuers.

He thought about the plan all winter. He thought about it when he helped the squaws dig paths in the snow after the biggest snowfall of the year nearly buried some of the horses and there was a shortage of wood and fuel. He thought about it when he cut shoots from the cottonwoods for the horses to eat: the bark was frozen so hard that it cut their mouths.

Pedro felt sympathy for the horses. Their coats became long and rough and matted with burs. With their bony hips protruding and their bellies swollen with barks and sticks, they were the most downcast creatures he had ever seen. He wondered if they would ever recover in time to carry him when the winter ended and he attempted to put his escape plan in motion. The plan was built about the vision quest. Pedro still believed it the best plan anybody could devise. He wondered why no other captive had ever thought of it.

Creek Water had told Pedro about the vision quest, the sacred search for power that every young warrior makes. Pedro knew what was expected of him. Clad only in breechclout and moccasins he must depart at night and walk to a place a mile or so from the village. There for four days and nights he would smoke and pray in solitude for power that might be used for good. He must go alone. No one would come near him. He must fast, taking no food. When he received his vision, it would come to him in a dream, and there would be some expression of nature such as the howl of a wolf, the screech of a hawk, or the moaning of the wind.

"It may take you longer, since you have lived most of your life with the white strangers," Creek Water had told him. "Tell me about your religion."

Pedro told him in detail the story of Christ's crucifixion and its special significance to man. When Pedro finished, a muscle twitched in Creek Water's face.

"I heard all this once from a white missionary who spoke to us at a peace conference on the Rio Brazos. When he told us that the white men had killed their savior, I was surprised. But I changed my mind later, after I became better acquainted with them."

Creek Water had reached for his pipe and his beaded tobacco pouch. "If you do not receive your vision within four days and nights, you should abandon your quest and try again later. But it will come. When it does, keep it secret. Do not reveal your new power to any man without the consent of your new guardian spirit. Once you have your new power, you may use it for many things. The greater your power, the greater will be your prestige."

In the dark of the tipi, Pedro reviewed his plan again. Four days and four nights. He must go alone. No one would come near him. What a priceless opportunity! The usual restrictions would be relaxed. He would be free to leave the lodge alone at night and no one would challenge him. He would conceal the cached food in his breechclout and go straight to the herding grounds and take two horses that would not be missed. He would ride by night and hide by day and since he would not be missed for four days, he should have all the headstart he needed. After two weeks of hard riding in a straight southeast direction he should reach the Texas settlements. Then it would be easy to find the rancho.

But he knew that even the best plans sometimes go awry. Thinking of Tito's fate, he bowed his head in the darkness and asked again for the help which had always sustained him.

Spring came and Yoo-ah-noo-eh, the south wind, swept warmly over the land. They were now camped in the Tanima country. The thorny mesquite trees put on gay costumes of elliptical leaves and decked themselves in veils of pale greenish yellow blossoms with pendants of long slender beans, reminding Pedro of the carob trees in the south of Spain. The time had come to make his break for freedom.

Creek Water was away on a council mission. Pedro told Old Sore he wanted to start that night on his vision quest. He hoped Old Sore would believe that he was sincere. Without a word, the old man collected a buffalo robe, bone pipe, quantity of tobacco, and a fire drill. He put the smaller articles in a buffalo-horn case.

When it grew dark Pedro bathed in the river. He withdrew his cache of dried buffalo meat from the hollow tree and secreted it in his breechclout before returning to the tipi. His body tingled with excitement and fear. He had waited so long for this night.

Wearing only his breechclout and moccasins, as Creek Water had instructed him, he picked up the buffalo horn of religious material.

Old Sore watched him from a corner of the tipi. The flames from the fire lit his bony face in mahogany hues. The old man sat very still, like a Comanche Buddha. He seemed almost dozing. For a brief moment, Pedro felt kindly toward his aged tutor. He was almost ashamed to be running off. But this was no time for regrets. He drew a long breath and took one final look around the lodge. Then he stooped beneath the flap and went out into the night.

He walked slowly through the moonlight, his moccasins noiselessly trodding the dewy grass. Every lodge glowed red from the fire within it. He paused a moment to listen to the night sounds. Children were crying, mothers were soothing. Everywhere there was conversation and laughter as people visited, feasting and talking. Occasionally the wild, eerie wailing of some family of mourners rose on the far fringes of the village like the baying of wolves, then died away in poignant lamentation. Pedro drank it all in and was surprised to feel a strange regret. It was the last time he would ever see or hear it, he told himself. He would never forget it.

He angled cautiously toward the tribal herding grounds on the outskirts of the village, a rope end in his hand. He had never been allowed here alone before. He watched cautiously for night herders.

In the moonlight, he saw hundreds of horses, heads down, night grazing on the open plain. He heard them stamping and switching their tails and biting off the grass with a soft crunch as they shook their heads and took an occasional step forward while they browsed. Some raised their heads when he approached, blowing the air out of their nostrils in mild surprise; then went on grazing.

Pedro was eying the nearest animals speculatively when a familiar voice, deep and scornful, spoke behind him.

"Are you lost, *español?*"

Pedro whirled around. Old Sore, astride the old pony, gazed down at him sardonically. Reared back to his full height against the moon, the tall old man looked like the manifestation of doom. His bow was in his left hand and his quiver hung conveniently over his right shoulder.

Pedro could only stand and stare. His heart beat so madly that he felt choked.

Old Sore spoke again in deep, taunting tones. "Most of our young men seek the area behind the village when they go on the vision quest." He pointed sternly to it with an outstretched arm that looked long as a tipi pole.

"And I am surprised that Creek Water did not instruct you better concerning the fasting. A young man does not take food on the vision quest. Some of it dropped from your breechclout when you left the tipi. I stepped on it when I got up to go outside."

Pedro fought down his terror. Did Old Sore really think he

was stupid enough to bring food on the vision quest and seek the herding grounds as a suitable place to make contact with the Great Spirit? Or was Old Sore aware of his escape intentions? There was only one way to find out.

"Thank you, grandfather," he muttered. Reaching both hands inside his breechclout, he threw the dried buffalo meat onto the grass. Then, with his heart still thumping, he turned and began to walk in the direction Old Sore had indicated. Remembering the fate of Tito, Pedro expected at any instant to be knocked flat on his face by an arrow ripping through his back.

But none came. Instead, there was a peculiar sound behind him, the sound of slurping and sucking and lips smacking. When he finally summoned the courage to throw a furtive look over his shoulder, he saw that the ancient had crawled off the pony and, squatted on the grass, was greedily munching the food Pedro had discarded.

Pedro had no difficulty analyzing his failure. He did not know enough yet to get away. He did not even know enough to start.

For three days and nights, Pedro fasted. But he did it from necessity, not because the vision ritual required it.

He carved from red cedar a small, crude likeness of the Holy Mother and prayed before it daily. Although he had prayed for success in his escape effort and it had not been granted him, he had been protected in his failure. Perhaps this was not meant to be the time for escape, perhaps his opportunity would come later, after he was better prepared.

On the second night Pedro dreamed he had a visitor. It was his mother. She bent over him and kissed him lightly, a look of tenderness in her eyes. She seemed very close and very real. "Pedro, keep up your courage," she said. "Do the very best you can." But when he reached for her, he awoke to find her gone.

Remembering the manner of her death, he threw off the buffalo robe, and assembling his Comanche religious articles, walked weakly back to the village. Not sure of how he would be received, he decided to act boldly, as if his mission had been genuine and he had nothing to conceal or fear.

He entered Creek Water's tipi in the dark and helped himself from the family cooking pot. He was very hungry. One of the squaws awakened and got him a slice of buffalo meat from a parfleche trunk. Grateful, he whispered his thanks and went outside. As he chewed hungrily in the darkness he realized that kindness was not restricted to those of the Christian faith. Some Indians understood it, too.

In his own tipi, he found Old Sore snoring loudly. Pedro got to bed without waking him and slept until midmorning. When he opened his eyes Old Sore was gone. Facing the old man was put off for a while. After eating dried venison and sand-plum cake, Pedro tumbled back upon the robe and slept the day through, waking just in time for supper.

Everyone in Creek Water's lodge treated him with respect and consideration. No one pressed him for the details of his search for power. They all seemed to assume that he had found it.

When he returned that night to his tipi, Old Sore was twisting a cedar stick into flame in the firehole. With painful effort, the old man stood and turned around, a sour look on his face. He grunted once and stared petulantly at Pedro.

"Indian's weakness is his trail." Old Sore barked gruffly, "Tomorrow we work on trailing. I show you how to follow trail, how to hide it."

Pedro knew he was safe. Apparently the ancient was his old irritable self again.

That night, Pedro lay in the darkness and thought of the mistakes he had made. He needed instruction on how to hide his trail better, how not to leave it littered with cached food.

He decided that his best chance to escape lay in doing exactly what Creek Water and Old Sore wanted. He would learn so thoroughly to be a Comanche that when he did make his break for freedom he would know as much about where to go and how to survive as any warrior in the band. He would learn to think like a Comanche. Then he would know what his pursuers were thinking and that would help. As he turned the new plan over in his mind it seemed so promising that he felt a secret exultation about it. Finally he closed his eyes and pulled the robe up around him. Soon he was asleep.

9 · The Joy Riders

Pedro was awakened late the next morning by somebody trodding solidly on the ground near his face. The trampling was accompanied by the faint clink of tiny bells.

As he opened his eyes, Pedro saw moccasins with polecat fringes and strings of blue beads and small metal jinglets sewn into the heel. Creek Water stood looking down upon him with piercing eyes.

A spasm of fear settled around Pedro's heart. The man's look was so deep and searching that Pedro felt hemmed in by guilt. Conquering a shudder, he got hold of himself. It would not do to show fear of any kind.

He shook his head to clear it and rose to his feet. "Won't you sit down, father?" With his hand, he designated a spot by the firehole.

Creek Water sank slowly and ponderously to a sitting position, crossed his legs, and waited in dignified silence. Pedro sat facing him. He hoped with all his heart that Old Sore had not told the chief what had happened. He knew that Creek Water would not ask him to reveal the source of his power because its identity was a life-and-death secret.

Creek Water's eyes, bleak and discerning, seemed to bite into Pedro's enforced calm. "You will need your new power for many things. You must learn to use it when you need it, for hunting, raiding, the warpath, to cure disease. You must be grateful for the help it can give you. You must be unselfish about it, as the spirits were unselfish when they gave it to you. You must use it to help a friend."

Pedro's fear subsided. Creek Water believed he had found his vision; he was teaching him how to derive power from it.

"Now that you have it, you can be a better Comanche," Creek Water went on. "Medicine is power and you must handle power carefully. Your power may be so strong that you will want to share it with a friend. If this happens, you must not approach the friend yourself. It is best to have your wife do this for you. We must soon look about for a wife for you."

Pedro felt his stomach puckering. He tried not to let his dismay show.

"Thank you, father."

Creek Water stood, his heel jinglets tinkling suddenly. He wrapped his gray wolfskin robe about him and stalked out with slow and solidly planted footsteps.

Pedro's new training started the next morning. He and Old Sore rode several miles west of the village to a spot where yellow wildflowers ran down the slopes to a big cottonwood growing in a draw. Black thatches of sand plum, dead from the winter freeze, lay everywhere.

"One Indian traveling alone has no fear for his rear," the old man began solemnly. "He knows how hard it is for an enemy following him to work out trail of one man on horse. And Indian traveling alone never makes fire or sleeps by fire. He is never afraid because he has all the advantage. He can watch for enemy behind him. If they sight him, he hides in rocks and thickets until dark. Then he gets on his horse and rides all night, putting many miles between himself and his enemies."

Pedro became more attentive. This sounded useful. It was the product of a lifetime of Indian living, by one who had no peer in its application. If Pedro learned it well, it might get him home many years faster than his present rate of progress.

"But a traveling party of warriors leaves too much trail." Frowning bleakly, the old man pursed his thin lips and pointed in several directions on the ground. "They fear the enemy will surprise them, wipe them out. And surprise always comes from the rear. When a war party is returning from a raid, they care nothing for advance guards but always put out the best warriors as rear guards. They travel high places so they can watch for pursuers. That is why one man is bold about his trail but a war party fearful about theirs."

Pedro permitted himself a tiny thrill of jubilation. When he made his break for freedom, he too would be alone. Unless he could find Roberto and take him with him. He was hungry to hear more about how to elude pursuers.

But Old Sore, bending his head so that he could better scratch his unmutilated ear, seemed more interested in the viewpoint of the pursuer.

"Indians travel by landmarks, *español,*" he explained. "We never get lost because we watch for unusual things which mark the trail—hills, valleys, rivers, timber, waterholes. The first thing a trailer does is locate a series of landmarks by which enemy is traveling. Then he is able, when entering valley, to tell the exact spot where the trail will leave it. The party ahead will twist and double, mix up the trail, but pursuers pay no attention to that. They watch only landmarks. They will go at once to the next landmark, pick up the trail there, and save much time."

Guiding his pony with his knees, the old man swiveled his head left and right, scanning the prairie for sign. Soon he slid off his horse and motioned for Pedro to dismount. He squatted, studying a cluster of dry horse droppings.

"A party stopped here many days ago. A trailer needs to know many things—from what nation the party ahead is from, how many men are in it, how long ago did they pass."

He showed Pedro that if the grass were pressed downward

by a horse's hoof during the dry season, the grass would retain the direction of impress and grow more yellow each day. Thus it was easy to judge from the degree of yellowness how many days had passed since it had first been trampled upon. Confirming this calculation, he broke off several strands of the trampled grass and tasted them to learn how much of their natural juices they still contained. As Old Sore worked, he patiently explained his findings, and Pedro listened avidly.

Old Sore found a moccasin print. Stooping, he studied it carefully.

"This party was from Penateka or Wasp bank. Trail twenty days old. Three horses. One mare." He picked up some of the dried horse dung and carefully broke it open with his hands, sniffing at it. He noticed the moisture and peered at the contents.

"Sometime *nah-ro-eep*, horse droppings, tell much."

He explained to Pedro that the contents of the dung showed the region from which the animals last came. Did the dung contain buffalo grass, gramma, mesquite, or sacatan? A different grass grew in every region and it was easy to recognize the region and identify the tribe from the content of the dung. If the dung contained barley, Texans had probably been over the route. If maize, the riders were probably Mexican.

Old Sore leered triumphantly up into Pedro's face. "When I was a young man, *español*, your Anza tried to surprise us and hit our camp. He marched at night and hid by day. But we crossed his backtrail and discovered who he was by the droppings of his horses. They contained corn, so we knew we had Spaniards after us."

Pedro still didn't understand how Old Sore had determined the sex of the four animals which had passed nearly three weeks before. The ancient pointed to the faded imprint of the horses' feet that indicated the attitude each animal had assumed while urinating. The males had stretched themselves and ejected their urine in front of their hind feet, the front hoofs of which were more deeply imprinted than the rear. The female had ejected to the rear of her hindprints.

Trailing fascinated Pedro more than anything else he learned. Old Sore taught him to know every mark on the ground, who made it, how old it was, why it was important. Unless he was familiar with all this, he could not hope to hide his own trail or follow that of another. If he could not read the signs of game animals, he might starve.

Insisting upon constant practice, the old man halted the old buckskin whenever the trail offered a difficult challenge and made Pedro get off the mule, solve it and explain his reasons. Pedro stored every detail of the old man's teaching in the pigeonholes of his orderly mind. Soon he could read trail as authoritatively as he had learned to translate German at the Royal Academy.

Spring ripened into summer, and they rode every day. One morning they passed over country that was rough and broken. When they came to a grassy spot along the river, Old Sore jerked his pony to a stop, muttering toothless obscenities. He leaned over and began to pick fresh sandburs out of his long, buckskin leggings.

"In the days when I was young and we were moving about, there were no brier weeds, no stickers, no burrs in this country," he grumbled. "Children, as well as their parents, went nearly everywhere barefooted. All that we could see on the prairie then was grass. When camps were pitched, we would make our beds on the grass. The air was always fresh. We wore no headshades. We did not mind the weather in those days."

Pedro was careful not to let his face show his amusement. Old Sore's loyalty to the old days was so absolute that it extended even to the surface vegetation. Despite the daytime heat, the old man was always dressed for winter. He usually wore leggings and draped a faded blue blanket or a stale-smelling buffalo robe about his wide, bony shoulders. He straightened and detached with difficulty the last sandbur from his withered fingers. He scowled at Pedro.

"Today we hunt antelope, *español*. Remember that hunting is serious work. If a man knows how to hunt well, his family will always have food, shelter, and clothing. If he doesn't know how to hunt, life for his family will be very hard. They might starve."

Pedro strung his bow and swung it over his shoulders. A man trying to get away across this desert might starve too, unless he knew how to do some hunting along the way.

They found the first herd of antelope grazing quietly on the high, dry prairie, several leagues off. In the distance, the tiny animals looked no taller than greyhounds. Their bodies shone reddish, inclining to yellow on the sides and white on the belly. Old Sore showed Pedro how to make the approach. They had hidden their mounts in a grove of blackjacks and were crawling on their stomachs when Pedro tried to steal a look and was seen by the herd. Instantly, their stub tails blurred whitely in the sunshine and every head was raised. However, they did not panic. They were still out of shooting range.

Old Sore glared at Pedro. "We'll never get close enough to shoot them now," he whispered bitterly. "That ridge over there would have hidden us and we could have crawled right up on them if they hadn't seen you. Now everything is changed. As soon as we disappear from sight to begin the stalk, they will change position, too. When we get there we will find nothing to shoot at. Perhaps we can still get one. Let's lie still in this grass."

Old Sore waited a moment. Then he turned carefully on his side and thrust one long shriveled leg into the air and wiggled his moccasined foot. Again thirty stub tails flashed in the sunshine like tin pans. The antelope began to crane their necks inquisitively and to approach closer and closer as if drawn to the spot by a hysteria compounded of both curiosity and terror. Soon they came so near that Pedro could see their small, frightened faces and their prong-shaped horns through the grass.

The sudden twang of Old Sore's bowstring sent them flying, but one remained on the prairie, kicking in its death throes, an arrow buried in its side. Old Sore helped Pedro butcher it at once, explaining that it would be unfit as food unless the viscera were removed immediately. He also taught Pedro to know the antelope's track, sharp at the toe, broad and round at the heel.

"Antelope's flesh is tender and juicy all year round," the old man said. He explained that should a hunter, suffering from lack of water, see a herd of antelope on the desert, if he did not alarm them they would eventually lead him to some hidden spring or a tiny pool of rain water, caught in the basin of a rock. He said one reason antelope were so plentiful on the high prairie was because the does were very motherly, frequently giving suck to the young of other dams killed by hunters as well as to their own young.

They got close enough two days later for Pedro to try a long shot that missed.

"You shut your eyes, _español!_" Old Sore scolded. "Some men are hunters. Others are not. A few who are not can be taught. Tomorrow we'll hunt red deer. We'll see if you can learn."

Pedro Pavón learned. He learned that the best time to take red deer was while they were feeding early in the morning or just before dark. He learned that the best way to stalk them was across the wind. They grazed with their heads turned away from the wind so that they could watch for an enemy from that direction, and depended on their noses to warn them of his approach from behind.

Vision is the red deer's keenest sense. Pedro stalked and

killed his first buck by observing Old Sore's warning to make
frequent halts and remain perfectly still when the animal heard
him. They were hunting half an hour before sunup when Pedro
saw the buck feeding in a pocket of grass thinly sheltered by
cottonwood and cedar. At once Pedro began the stalk; Old
Sore was right behind him. When Pedro's hip brushed a grass
clump, making a slight noise, the buck flirted its white tail and
raised its head to look about. Pedro froze. Unable to see him,
the buck resumed grazing.

Reaching cautiously over his shoulder, Pedro extracted an
arrow from his quiver. Noiselessly, he fitted it to the bow. He
dreaded Old Sore's censure if he botched any phase of the
operation, and longed for a bit of advice from the old man that
might help him bag the buck. But Old Sore remained silent.

Pedro hesitated, striving for self-control. He wanted so
badly to kill the deer that he wished he had it by the horns so
he could wrestle it to the grass and draw his knife across its
throat; that seemed a surer method. The buck took another
step forward, and with his head down nibbled at a grass clump.
Drawing a short breath, Pedro drew the arrow back, sighting
at the animal's chestnut flank.

Chook!

The buck plunged and fell as though straining against an in-
visible rope tethering it to the spot. Pulling itself up gamely, it
stumbled forward a few steps and collapsed again. Its antlers
tore up the grass, its feet threshed the air as it tried to flee the
force that had felled it.

"Yehh!" whooped Old Sore.

Pedro looked down unbelievingly at the quivering corpse
and the soft eyes glazing in death. He felt an enormous sense of
triumph and pleasure.

Old Sore made Pedro stop and offer a prayer to the dead
animal. "This deer might become your guardian spirit," the
old man pointed out. "A deer has much power for both good

or evil. It has power to cause disease or cure it. It has power in love affairs. If it likes you, it can warn you when to run. It can help you run very fast. Of all the things that tread the ground there is nothing that can beat it in running."

Although Pedro believed no part of Old Sore's supernatural interpretation, he pretended to. His mind was filled with the sheer delight of the hunting. It was such a completely satisfying art. He had not only made the stalk and killed the buck himself, he had also built the arrow that pierced its heart. Afterward he would skin and dress the animal himself, pack it home, and contribute it to Creek Water's family larder. Pedro looked forward to eating it as a change from the buffalo diet. Old Sore had told him that no meat tastes quite as good as fresh venison from a red deer one has killed himself.

Some of his joy in the kill was lessened when he returned to the village that evening. As he proudly unloaded the dead buck from his mule, three young braves, Hairy Belly, Hugger, and Frothing Buffalo, came up to him. With arms folded across their chests, they stared sternly, then finally walked off abruptly without saying a word.

"Don't pay any attention to them," counseled Porcupine Woman as she began to cut up the meat. "They're jealous because Old Sore is teaching you and because you are learning so fast."

Next day they hunted red deer again. Old Sore taught Pedro to be selective. He explained that when the males began fighting for the females in late fall, the whipped bucks were run out of the herd and became extremely fat. They were the ones the hunter sought because of the exquisite flavor of their flesh. The victorious bucks, grazing with the does and burdened by the cares of fatherhood, grew thin and were not worth killing because their flesh was stringy and tough.

Old Sore showed him a tiny, big-eared fawn sleeping alone in a grass clump. The old man explained that the speckled infant has no scent, so it is hidden by its mother in a spot where it will not be seen. In silent obedience, it lies quietly and safely alone with hungry wolves prowling all around it. Its mother, enjoying no such immunity, retreats to a nearby thicket to make her bed alone and take her risk apart from her young.

Pedro's vision in the open was now sharper than Old Sore's. He thought his hearing was keener too. But one afternoon when they were resting beside the trail, Old Sore suddenly took his catbrier cigarette out of his mouth and clapping his lone ear to the ground, listened carefully. Pedro listened too, but heard nothing.

"What is it, grandfather?"

Old Sore's only answer was to look north.

Soon Pedro heard at a distance the faint drumming of approaching horses' feet. Old Sore sat up but never moved. Six mounted Indians galloped past, taking a slight circuit away from the trail to avoid coming near. Their ponies were sweating and blowing. They were heavily armed with bows, arrows, and lances, but they wore no paint. They did not wave or try to communicate in any way.

"Kiowas," barked Old Sore laconically, and went on smoking. Pedro knew the Kiowas were allies of the Comanches. With envious awe, he wondered how long it would be before he too could hear as well as his aged, one-eared companion.

With the arrival of August, a lassitude settled over the land, and when the black-tailed deer came down from the north to select their autumnal homes, Old Sore showed Pedro that the best time to take them was at noon when their tracks could be followed to where they had lain down to enjoy a siesta on some densely cedared ridge. The blacktails always selected the ridge's lower slope where the rise became so precipitous that they could see everything on the plain below and nothing could see them from above. If anything approached, a small landslide of gravel or loose rocks would be launched and give them warning. Old Sore and Pedro hunted as a team, one detouring widely to approach from leeward of the deer, the other advancing from windward. When the blacktails scented the man to windward, they got up and walked quietly downwind, almost treading on the huntsman waiting for them there.

September came with a russet glow. Heavy frosts began to whiten the tan grass. Pedro learned that elk began moving early in September, traveling mostly at night. When journeying unmolested they always walked in single file, one behind the other, and were easily tracked. He came upon such a trail one afternoon, and following it, surprised a herd of the big, noble-looking beasts feeding. Hearing him, they huddled like frightened sheep and gawked at him with fear as they formed a widening wedge around their leader.

When Pedro knocked down the leader with an arrow, the others did not flee but collected stupidly together as if to hold another silent conclave. Old Sore magnanimously left his bow on his back, so Pedro quickly shot another and proudly packed the choice meat back to the village.

Pedro was learning with a hungry eagerness. He learned how to approach game patiently and noiselessly, how to use vegetation and the physical features of the land for concealment, how to track, surround, and make adjustments for the wind. His memory was keen and he rarely repeated his mistakes. He lived constantly outdoors, and becoming accustomed to the Comanche meat diet, grew lean, brown, and wiry.

The village moved every two or three weeks and Pedro roamed the land on all sides without ever missing a cutoff or a trail. He acquired an intimate knowledge of every canyon, stream, and landmark. Whenever he heard a warrior talk about what lay in the distance he listened, thoughtfully hoarding the information against the day he would make his next bolt for liberty.

He knew that he was still being watched. Creek Water

never permitted him to ride anything faster than the mule, unless the herdboy Arrow Bush was along as well as Old Sore. Other hunting parties moved constantly around them. Pedro paid no attention. He knew that he was still many months from accomplishing his goal. He directed all his energies toward enjoying the hunts and mastering each new lesson presented by his white-haired tutor.

One night just before the coming of Toh-muh, winter, Old Sore dug into his medicine bag and found a small drum. Soon Pedro heard him singing outside. The old man's deep voice seemed to come from way down in his moccasins, pulsing strongly on the prolonged notes, then trailing downward at the end. He was lying on his back in the grass, supporting the drum on his stomach while he sang.

"What are you singing, grandfather?"

"There are no words to this song, *español*. It is just singing. This song belonged to my father. I paid him three packdogs for it. That was before we had many horses."

The old man sang a little more. Then he sat up, a restless look in his weak old eyes. It had just grown dark but a big moon, round and golden as an orange, was rising out of the sage on the eastern horizon. Soon there would be plenty of light.

"*Español,* this is the first time in years I've felt like singing. I dreamed last night of my youth and of how long it has been since I have done any of the high-spirited things I did as a boy. Then I thought of you and how you haven't had much fun either. I've been trying to help you learn to ride but you can't learn properly the way we've been doing it."

Old Sore's eyes flattened into cunning little slits. "Find us some ropes, *español.*"

Although he didn't understand, Pedro found the ropes. They waited until the village was asleep. Then they left the tipi, each carrying the ropes and a small elm saddle. They walked quietly, making no noise. They had gone fifty paces when a woman's voice spoke softly behind them.

"Where are you going, grandfather?" it asked.

Startled, Pedro jumped. Old Sore looked around, scowling. Then they recognized her. It was not a woman at all. It was To-a-nick-pe, "The Boy," who had ridden so well that day when Wolf Milk and the young men were practicing their feats near the river. Pedro made no answer because he did not know where they were going. Old Sore did not answer either. Pedro guessed the old man did not want her along.

Pedro saw that she was carrying precisely what they were carrying, a saddle and spurs in one hand, a rope in the other. "Please let me go with you," the girl said. "I often go joyriding by myself. But it is lonely. I would rather go with you."

Old Sore stopped. He looked around sourly as though the girl's joining them had endangered his medicine. He said, "All right. But first I think we had better pray to the moon god. She's the guardian of the raid. She must also be the guardian of what we're about to do."

He took his longest rope and made a ring of it on the ground. They all sat within it. The old man produced a small pipe made of elk bone. Quickly he filled it, lit it, and blew smoke toward the moon.

"Mother," he prayed simply, "if it be your will, bring us many horses." He arose and picked up his rope.

"Thank you, grandfather," To-a-nick-pe murmured. Old Sore grunted and stalked on ahead. To-a-nick-pe walked silently with Pedro.

As they walked, Pedro studied her out of the corner of his eyes. Her lips were thick and coarse. Her nostrils were broad. Her hair was banged to her eyelids. She had an odor, but it was not a bad one. To-a-nick-pe just smelled of horses.

They passed quietly among the tall white tipis standing in irregular fashion on the prairie. The tipis were dark and Pedro knew the occupants were sleeping. Occasionally a dog rushed at them, barking noisily, but this was so commonplace that no one paid any attention.

Picketed near some of the tipis were the owner's favorite horses. Pedro knew about these horses. They were either buffalo horses, trained to follow and crowd the great, galloping bulls on the communal hunts, guided only by the pressure of their master's knee, or they were warhorses, noted for their speed, intelligence, and stamina. Pedro had seen the warriors tending and petting them in the daytime. Old Sore had told him that most of the warriors loved their horses more than they loved their wives.

Suddenly Old Sore and the girl darted like ghosts among the lodges, pulling up picket pegs and accumulating horses. As fast as they collected one horse, Old Sore tied it to the tail of another with one of the short ropes he had brought along. He put a rope around the jaw of the front horse and handed it to Pedro, who discovered he was leading the whole string. Proud and thrilled and a little frightened to be escorting these tribal bluebloods, Pedro clutched the lead rope tightly. The animals were well-behaved and gave him no trouble. Soon he was leading nine.

Pedro's heart began to hammer. What was it all about? This was a risky business. Comanches did not steal from Comanches. If an owner awakened and found his pet gone, somebody might be hurt.

He turned anxiously to To-a-nick-pe. "What do we do if we are discovered?"

She brushed the bangs out of her eyes and whispered back, "Jump off and scatter. They'll never find us." She made it sound exciting.

Old Sore and the girl knew how to handle the sleek beauties. Soon they passed a mile beyond the limits of the sleeping camp and came to the open prairie, a sea of moon-bathed grass.

Here they bridled and saddled three of the nine cavaliers in their string. Old Sore knew what to do with the remaining six. The lead horse was brought around and tied to the tail of the hindmost, forming a circle. They began to graze that way.

Old Sore, To-a-nick-pe, and Pedro each mounted one of the saddled horses.

Riding side by side like three men, they first trotted slowly over the stretch they had chosen, examining it for prairie-dog holes and buffalo wallows. The surface was level as a floor. Then the riding began and Pedro discovered why they had come.

He had never ridden such horses. Heads erect, ears cocked intelligently, these tribal aristocrats seemed to relish the nocturnal adventure as much as Old Sore and the girl. Pedro was on a buckskin with black mane and tail. He could feel it gather itself in a crouch, its long, lean muscles mobilized and ready, its hide warm between his knees. When Old Sore made a little sucking noise with his lips that sounded like kissing, all three horses shot out flat, like arrows from the bow.

It was like riding a low cloud. The buckskin was sure-footed, and ran smoothly and powerfully, negotiating slight dips and inclines with ease.

Pedro's eyes watered and stung. Soon he was breathing fast. He could feel the blood coursing through his veins. His nostrils were wide open as he drank in the cool night air. He felt an ecstasy he had never known. He loved the full-speed galloping in the face of the strong south wind.

Old Sore had straddled a pinto gelding. With his fretful face low over its mane and his heels in its flanks, the old man rode with as much abandon as either Pedro or the girl. But it was the girl who rode the most skillfully.

She did everything at full speed, yipping shrilly. Sure of herself, she slid from one side of her racing mount to the other, her small, hard body out of sight except for one moccasined heel on the cantle of the juniper saddle. She rode standing, legs spraddled, arms outspread for balance. And later, when they changed horses, she spurred the fleet piebald she rode into a dead run, and leaning almost to the ground, picked up from the grass one of her own moccasins and flourished it triumphantly in the moonlight.

Tired finally of the joyriding, To-a-nick-pe coiled a rope over her arm and, riding into the midst of the tribal herd, she lassoed a wild sorrel. The animal reared and plunged but Old Sore dismounted, grasped the lasso, and advanced down it hand over hand until he got close enough to place one hand on the sorrel's nose and the other over its eyes. Then he breathed into its nostrils until it wiggled its ears and grew quiet.

With Pedro's help, they got the girl's saddle on securely. She leaped into it with a cry and Old Sore turned the foaming sorrel loose.

It ducked its head and erupted, grunting like a lion. First it bucked in circles, landing alternately on front and hind feet. Then it twisted its body into a crescent, almost touching the ground with first one shoulder then the other, and Pedro could see the moonlight shining on its belly. It humped its back and came down hard with all four legs stiff. But it could not dislodge the screeching girl. She stuck to it as though she were a tick inside its ear. Soon the sorrel slowed down and began taking long jumps straight ahead without any twists or rearing. Finally it quit, raising its head and trotting wherever the girl guided it.

They rode for another half hour, then rubbed down the noble beasts with grass, tied them together again and led them quietly back to the village. Now the moon swung at the zenith of the heavens and the lodges loomed whiter than ever.

Stealthily, Old Sore and the girl cut out first one animal then another, staking them out near their home tipis. Pedro marveled at how unerringly they knew which horse belonged to which lodge. With Old Sore directing him, Pedro staked out the buckskin himself, thinking, When I do make my escape dash, I would like nothing better than to leave on this one.

"Thank you for fun," To-a-nick-pe told them as she turned off to go to her tipi.

Pedro liked her politeness. He had never seen a girl like her anywhere, in Spain or among the gypsies. He liked the way she stayed to herself. She had made no romantic overtures of any kind. Apparently, horses were all she was interested in. Pedro wondered, would he ever learn to ride half as well as she?

10 · The Yamparika Girl

Old Sore said, "Some shields have strong power. They give spiritual protection, as well as battle protection. If a young man wants his shield to have power, he asks a man with a medicine shield for some of his power, or he can ask a medicine man to get the power for him."

The early morning sun was casting oblique shafts of light among the tipis. The old man was helping Pedro make a shield from the shoulder side of an old buffalo bull. They heated and steamed the green hide over the fire to thicken it. Then, while it was still hot, they fleshed it by rubbing it across a rock. The old man had cut circular patches from the hide and stretched them—flesh part out—over each side of a wooden hoop. Now he was sewing the big, round patches onto first one side of the hoop then the other with rawhide thongs, his ghoulish face clenched in a frown of concentration. While Old Sore rested between sewings, Pedro packed the space between the two perimeters of patches with turkey feathers and horsehair.

"You must never bring this shield inside a tipi if it has power," the old man warned. "If somebody with greasy hands touches it, its power would be broken and you would be wounded the first time you used the shield in battle. You must keep it at least three arrow shoots from camp."

Pedro thought it foolish to keep a shield half a mile from camp. What if a surprise attack hit the camp? But he had long ago learned not to argue with Old Sore.

"After you take a man's part in battle and do the things that belong to being a man, I will help you make a lance," the old one said. "But owning a lance is too big a responsibility for you now. Only a brave man carries a lance because he must fight hand to hand. He cannot retreat. He either kills his opponent or he gets killed. If a lance carrier ever retreated he could never face his warrior comrades again."

Old Sore gestured proudly toward his own seven-foot lance that lay on his weapons platform near the tipi. "That lance has power. It's a medicine spear. It once killed five Apaches who shot my horse and charged me on foot. I haven't fought with it for forty summers but it is still hot. Its medicine is still strong. No enemy can face the power of that lance and live."

Footsteps approached, slow and solidly planted down. Creek Water walked up with his pigeon-toed gait. His gray wolfskin was wrapped closely around him. He stood with bowed legs and moccasined feet slightly spraddled, his face impassive, his sharp eyes fixed solemnly on Pedro.

"My son," he began. "You now hunt so well that you would keep a wife busy skinning and dressing the game you kill. Every lodge should have a woman in it. I have told you that our young men often marry at an early age. You have no horses and no plunder with which to buy a wife. So I have brought you a wife who is ready to start cooking for you, bring your wood and water, pack your game, make your clothing, raise your children. Her husband was Medicine Breath. He was killed in battle with the Tuhksees. Here she is."

A woman stood behind Creek Water. Pedro stared at her in horror. She was fat and flabby and several years older than he. A fiery new moon was painted over each eye and a full moon in the center of her forehead. She squinted ferociously at him. He frowned and felt his nostrils pursing. Although she stood well away from him, she smelled faintly like a sewer ditch.

Pedro's small body straightened. His back stiffened with

pride and loathing. He was Pedro Herraro Vicente de la Pavón, member of the Spanish royal family, descended directly from Ferdinand the Catholic king, and a savage was telling him that he must marry this smelly hag. He drew a deep breath and looked defiantly at Creek Water.

Then he remembered with whom he was dealing. Creek Water was the most powerful chief in the band. He was widely respected for his judgment in council as well as for his feats in war. Pedro thought of how much he owed to this man. But for Creek Water, he would still be a slave in Belt Whip's tipi with no prospect of ever escaping; he might not even be alive. He spoke slowly, choosing his words with care.

"My father, you are right. Every lodge needs a woman in it. But I have not been thinking about marriage. I have been busy learning to be a better Comanche. Now that you bring this woman and I do think about marriage, I think that when I marry I will want a younger wife, one who has never shared a lodge with another husband. This woman is much too old for me."

No change showed in Creek Water's face. For a moment they stood confronting each other in the morning light outside the tipi. The chief's black eyes bored into Pedro's. Pedro stared fearlessly back at him.

Then a tiny shred of emotion showed on Creek Water's usually unfathomable face. He looked at his adopted son with a flicker of something that might have been pride, pride in the boy's bold spirit and regal bearing. Pedro again was reminded that Comanches admire courage and that a captive fares better among them by occasionally exhibiting it.

The expression went out of Creek Water's face. "I will think about this," he said, gravely. He left, taking the woman with him.

But Pedro had a premonition that the issue had not been resolved, only postponed.

A fortnight later, the shield was finished and Pedro and Old Sore took it out on the prairie to test it. They set it up at an angle. It was round and stood a little above Old Sore's knee. Backing off, they shot at it with arrows, and with a bullet from Creek Water's ancient musket. Both glanced off the shield. Old Sore knew how to make a shield. Then they laced buckskin strings through each side so it could be fitted speedily on Pedro's arm. "Now," said Old Sore, grunting with satisfaction, "we will teach you how to use it."

Old Sore enlisted two other old men from his smoke lodge, where the aged warriors gathered to smoke and gossip. The three of them placed Pedro fifty paces away. Using blunt arrows, they shot at him. Old Sore trained Pedro in warding off arrows. Pedro ducked behind his shield and moved it in a wavy motion, slanting it slightly so the shafts struck it at an angle and bounded off. Old Sore had sewn feathers around the rim of the shield. When Pedro shook the shield, the feathers rippled, disconcerting the aim of the enemy.

The old men shot faster until the arrows came in torrents. Twice Pedro was knocked down by blunt shafts that got through his guard. One struck him squarely in the forehead, stunning him. As he lay groggy and bleeding on the prairie, he reflected that had the shaft struck lower, he might have been blinded. After they revived him, the old men renewed the practice. It was sport to them. Each time an arrow got through, they shouted with delight. They gave Pedro no rest.

Day after day, he worked at fending off shots. He doubted if this instruction was necessary for his escape plans but again he had no choice.

"You must secure spiritual power for your shield," Old Sore advised. "Take it to Much Saliva. He is a powerful medicine man. Ask him for a share of his power. His medicine is the long-legged owl that lives with the prairie dogs. Much Saliva lives at the north side of the camp near a prairie-dog village.

Smoke with him and he will give you some of his power."

On his way to Much Saliva's lodge, Pedro came to the northern border of the village. Beyond it the grass was dotted with small prairie-dog burrows. Children were trying to catch the tiny yellowish-gray animals before they scampered into their holes.

A childish scream of terror pealed out from among the burrows. One of the children, a naked boy of about three, struggled to stand, but he was weighed down by a rattlesnake coiled about his arm. Drawing back its head, the snake struck the boy repeatedly. The child's screams only seemed to excite it to further strikes.

Pedro raced to the scene, carrying his new shield on his arm. The snake, thick-bodied, with dark, diamond-shaped blotches running the length of its back, saw him coming. Pedro heard the deadly singing of its rattles.

The snake hissed and blew at him. Its head swung from side to side, following Pedro. Then it struck—but Pedro thrust up the shield. He heard the snake's head strike the shield's surface and felt the force of the blow.

Pedro grasped the snake by the end of its tail, feeling the horny interlocking joints which gave the rattler its name. The snake exuded a musty odor, like rotting cloth. Pedro jerked with all his strength. The reptile slid off the boy's arm and then Pedro felt the heavy scales of its smooth, tan underside against his own bare skin.

The snake dropped to the ground. Before it could recoil, Pedro drew his bow and beat it over the head. Its body still writhed in slow, flat contortions. Its rattles buzzed feebly and were still.

The child's mother, hearing the screams, ran to the scene. She was a buxom young squaw, wearing silver earrings that jingled noisily as she ran.

She snatched up the shrieking boy and examined his young

body, gasping in dismay at his wounds. Pedro saw the double fang marks of three bites, two on the child's left arm and one on his back. He knew those bites could be fatal.

Other women from the village were staring at the boy. One of them ran for a medicine man, who came at once. After lighting his pipe with a coal from the fire and blowing smoke to heaven, earth, and the four directions, the medicine man began to growl like a bear. He tied a bundle of black crow feathers to the child's foot and coughed violently as though to disgorge the evil spirit in the snake.

The doomed boy lay whimpering on a buffalo robe. The area around each of his wounds was beginning to swell and turn black.

Realizing that the lad would die quickly, Pedro hurried into action. He had seen a mule driver bitten by a snake during the long trek to Don Luis' rancho. He remembered the remedy.

First he broke off several of the brownish needlelike points of a nearby yucca plant, then he elbowed his way into the circle around the child. The medicine man glared at him, but moved back. The distraught mother looked imploringly from Pedro to the medicine man and back to Pedro again.

Quickly Pedro jabbed the sharp ends of the yucca deep into the swollen areas around each fang wound. The child shrieked with pain but black blood gushed out of the punctures, staining the grass and carrying off some of the venom. With his mouth, Pedro sucked each wound to promote bleeding, then spat the dark, poisonous blood out onto the ground. Finally, he applied a poultice of prickly-pear leaves. Although the mother did not understand what Pedro was doing, she seemed to sense that he was helping her son. With low, soothing cries she tried to comfort the screaming youngster.

Pedro rose, exhausted by the strain. He looked down at the boy, who now lay in a stupor. The mother picked him up and, crooning to him, carried him inside a nearby tipi. As Pedro looked after her he noticed the lodge. It was large and commodious. Clusters of blue circles had been painted on the outside, and there was a small platform for the owner's weapons. Obviously the owner was a warrior. His weapons were gone, signifying that he was absent on a hunt or raid.

"Who is the boy's father?" Pedro asked.

"Coby," an old woman answered. "He has taken more scalps and stolen more horses than any man in the band. He is the leader of the Crow Tassel Wearers." Pedro had heard of the Crow Tassel Wearers. They were the bravest of all the warrior societies. War was their business. They dedicated their lives to it.

Pedro walked to the river to wash out his mouth, carrying the shield with him. Then he found the lodge of Much Saliva, the medicine man to whom Old Sore had directed him.

The man huddled in the tipi was the medicine man who had been summoned to attend the bitten child. At the sight of Pedro, he arose, muttering. Angrily he drove him out of the lodge.

"You should not have offended him like that," Old Sore advised him when he returned to his tipi. "Much Saliva is powerful. If he wants to, he can paralyze your legs or cause you to lose your mind. Medicine men can use their power for evil as well as for good."

Pedro did not share the old man's fear of Much Saliva's sorcery. He did not care if he never got spiritual power for his shield. All he wanted it to do was ward off enemy spears and arrows.

"The child would have died quickly had I not helped it. He may die anyhow. But at least I prolonged his life." He wondered if anything he did would ever please Old Sore.

Picking up his soapstone ceremonial pipe and a pinch of tobacco, Old Sore limped out. Pedro knew he was bound for the old men's smoke lodge where he would smoke and talk with the other old men of the band.

Pedro had begun to strip off his leggings when the lodge flap parted and a Comanche stepped in. Behind him came a plumpish young squaw whose silver earrings jingled softly. In her hand she held a beaded toilet case made of buffalo hide. She was the mother of the Indian child who had been bitten by the snake. The man must be her husband, Coby the warrior.

The Comanche stood very still, his lightly molded body throwing off the same reddish hue as the soil. He had the broad brow and flaring nostril of a fighting man but seemed very young to be so renowned in battle. On his face was an expression of deep loneliness.

"I am Coby," he said with simple dignity. "This afternoon you saved my son from the snake. Now we are brothers." His speaking voice was pleasingly vibrant and melodious.

"We will always be brothers," Coby continued. "You are new here. All our customs may not be known to you. A man loves his brother. He is generous with him. He wants to give him everything he can. Sometimes he sends him his wife as a gift. Tonight I am letting you have my wife. Before the moon goes down she will return to my lodge." He gestured behind him to the woman, then turned his back and walked out.

Pedro stood silent, staring at the young squaw. What odd customs these Comanches had! Would he ever understand them entirely? The fire in the tipi floor crackled and snapped. Shadows from its flames danced on the interior lodge wall.

The young woman walked over to Pedro's pallet and dropped gracefully to her knees, her moccasined feet and lower legs turned under her buckskin skirt.

Pedro felt himself blushing to the roots of his hair. "How is your son's health?" he asked.

Coby's wife kept her eyes cast decorously downward. "Our

son is better. He slept an hour ago. He will live. We are both very grateful to you." Her voice was husky with gratitude. Pedro swallowed uncomfortably and licked his lips. The back of his neck grew hot. Despite his ignorance of Comanche mores, he felt that Coby and his wife were respectable people by Comanche standards. What they now sought to give him must be socially correct. How could he reject this gift without offending the givers?

"What is your name?" he asked.

"Kildee." The squaw's gaze was still fixed on the ground.

Pedro collected his thoughts, choosing his words carefully. "Return to your lodge. Tell Coby that I thank him for his generosity. Tell him that I know he could not tender me a greater gift than this. I am deeply honored. I shall not forget it. Tell him that his friendship is all the gift I want. He could not give me anything more dear." Pedro could feel his ears burning and the arteries in his throat pounding.

The Comanche woman looked at him, puzzled, then got to her feet. Picking up her toilet case, she ducked beneath the tipi flap and was gone.

Shortly afterward, Old Sore came in. Pedro waited as the old man carefully put his soapstone ceremonial pipe into the deerskin pouch lashed to one of the tipi poles. Then he told him of the visit of Coby and Kildee.

With a long, bony hand, Old Sore picked at his nose as he listened.

"What's the matter with you, *español?*" His deep voice was scornful. "Was the woman not acceptable? Did she not smell good enough? Coby won't like your refusal. Brothers are close comrades. They always help each other in everything. An older, unmarried brother gives his younger brother much helpful advice. If they are both married, they lend each other their wives. If not, the older brother always accommodates his younger one by sending him his wife. He will expect the younger brother to do the same when he marries. This relationship also applies to two close friends. Coby has no brother. Since he now calls you brother, he will expect you to act like one."

Pedro did not answer. Bewildered, he lay down on his robe. What was the use of having gained a friend if he had offended and lost him the same day? Nobody needed friends worse than he. For a long time he lay awake, worrying.

He was still brooding the next evening when he rode with Creek Water to the central meeting place of the village to participate in the hunting dance. Cold Bull, Creek Water's friend, had invited them. The dance was to be near his lodge. The whole village was excited about the approach of the autumn buffalo-hunting season.

Shrill cries and the sound of blows broke out ahead of them. A woman bolted out of a lodge door screaming with pain. Behind her, moving as nimbly as a goat despite his great bulk, ran the biggest and fattest man Pedro had ever seen. Almost globular in shape, he held a strong elmwood bow clutched in his right hand. Overtaking the woman, he struck her from behind with the bow and knocked her flat. Dazed, she got to her knees in the sand.

"Don't go slinking off like a dog when I speak to you. When I tell you to do something, run!" The fat man gave her another clout.

The woman shrieked afresh, trying to rise; red welts blossomed on her face and neck.

"Stop that yelling!" The man swung the bow again with all his strength.

The woman tried to stifle a pain-crazed howl. Clawing herself up, she got to her feet and reeled into the lodge, moaning as she went.

Anger surged through Pedro like a flame. His hand sought

the handle of the knife in his breechclout. He would enjoy carving great scallops of flesh out of this monster. It was unfortunate he had only this knife and not a butcher's cleaver. Then reason overcame impulse. "It's not your fight," he told himself. With an effort, he conquered his rage.

A pinto mare staked out nearby raised its head and nickered softly. With a complete change of mood, the fat man stooped and snatched up a handful of prairie grass. He walked to the mare's side and rubbed her with the grass, caressing her with his big hands, speaking to her in the most tender and endearing way.

Pedro turned to Creek Water. "Father, who is that man?"

"He is called Paunch," Creek Water said, "He's the richest man on the plains. It is said that he owns three thousand horses. He has so many that he has to hire herdsmen to watch them. He would do anything to obtain more. And yet he is so fat that he cannot ride a single one."

Pedro eased his slight weight in the saddle. "If he already has so many, why does he want more?"

"Because he still doesn't have the herd he wants. He yearns for a herd that belongs to a wealthy New Mexican trader who lives beyond the country of the Kwahades near a fort called Union. The trader's name is Tafoya. His horses are said to be so fast and so beautiful that many tribes have attempted to steal them. But he watches them so closely that all have failed. They are kept in a strong stockade and heavily guarded. Paunch has sent so many raids against that stockade that he is despised by the wives of our warriors slain on the raids."

They arrived early at Cold Bull's tipi. Cold Bull, Pedro was surprised to discover, was an old man more than sixty years of age. He sat outside his lodge with his three young wives, the oldest of whom looked no older than twenty. They seemed very fond of the old man and sat caressing him and combing his grayish hair with a porcupine tail brush. Pedro could tell from the benign, satisfied look on Cold Bull's face that he enjoyed it.

When Cold Bull saw Creek Water, he got up and greeted them. "Get down, brothers."

Pedro staked out the horses and soon afterward the dance started. Music was provided by two drummers and several singers. Light came from a roaring fire. It was a big dance. The people seemed joyful about the coming hunt, with its promise of excitement, feasting, and social activity. Everybody seemed hungry for fresh roasted buffalo tongues.

Men and women lined up and faced each other. This was Pedro's first participation in a tribal dance. His long leggings and extra blue blanket felt good in the crisp November air. When a woman crossed over and selected a male partner, Pedro watched carefully to see how the man moved his feet, his arms, and his body. Partners clasped each other around the waist. Otherwise their bodies did not touch. It looked easy. The voices of the singers rose above the booming of the drums.

A girl crossed over and stood in front of Pedro. Squat and broad-nosed, she wore bits of red flannel in her black hair. Pedro joined her and they danced. He had no trouble doing the steps, and soon found himself enjoying the dance.

"You dance well, Little Singer," his partner commented. Her voice sounded familiar somehow. She smelled like the sweat under a horse blanket.

"I don't dance as well as you ride," Pedro replied and To-a-nick-pe, the tomboy, smiled at the compliment. It was the first time he had seen her plainly. He liked her even if she did smell of horses.

Another girl among the dancers came gliding up to face a young man standing beside Pedro. The small bells on her moccasins jingled musically, the resplendent fringes on her buckskin skirt swayed with every motion of her graceful body.

The blue beading across her high, straight neckline sparkled in the firelight.

This girl reminded Pedro of a young tumbleweed tossing lightly about in a high wind. Her moccasins, with their long fringes running from lace to toe, seemed barely to touch the ground.

Like every other young man in the vicinity, Pedro watched her closely. She had narrow, finely arched black eyebrows. Her nose was straight and well molded, her chin firm. Her nostrils were not broad. Once when she passed Pedro at close range, he caught her scent. It made him think of sweet-smelling leaves.

For a moment he stood staring after her. Something nagged at his memory. Then he recognized her. She was the young girl who had comforted the captive white children back on the Kweetacooeh and later had listened to him play the comanchero's guitar. *Ai!* How she had ripened! Tall and stately, with a well-rounded shape, she moved like a queen.

"Who is that girl?" he asked To-a-nick-pe.

"She is called Willow Girl. She's the daughter of Wallowing Bear, a Yamparika peace chief. Her band generally camps north of the Peeahoonoo in the northern part of our country. They used to raid far beyond that stream. Two years ago some of them joined our band. Her mother is Cheyenne and very strict. Many of our people make fun of them because of their customs. They don't wear much paint. Their women won't eat horsemeat. They won't eat anything without washing. They bathe at all seasons of the year. They even break the ice to bathe. Why? Do you like her?"

"Like her?" Pedro snorted and drew himself up. "I don't even know her." He was provoked with To-a-nick-pe.

"Why don't you pick out a fullblood Comanche girl when you fall in love?" To-a-nick-pe persisted. "This one's mother is part Cheyenne."

Pedro felt a flush of indignation. Even these savages placed a social stigma on an interfused pedigree.

As he watched the Yamparika girl she seemed conscious of his stolen scrutinies. Once when he looked her full in the face, she dropped her eyes and ignored him.

Pedro finished dancing with To-a-nick-pe. Then, returning to the men's line, he stood directly opposite the Yamparika girl, hoping she might choose him next for a partner. But three other young men had the same idea. Crowding around, they jostled one another for the most favorable position. She paid no attention whatever to any of them, choosing instead a young man who wore a string of elk's teeth around his neck.

At midnight the dance ended. The sky clouded over and the north wind had a bite. The people began returning to their tipis. While Creek Water lingered to talk to Cold Bull, Pedro got the horses. All the way home he thought about the Yamparika girl. He almost forgot that tomorrow he and Old Sore would be off on a buffalo hunt.

11 · Ultimatum

"There they are," Old Sore grunted, peering keenly into the distance. At first, Pedro saw nothing but miles and miles of rolling brown prairie broken by an occasional arroyo, canyon, or butte. It was barely daylight. Long swaths of white frost coated the ground.

Suddenly Pedro saw them. From where he was they looked like a long black line along the edge of the horizon.

"Your Anza called them crooked-back cattle, *español,*" muttered Old Sore, "but to us they are a gift from the Great Spirit. We use every part of the buffalo except the skull, spine, and rump. We even use his dung for fuel, his paunch for a waterbag, and his sinews for thread and bowstrings. We make spoons, cups, and bows from his bones, horns, and hooves. Besides, he is a part of our spiritual life."

As they waited in line while the leader of the hunt talked to the scouts, Pedro felt hostile eyes upon him. A young brave had ridden up on his right. He had dark, shaggy hair, cruel lips, and an arrogant stare. With him rode a number of his friends and they seemed hostile too. Pedro saw Wolf Milk among them.

"He is fit only to work with the women," one of the braves remarked with a sneer. "That's where he would be now if Creek Water hadn't adopted him."

The shaggy-haired one had never taken his baleful eyes off

Pedro. Finally, he said to his comrades, "Look at his pale skin." Actually Pedro's skin was almost as dark as their own. "And look with what a proud air he holds himself."

At that moment the signal was given for everybody to move forward. The taunting stopped. The young men dropped back.

"Think nothing of what they said," advised a man on his left. "That bushy-haired one is Yellow Stirrup. He is Wolf Milk's cousin. He is the most quarrelsome young man in the village. The others just follow him."

As they moved closer, working against the wind, they formed a semicircle around the herd. Pedro saw the great woolly-maned animals, heads down, feeding on the prairie in as bovine a manner as a herd of domestic cattle on an acacia-dotted pasture in Granada. When would they start running? He quivered with excitement. Old Sore had told him that buffalo saw very poorly. Because of the thick mane that hung down over their eyes, they depended chiefly on their sense of smell for guidance, following one another's tracks when running.

"Watch the ground under your horse and be careful," the old man warned in a hoarse whisper. "There is little danger from the buffalo. But your running horse may step in a prairie-dog hole and fall. That's the quickest way you can be killed hunting buffalo."

They stopped to discard all their clothing save their breech-clouts and moccasins. The dawn air was icy but Pedro was too excited to care. Creek Water had lent them fresh horses for the chase. Old Sore had shown Pedro how to pass a rope around his horse's body behind the forelegs, and thrust his bare knees under the rope, leaving both hands free for the shooting. They all rode bareback on the hunt.

Pedro drew the cold air deeply into his lungs. This was far better than being stranded with the women and the pack animals back at the hunting tents.

Quietly they maneuvered until they were within bow-and-arrow range of the nearest bulls. At the firing of a musket, the chase was on. Pedro felt his horse almost jump out from under him in its eagerness to be off. Cold air rushed past, chilling his nearly naked body. The buffalo wheeled and began running, their short tails suspended ludicrously behind them. With small puffs of white vapor blowing from their mouths with each panting breath, the beasts looked as if they were driven by steam engines. Dust swirled and the prairie shook from the rhythmic pounding of thousands of hooves. Pedro felt an exhilaration and excitement he had never dreamed of before. Now he understood why his horse had been in such a ferment waiting for the chase to start.

Everybody had fun but the buffalo. Pedro could see them running strongly, the shaggy, massed bodies pouring in undulating brown waves over the crest of a small butte. They seemed to run more from instinct than from terror. The hunters, their faces intoxicated with pleasure, gained steadily on the galloping beasts. Pedro could taste dust on his tongue and feel it sting his eyes. The shrill cries of the hunters rang in his ears. The earthy smell of freshly torn turf filled his nostrils. The pounding of all the hooves, buffalo and horses together, swelled into thunder as the hunters rode up on them. Then the men separated, each becoming involved with a segment of the fleeing herd. Old Sore was not in sight.

As the climax of the hunt approached, Pedro was conscious only of massive movement and felt himself to be but a small, unimportant part of the tremendous spectacle. No wonder the Comanches regarded a buffalo hunt as something important. It was easy to see why so much tribal ceremony and social activity was built around it.

The young calves ran like the wind. The bulls and the cows just loped, their backs humping awkwardly. Grunting with effort, Pedro's horse tore along at full speed. Pedro was surprised to see the fleeing beasts divide on each side of him as they veered off to become two herds. It was time for his bow. He was here to kill, not to look. As his heart pumped furiously he got his arrows ready, careful not to drop them.

"You must kill as quickly as possible," Old Sore had told him. "If a buffalo is overheated from too long a chase, his meat will spoil before it can be cured."

Pedro rode up on the bulls from the right and began to shoot. Leading the running target, he tried for the soft spot between the last rib and the hip bone. It was there that the heart hung low, Old Sore had explained. To Pedro's surprise, it was not necessary to steer the gray horse Creek Water had lent him. Pedro had only to point the horse in the direction of the beast he was after. With a burst of speed, the highly trained gray would promptly put him within point-blank range of the quarry. Pedro began to feel a warm affinity with his mount. To shoot off the back of a horse that understood a hunt as well as this one was a joy.

Pedro shot coolly and fast, burying his shafts in the right flanks of the great beasts. Dust coated his tongue, and the smell of his horse's sweat was in his nostrils. He heard the mad bawling of wounded bulls as stone-tipped arrows drove home. Sometimes the bulls stumbled and fell within a few steps. At other times they staggered but kept going with decreasing speed, whereupon Pedro's mount would slow with them, keeping them on target. One wounded beast turned and tried to gore Pedro with its short, curved horns, but the gray easily avoided it.

After a sprint of half a mile, the horses began to breathe hard and slow down. Old Sore had told him that if the herd was not overtaken in two arrow shoots before the killing started the chase had better be abandoned. A running buffalo has great vitality and although he moves only two-thirds as fast as a horse, he can run much farther.

They jogged their blown mounts back to the scene of the kill, where identification of each slaughtered animal was made from the mark left in it by the hunter's arrow. Pedro's mark was found on four dead bulls and on a fifth that was wounded and had to be killed. It was excellent shooting for a young man on his first hunt.

Creek Water was not there to see it, having left for a council three days distant. Old Sore helped Pedro start the butchering until Creek Water's wives arrived.

"You should have killed the fifth bull too," the old man grumbled as he wiped his bloody hands on his deerskin shirt. "This arrow you made was defective. See? You did not wing the feathers properly. Too much glue on the split stems."

At the Buffalo Tongue dance back at the village, Pedro sat in the half circle of hunters. The smell of the juicy tongues roasting drove him to maddening hunger. Soon the pink meat was done to a turn. The women served the first roasted tongue to a hunter from the Wasp band who had shot seven bulls. They gave the fourth one to Pedro and he felt a fulfillment he had not known for years.

The dance broke up just before noon and Pedro rode Creek Water's gray to the nearby herding area and freed him. He was walking back among the tipis along the river when he saw them ahead, waiting for him. There were six of them, Yellow Stirrup in front, Wolf Milk behind him. He knew they were after him for breaking Wolf Milk's nose in the persimmon grove.

Pedro felt his hands shaking and his insides knotting. He knew their motive. They would try to taunt him into an impulsive act so they could kill him. He looked about him for the sight of a friend. He saw nobody except a couple of squaws fleshing a hide and some children playing in the river sand. He feared what lay ahead.

Then he remembered Creek Water's advice. "Do not turn

around." He walked boldly down the path toward them. When he sought to pass them, Yellow Stirrup stepped in front of him.

"You are not a Comanche," Yellow Stirrup said passionately. "You are a stranger who has come uninvited among us to live in a country that does not belong to you. Yesterday you visited our best hunting grounds. You were fortunate. The buffalo ran into your arrows. You destroyed many of the animals the Great Spirit intended for Comanches to kill. Leave this village at once or I will take your life."

Another young man behind Yellow Stirrup spoke. "You think that because a Comanche adopted you, that gives you the right to look and act like a Comanche."

Another pointed derisively at the simple lines of olive green Pedro had painted down his cheeks. "You don't even wear paint like a Comanche. You wear it like a Ute. What's the matter? Aren't our painting customs good enough for you?"

Yellow Stirrup whipped out his knife. "I see your ears are whole yet, in spite of the cactus spines our squaws ran through them. You heard me tell you to leave this country forever. But you are not going to leave it until I've notched your ears, so that I may know you next time I catch you."

Pedro stood very still, focusing his senses and his wits. Yellow Stirrup's knife did not frighten him. He knew half a dozen ways to take it from him. Best to let this surly fool talk. When he had talked out most of his hate perhaps he would cool off.

"Look how straight and proud he stands," Yellow Stirrup sneered. "What has he to be proud of? He does not have a drop of Comanche blood in his veins. He is not even a mixed-blood Comanche."

Pedro could feel his face flush. Why were his enemies always going out of their way to taunt him about not being of pure blood? In Spain he was spat upon because his noble blood had a gypsy strain. Here they despised him because he was not pure Comanche. What was wrong with his blood that everyone so despised it?

Triumph gleamed in Yellow Stirrup's eyes. At last he had found a way to goad this white youth.

"Hear this, you Worse-Than-a-Mixed-Breed. I forbid you to consider yourself a Comanche any longer, or to hunt any more on our domain, or to dance any more with our young women. If ever again I catch you doing any of these things, I will take your life. I will drain out all your black adulterated blood and spill it on the ground."

Pedro's pulse began to race. A deranged music began to sound in his head. He crouched. This villain deserved far more than just being deprived of his knife. He deserved to have his heart cut out. Pedro's leap was fast as lightning.

Whap!

Yellow Stirrup reeled from the stinging slap. Recoiling, he charged and slashed underhanded at Pedro with his knife. With incredible quickness, Pedro withdrew his body, turning it to the right. As the knife went past his bare stomach, he caught Yellow Stirrup's wrist with both hands, pulled him in the direction he was going, unbalanced him, and in a flash twisted the knife out of his hand. It fell to the ground.

Pedro stepped in with his little stone knife, thrusting upward. He could feel the knife bite in, feel the weight upon it. When he leaped back, Yellow Stirrup, his face distorted in stunned disbelief, was bent over, his hands wrapped about the deep gash in his side.

Pedro kicked Yellow Stirrup's knife behind him, and whirling, faced Wolf Milk and Yellow Stirrup's other friends, knife in hand. Motionless, they stared at him for a moment, then at the red tip of his knife, then at Yellow Stirrup kneeling on the sand. Surprise flooded their faces.

Pedro was astonished at how easy it had been. Old Cavo's instruction had been sound. Pedro's own lack of practice had probably saved Yellow Stirrup's life. In his rage he had missed the artery, inflicting only a deep side wound. How red was the blood that spewed out of Yellow Stirrup, the pure Comanche blood Yellow Stirrup had been so proud of! It stained the wounded man's fingers and formed tiny crimson puddles in the sand at his feet.

Pedro was relieved and exhilarated, as if a painful boil had been lanced and the poison drained out.

But a feeling of guilt washed over him. Yellow Stirrup had received exactly what he deserved. Still, a small voice deep inside Pedro kept saying, "Thou shall not kill." He had tried to kill a human being, failing only because he had been awkward. He had lived among these people so long that he was copying their cruelty and violence. Every step of the way back to the lodge, he thought about what he had become.

Outside the tipi, he paused and looked down at his hands. Feeling suddenly sick, he leaned over and vomited. Then he fled inside, found his little cedar shrine and dropping to his knees, made the act of contrition as perfectly as he could. "Oh my God, I am heartily sorry for having offended Thee. . . ."

The lodge flap lifted. Old Sore, ducking grotesquely because of his great height, hurried in, moving faster than Pedro had ever seen him move before. His usually bilious face was stamped with concern, a new emotion for him. An angry hum of voices arose outside.

"Yellow Stirrup's relatives and friends have come after you," Old Sore said. "He probably won't die but they are angry because you aren't a Comanche. It's a bad thing when a captive cuts up a Comanche. There's always trouble over it."

Hurriedly, the old man began to daub on his blue war paint. The noise outside redoubled. Dogs began to bark. Pedro heard somebody outside say in muffled tones, "Let's go in and take him."

Old Sore picked up his seven-foot lance. Facing the lodge

door, he began singing his war song. His harsh, jangling old voice rang out strongly. Although it screaked a little on the upper notes, there was no doubting his intention. Despite his feebleness, Old Sore intended to fight.

Shaken, Pedro stood by him, bow and arrows ready. He wished with all his heart that Creek Water was in the village. It seemed so stupid to die for knifing a villain like Yellow Stirrup.

Then a new voice spoke just outside the lodge door, a rich, low-pitched melodious voice. "Whoever tries to fight him," it said, "will have to fight me too." It was the voice of Coby, the warrior.

Everything became quiet. Coby knew the leaders of the group personally. He called them by name, told them the attempt would have to be stopped.

"I've talked to the other young men who were with Yellow Stirrup," he said. "They've acknowledged that they started the trouble and that Yellow Stirrup was the first to draw his knife. My friends, what is anybody—even an adopted person—supposed to do when six people threaten him and one of them draws his knife and tells him he is going to notch his ears? Would you have him run?"

Coby kept on talking, calmly and logically, and so great was his reputation as a fighter that Yellow Stirrup's friends gradually forgot their wrath and went home.

Coby walked into the lodge, his bow and arrows on his back, his short warclub of flint sticking out of his breechclout. His somber eyes fell upon Pedro.

"Brother, you were right. This is what makes a man—to fight and not to be afraid." He came up to Pedro, put his arms around him, and hugged him affectionately. Then, as suddenly as he had entered, he left the lodge.

"What happened out there today to make them so angry?" Old Sore growled, leaning his lance against a tipi pole and starting to wipe off his paint. "The last time I saw you, you were full of roasted buffalo tongue and had started after the horses."

Pedro told him.

Old Sore grunted. *"Español,* you've done well lately. Shot four buffalo and should have shot a fifth. Knifed Yellow Stirrup, who has needed it for a long time, but failed to kill him. Now you're so well known that all the girls in camp will try to sleep-crawl this tipi tonight. To elude them, we'll probably have to roost in the trees, like turkeys."

Pedro paid no attention to the old man's jesting. Something swelled in his breast, something proud and grateful and heart-warming. It was good to have a friend like Coby in this wild country, a friend who would die for him if necessary. A great humility that Pedro had not felt in his more than two years with these wild people swept over him. He wet his lips and looked down at his moccasins. His loneliness had been almost as hard to bear as his mistreatment.

Then his heart sank. He had forgotten to thank Coby. His new friend could not help but think him ungrateful. With another stab of conscience, he remembered that he had forgotten to thank his old friend too.

"Thank you for helping me, grandfather."

The old man shot a proud look at his lance. An old-style weapon, it had a chipped stone head and a single feather attached to the end of its shaft.

"Don't thank me. Thank that spear," Old Sore said. "That's a medicine spear. Yellow Stirrup's friends didn't want to face the power of that spear."

Early the next morning, Pedro hung a bundle of arrow shafts outdoors to season, and straightened to look at the prairie sunrise. The sparkle of the sun's flat rays on the frost-laden buffalo grass was a sight that always moved him.

Moccasin steps, slow and measured, sounded behind him,

and Creek Water walked up, quirt in hand. Reaching within
his gray wolfskin robe he offered Pedro tobacco, explaining
that he had secured it from a Kwahade at the council. The
Kwahade had got it from the New Mexican traders.

"Thank you for tobacco," Pedro said. He rolled an oak-leaf
cigarette, lit it from the nearby breakfast fire, and inhaled cautiously, resigned to the fact that Indian tobacco is so heavily
mixed with crushed sumac as to be almost unrecognizable. But
the minute he savored this, Pedro breathed it heavily and
luxuriously into his lungs. It was real tobacco.

Suddenly he stiffened, on guard. Creek Water would not
give him tobacco unless he wanted something in return. Tobacco was too scarce.

Gravely, Creek Water looked at him, his shrewd eyes slitted
against the morning sun.

"My son, I have heard about the buffalo hunt and about
your fight with Yellow Stirrup. You are fast making yourself
known as a hunter, a fighter, and a man. It is now more fitting
than ever that you should have a woman to look after your
property, clean the game you kill, take care of your lodge. You
said you wanted a young wife. My friend Diving Duck will
give you his daughter. His daughter is young and unmarried."

In a panic Pedro thought of Diving Duck's daughter. At the
hunting camp he had seen her feasting from the entrail of a
buffalo, her dirty hands red to the wrists in the dead beast's
blood. Pedro got hold of himself, remembering again that if it
were not for Creek Water he would still be Belt Whip's slave.

Choosing his words carefully, he replied, "It is true, my father, that I will want a young wife when I marry. But before I
select her, I will want to see her myself and judge myself
whether I want her in my tipi."

Creek Water's massive jaws hardened. "Everything has already been settled between Diving Duck and me. I have told

him that you would take her. The young woman has agreed to the marriage. I can do nothing else now but bring her to your lodge. Her mother is helping her pack."

Pedro straightened and looked Creek Water squarely in the eye. A chief isn't accustomed to being argued with; he knew that well. Nevertheless, before he'd be rushed into a marriage with Diving Duck's odorous daughter, he'd go back into slavery. He'd even risk death itself.

"Father, you have been generous with me. I owe you much. Most of all I am grateful to you for making it possible for me to learn to be a true Comanche, to hunt, to fight, and to think like a Comanche. I am thinking like one now. Here is what I think. I want to be free to choose my own wife, like the other young men of the village. As you did when you were a young man and you were first married. I will not marry Diving Duck's daughter."

The war chief of the Cuchaneos stood, bowlegged and impassive. Nothing moved in his sculptured face save his glittering eyes as he and his adopted son stood staring at each other while the long shadows of the tipis crept across the land.

Creek Water said soberly, "I will tell Diving Duck that we won't take his daughter now. We will wait."

Then he shifted his pigeon-toed feet and his hand tightened on the butt of the quirt. His bronzed face turned bleak and Pedro knew that further talk between them on this matter was over forever.

Creek Water's voice was edged with impatience. "But we will not wait any longer than the spring moon. If you have not chosen a wife by then, I will chose one for you."

He turned and walked away among the forest of tipis, his buckskin leggings squeaking with each step he took, his heel jinglets tinkling ominously.

Uneasy, Pedro watched him go. He tried to fight down his panic. Time was closing in on him. Only four months' grace.

He doubted if he would be ready to make the escape effort in four months. Although he knew the terrain where he and Old Sore had camped and hunted, he was ignorant of the geography beyond. Every time he asked Old Sore about the distant domain, the old man grew tight-lipped and silent. It seemed to Pedro that they were all in league to hold him here. He did not want to make his bolt for freedom until he knew exactly where he was going and how far. He did not dare fail this time. And yet if he started too soon, he knew he would fail.

He plucked one of the arrows out of the curing bundle and began to wing it with turkey feathers. If marriage would save his life and let him buy the precious time he needed, perhaps marriage would be wise after all. Still, he was torn with doubt every time he considered it. He knew the inflexible attitude of his church concerning marriage. A man did not embrace it lightly. Marriage was for life. He doubted if the Blessed Mother would look with favor upon a union consummated in expediency and dissolved a few months later when the husband ran off. Besides, there were no vows, no ceremony in a Comanche wedding. The husband and wife just started living together. How would the church like that? But he might not have any choice.

He kept working on the arrow, binding the feathers to the grooves on either side of the shaft with glue and threads of sinew. He was nearly eighteen, old enough to marry by Comanche standards. Some Comanche boys married at sixteen. Most of all he dreaded the kind of a woman Creek Water might choose for him. Then he thought of the girl he had seen at the hunting dance. Willow Girl was her name, To-a-nick-pe had said.

He remembered the kindness she had shown the terrified captive white children on the Kweetacooeh. He had found her scent most pleasant.

With his little stone knife Pedro notched the front end of the arrow and set a flint head in it, slanting it at right angles as Old Sore had taught him so it would pass through the horizontal ribs of an enemy. Marriage to the Yamparika girl might not be so distasteful. Surely he could bear it for a few short months.

Perhaps he should find Coby and seek his advice about how to win her. Coby was his friend. He decided to talk to Coby at once.

"Forget about that girl, brother," Coby advised him. "Every buck in the band is trying to win her. Her father will probably give her to the man who gives him the most horses. You have no horses. I would give horses to you for a wedding gift but that would not be respectable. Besides, I could not give you enough. The bidding will be high for that girl. Find another girl."

Pedro nibbled at the dried venison Kildee had placed before him. "Brother, I don't understand why Creek Water wants me to marry so quickly. Why does it mean so much to him?"

Coby's sad eyes held Pedro in their melancholy stare. "He probably thinks that a wife and family will make you more satisfied with Comanche life. He probably reasons that marriage will make you settle down, learn our customs, go on the warpath, distinguish yourself in battle, and do him great honor. Creek Water has no sons. He has great hope in you."

Pedro chewed reflectively. "I hope he changes his mind about finding me a wife. I don't want to marry anybody."

"He won't change," Coby predicted gloomily. "The thing for you to do is find one yourself before he chooses for you. The Yamparika girl is out of your reach. She's pretty. She's a good housekeeper, and she has a good reputation. But everybody's after her. People say that Two-in-a-Blanket has the best chance. He's the best dresser in the village. He has a way with the women. Find another girl."

Pedro fell silent. How could he tell Coby what he thought of all the others?

"I know what you are thinking," Coby sympathized. "All the other girls are dogs. It always seems that way after you've met the one you like."

Pedro nodded miserably. "How does one go about meeting other girls?"

"At the dances."

Pedro's platter was empty. Quickly Kildee appeared behind him and filled it again. Their small son who had been bitten by the snake a month earlier stuck his black head into the tipi flap. He looked solemnly at Pedro and withdrew. His arm was still scabbed and discolored but the swelling had gone down.

Pedro said, "I don't want to marry anybody, brother. But if I do marry, it would have to be somebody like the Yamparika girl. Either her or another one like her."

Coby said, "There isn't another like her."

Pedro nodded gloomily. "I know."

Coby scratched his scalplock and looked thoughtful.

"There's still another way. You could make friends with her brother or some other near relative. Give him a horse, or some arrows. After you do this and after you several times address him as 'our children's uncle' he would understand what you are after and he might help you. A brother can invite a friend to the family lodge."

Pedro brightened. "Has the Yamparika girl got a brother?"

"Yes." Then Coby's face fell again. "But Two-in-a-Blanket is courting him almost as hard as he is courting her. He practically lives with her brother already."

Pedro wiped the grease off his lips with his hand, then wiped his hand on the grass floor. Two-in-a-Blanket! What an appropriate name for a dandy. Already Pedro disliked the man.

With a sigh he rose and followed Coby outside. Coby took him to a small sandy hollow nearby where several large birds stalked nervously about on the ground, their great wings spread in the heat and dragging in the sand. Their beaks were fierce-looking and their legs feathered to the toes. They stared into the distance as though wishing they were free. Someone had staked them out on buckskin leashes attached to pins in the ground.

"What are those?" asked Pedro.

"Eagles," Coby answered simply. "I captured them from their nest in Ehsetoyahpe, the gray mountains, when they were young. When they are grown, I pull out their tail feathers to put around my shield. Eagles have great power in war. I've never been hit by an arrow or a bullet since I began wearing eagle feathers and attaching them to my shield."

Pedro thought, I'm like those eagles. Hungry for freedom. For a moment he permitted himself the fantastic wish that he could make an agreement with Coby's birds. He would slip over some night and free them if they would fly him to his uncle's ranch in Chihuahua and a reunion with his beloved guitar. On the way they would swoop down on Green Turtle's band, wherever it was camped, and pick up Roberto. Then Pedro smiled sadly. No sense in that kind of dreaming. It only made captivity worse.

"Thank you, brother, for food and advice," he told Coby.

"If you still want to meet some new girls, there's a dance tonight," Coby told him. "It's just a dance for fun. A lot of girls will be there. Anybody can go. In this dance, men can select the women they want for partners. If you want to go, I'll go with you."

"All right, brother." Discouraged, Pedro walked slowly back to his tipi. He did not want to go to any dance, or meet any new girls. But it would give him something to do.

12 · The Courting

Pedro and Coby sat on the ground in the circle of spectators, watching the dancers. It was colder and the robe about Pedro's shoulders felt comfortable. The cottonwood limb fire crackled and popped; the shadows of its flames flickered off the buff-colored lodgeskins. The smell of it was good in Pedro's nostrils.

This was a different dance from the hunting dance. This time the men did the choosing. Two long lines of dancers stood apart, facing each other. There were young men in one line and young women in the other. When the singing and drum beating began, a man would advance and place his hands upon the hips of the woman he wished to dance with. She would clasp him in the same way. The only dancing motion was a short sidestep with the left foot leading and the right foot following. When the music ended, the dancers parted, re-forming their original lines and waiting for the drums to start again so new partners might be chosen.

Pedro's eyes darted everywhere, inspecting every girl in the line. It was hard to see them from his vantage point on the ground. It was hard to smell them, too. The wind, blowing from his back, was wrong.

"There's one," Coby would whisper, "that small one with the orange circles on her cheeks and the tattoo on her forehead." Coby judged Comanche beauty by Comanche standards. The heavily decorated faces of his own kind attracted him. But Pedro saw them differently.

"No, brother," he would mutter cheerlessly. "She's a dog, too."

Pedro shifted his attention to the female spectators and saw Cedar and Caught While Mad seated among them. Despite the blanket Cedar wore, her stomach bulged outward. She was pregnant again.

Tired of scouting the females, he switched his eyes to the male line. One dancer caught his attention. Circles of silver wire swung from his ears and his cheeks were tinged neatly with vermilion. His buckskin jacket fitted without a wrinkle. The embroidered fringes of his moccasins were so long that they trailed a yard behind his ankles. The most noticeable thing about him was the way he wore his hair in two long, neatly knotted braids that fell almost to his knees. The braid ends, bound in beaver fur, leaped and tossed crazily as he whirled to the rhythm of the drums.

"Who is that one?"

"That's Two-in-a-Blanket," Coby said, "the one I was telling you about. He enjoys the company of the women but he's a warrior, too. He's always as ready to fight as he is to flirt."

Pedro studied him. Tall and slender, he danced with rhythm and grace and boundless stamina. He looked as if he could go on all night. At every lull in the dancing he dragged a small yucca-stalk brush through his carefully groomed tresses or plucked hairs from his smooth cheek with a pair of bone tweezers. Pedro snorted. The man obviously thought too much about how he looked.

Suddenly Two-in-a-Blanket thrust his brush and bone tweezers into his breechclout, tossed his braids back over his shoulders, and hurried toward the dancers. The Yamparika girl had arrived with her mother.

With her curiously graceful motion, she came up to the

dancing line. Her buckskin dress swished musically and her sleeve fringes swayed in the breeze. Pedro's head lifted, his dark eyes exploring every line of her. Her long black hair, parted down the middle, was brushed close to the head. There was a clean ranginess about her that he liked. Every motion and posture suggested dignity, modesty, and good sense. In her narrow face with its high cheekbones, excitement shone. She seemed eager for the dancing to start.

Pedro felt a quick fire coursing through his body. He shook his head, trying to clear his senses. No Spanish girl had ever moved him like this.

Why did he always feel excited and disturbed when he was near this girl? Their cultures were centuries apart. Yet he felt strangely drawn to her.

Pedro jumped to his feet and joined the men swarming toward her. He was a step behind Two-in-a-Blanket, who lagged another full pace behind a muscular brave with a turkey feather in his hair. This newcomer put his hands on Willow Girl's waist and triumphantly guided her about the dancing area.

His moment in the sun was brief. Two-in-a-Blanket soon replaced him. The girl smiled, showing two rows of perfect white teeth. She held up her arms so he could put his hands on her hips. Pedro watched them float smoothly back and forth. They might have been dancing partners for years. All eyes seemed to focus on these two who danced with such unity and grace.

Never missing a step, Two-in-a-Blanket several times gave his long braids a vigorous toss back over his shoulder. Everybody was watching those braids with their wrappings of beaver fur. Pedro watched them, too, despising the man's easy familiarity and grace.

Suddenly the end of one of the handsome braids detached itself and fell onto the sand behind Two-in-a-Blanket. False! thought Pedro exultantly. It was probably made of hair some woman had cut off in mourning. Boldly he walked up to the dandy's elbow.

"Brother," he said, pointing to the black plait upon the ground, "your hair is falling out."

Two-in-a-Blanket saw that Pedro spoke the truth. Blushing, he snatched up the severed coil in one hand and hurriedly left the line to repair the cleavage.

At last Pedro was face to face with the Yamparika girl. She was too polite to laugh openly at Two-in-a-Blanket's misfortune, but the corners of her mouth turned up slightly and her eyes twinkled.

Pedro held out his hands toward her hips. She lifted her arms and off they glided, in time to the singing and the drums. Light as thistledown, the girl followed his lead perfectly, evidently sensing his dancing intention through the feel of her fingertips on his sides. Pedro felt his heart hammering. This was the nearest he had ever been to her. Very much aware of the warmth and sweet smell of her, he wondered how she achieved her pleasant body fragrance.

Obviously she did not indulge in the gaudy facial decoration of other Comanche women. There was no paint on her face except for two slender yellow lines traced above and below her eyelids. Crossing at the outer corners, they accentuated the friendly little crinkles there. Her mouth, slightly protruding, curved pleasantly. Her lips were thin, her chin firm.

She danced with a detachment that Pedro found frustrating, however. Whenever he looked at her she modestly dropped her eyes. As they moved past her mother who sat in a circle of older women, Pedro saw the woman frown. He supposed it had something to do with the fact that technically he was still a captive. With an effort, he controlled the anger that flared up in him. Nothing must mar the only dance he had ever had with this girl. Earnestly he spoke to her.

"Where do you live, friend? I should like to see you again."

For the first time, she looked directly at him and he saw the ginger-brown cast of her slightly slanted eyes. Their depth added a slenderness to the bridge of her nose. Biting her lip and cocking her head to one side, she regarded him with a puzzled expression. Pedro feared that he had violated some convention. Then her face brightened.

"Aren't you the one who brought music out of the wooden gourd that day at the trading?"

Pedro nodded.

A warm expression came into the girl's eyes. Her lips parted. A look of wonder and bewilderment came into her face just as it had that night Pedro had played at the trading stall.

He explained that the "gourd" was a guitar and that back in his own country he had intended to make a career for himself by coaxing music from it.

"The guitar was my life," he told her simply. "When I was first captured by your people, I almost went mad because I did not have it. I felt like José Marín, a countryman of mine who was a prisoner in the tower at Madrid. They took his guitar away from him and put a forty-pound fetter on his ankle. Caged like a bird, he sang to ease his sorrow. This is what he sang."

In his youthful tenor, Pedro sang the first two lines of the old *copla* beginning, *"Cautivo y prisionero, canto mis penas. . . .* A captive in a prison cell, I sing the woes I feel."

The girl looked at him strangely, her face alive with a play of emotion he had seldom seen on an Indian's face. "I have never heard that kind of singing, friend." Her voice was low and expressive. "How many ponies did you pay for that song?"

Now it was Pedro's turn to look surprised. "Such songs are free in my country. Anyone may sing them at any time without having to pay for them."

"Our people respect the ownership of songs," she explained. "Thus a man will say before he sings, 'I am now going to sing my uncle's song,' or, 'This song belonged to a friend of my father who is long dead.' And he would mention the owner's name before he sang it. In the old days it was not unusual for a person to pay the value of one or two ponies for a song. A father would not think of teaching his son a song without asking for compensation. A person selling a song shares its magic power with the purchaser."

Pedro thought fast.

"Friend," he said, "I would like to learn some of your Comanche songs." He had in mind asking her to teach them to him. Coby had told him that in Comanche courtship, the boy and girl were not supposed to be seen together, although they sometimes managed to be in each other's company at night if the girl went for water and wood.

She said quickly, "That should not be difficult. Young men are allowed to sit with the singers around the drum and sing softly the tribal songs until they learn the melodies. These dance songs belong to everybody." Before she lowered her grave, downcast eyes Pedro thought he saw a hidden merriment in them.

Was she purposely teasing him? She seemed too candid and unaffected to be jesting—and yet he was not sure.

They danced past the circle of spectators and he saw her mother scowling more darkly than ever. What a vigilant old dragoness she was! As watchful as any Spanish chaperone he had ever encountered.

All too soon the singing and the drumming stopped. He felt the girl's hands release his waist. Pedro swung round, scowling at the drummer.

A shadow darted past him toward the girl and raised its arms. It was Two-in-a-Blanket, his counterfeit plait mended. Apparently the man had no shame. The music started up again, wild and rhythmic. The girl sailed off in the company of the dandy.

So this is love, thought Pedro. *Hola y hasta luego,* hello and goodbye.

Sighing, he went off to find Coby. As he walked, he tried to probe his feelings toward the girl. Did he desire her solely as a means of rescue from the matrimonial snare in which Creek Water had entangled him? Or did he love her for her own sweet self?

Coby sat alone, his robe drawn up to his chin, his melancholy eyes watching the dancers. Quickly Pedro told him what had happened.

"What shall I do now?" he asked miserably.

Coby looked at him with pity. "Brother, there's only one thing for you to do. It's always wise, if possible, to win the love of the girl. Go to her tipi after dark and stand around. When she leaves the tipi to go for wood or water, step toward her. Let her see you. If she's interested, she'll let you know through her actions and you can see her for a short time. Or you and she can agree then on a future meeting place. If she isn't interested, she'll let you know."

Next evening at dusk, Pedro went quietly to the vicinity of the tipi of Willow Girl's parents. The girl's own tipi, smaller than her father's, stood close by, but it was dark. As Pedro stepped cautiously around to the side nearest the doorflap, he stumbled over a man who was lying on the ground. Startled, he jumped back, his hand dropping to the haft of the little stone knife.

"Forgive me for treading on you."

The other sat up and fastidiously began brushing that part of his deerskin shirt Pedro had stumbled against.

"That's all right." He sounded haughty. Producing a yucca stalk from his breechclout, he dragged it through his carefully groomed hair.

Pedro sighed. Would he ever be entirely rid of the dandy? As his eyes became accustomed to the darkness, he saw other forms lying nearby. Probably other rivals. Discouraged, he lay down among them in the sand. It was cold and he had forgotten to bring a blanket but he decided to stay anyhow. She might come out while he was gone and he did not want to miss her.

When she did emerge half an hour later, her mother was with her. They went off into the darkness together.

The next night Pedro tried it again. Again he found his competitors scattered all about, some concealed in the sage, others hidden among the willows growing a short distance from the lodge door. This time the girl appeared alone. The resulting rush reminded Pedro of a herd of buffalo in stampede.

Two-in-a-Blanket was the first to reach her. He seized her and tried to throw his blanket around her, but she resisted, crying out in protest. Mortified, the dandy released her and she went back into the tipi.

Hope surged through Pedro. Perhaps the girl was not in love with anyone.

After another hour, he again grew discouraged and gave up waiting. Although he had not been rebuffed, he was not making any progress.

"I'll speak for you to her father," Coby offered next day. "Sometimes it helps to have a friend do this. I'll give him a present and remind him what a good hunter you are. I don't think it will do any good but I'll try. I think it is your place to let the girl know you want her. When so many suitors are courting her, a girl sometimes pays attention to the one who goes to some particular trouble to make his affections known. Have you ever thought about getting a flute or a hand drum and playing at night outside her tipi?"

Pedro shook his head. In Spain, lovers sometimes serenaded their sweethearts with guitar and song but he had never done it, nor had he ever heard of anybody serenading a girl with a drum. But this was not Spain.

"I know a woman who has a hand drum," Coby said. "It's the only one in the village. Maybe we can buy it." At sunset, he led Pedro to a lodge pitched a short distance away from the others. As they approached, they heard a dismal crying and howling.

Coby said, "That's her. She's in mourning. Her name is Mad Woman. Her husband, Standing Feather, was killed in battle against the Utes three years ago. She still mourns him every evening when the sun goes down."

As they walked up, Mad Woman ceased her wailing. Dignified and distinguished-looking, she took them to her tipi, set meat before them, and listened patiently to Coby's offer to buy the drum. She even let Pedro hold it. When he thrummed his fingers tentatively across its taut head, he was surprised at its soft resonance.

But she refused to sell. "It's so much company to me in the long winter evenings when I sing by myself," she explained.

Pedro decided to make a flute instead. Because he wanted to go beyond the usual simple Indian pipe that could play only two notes, the job took him six whole days. He made the flute from the soft wood of the sumac, cutting out a straight, round piece and splitting it lengthwise into two equal parts. He hollowed out each half cylinder, gluing the two together with gum and wrapping them tightly with buffalo sinew.

He cut six holes for his fingers and devised a mouthpiece so that sound was produced by blowing across the open end. With very little practice, he soon became able to play simple melodies, although the music seemed a wretched substitute for what he had in mind.

The first night after Pedro had finished it, he stole to the vicinity of the girl's lodge, put the flute to his lips, and began to play. At once he was aware of an Indian flute blown by another person lying on the ground nearby. As he paused to listen, Pedro admitted to himself that the doleful strains tootled by his competitor were pleasing in spite of the limitations of the instrument.

When the moon came up, the soft, harmonious tattoo of a hand drum broke from a sand-plum cluster near the door of the girl's lodge. Pedro could scarcely believe his ears.

Anger flamed through him as he recognized the sound. And when the increasing moonlight revealed the beater occasionally pausing to tidy his hair, Pedro was angrier than ever. Two-in-a-Blanket had somehow persuaded Mad Woman to sell him the hand drum.

Now the piping of the flutes and the throbbing of the drum blended together in one discordant jangle. Somewhere a nearby dog began to howl, and before long was joined by half of the dogs in the village. From a neighboring lodge an old woman hobbled out to scold the musicians and throw sticks at the nearest dogs.

Pedro got up and put the six-holed flute in his breechclout. Two-in-a-Blanket and the other flutist rose, too. The dandy looked with contempt at Pedro's homemade flute.

"Brother, how long do you blow on that passion pipe before your eyes fall out?" he asked. Pedro was too disgusted to reply.

When Pedro told Old Sore about his troubles that night over their late meal of dried buffalo meat and Indian potato roots, the old man screwed his wrinkled visage into a frown.

"Love songs are dangerous," he said with a grunt. "In the old days, if a man started singing them, or playing them on a flute, we sent for a medicine man to treat him."

Depressed, Pedro went to bed. Everything he tried had failed. How could he court a girl he couldn't see? And even if he could figure out a way to reach her, what could she possibly see in him? He had no ponies to give to her father, no warrior reputation. He was an adopted person without pure Comanche blood, looked down on by most of the tribe. His chance of winning the girl seemed much the poorest of any of her suitors. Yet he had to keep on. As a last resort he would have to try flattering the girl's brother. He might do that tomorrow. Before he closed his eyes in sleep, he heard the bark of many a distant wolf.

Two hours after sunup the next morning Pedro mounted his mule and rode to Wallowing Bear's tipi.

The father was gone but he found Long Hungry, the fifteen-year-old brother, standing knee deep in sandburs on a nearby hillock, his thin chest bared to the breeze, greeting the new day with song. Long Hungry's caroling was as spontaneous and joyful as the outpouring of the birds in the hackberry trees. Apparently it was his custom to greet each morn in this fashion. Pedro thought, I could stand anything from her relatives —even this—if I could somehow win her in marriage.

When Long Hungry saw Pedro, he obligingly cut his paean short, ending it with a shrill yell. "Get down, brother," he invited.

Pedro climbed off the mule, his hands shaking as he held out six new arrows. This was his last chance and he mustn't fail.

Long Hungry gazed with pleasure at the gift. His face, like his sister's, was expressive and full of feeling.

"Thank you for arrows." He ran his fingers up and down one of the smooth shafts. Pedro watched him hopefully. He had rubbed each shaft carefully for hours, polishing it with sandstone while smoothing it to perfect roundness.

Willow Girl's brother knew the purpose of the gift. "She's not here, brother," he said, honestly. "She got up early and went across camp to play double ball. My mother went with her." There was sympathy in his open countenance.

Pedro fought down his disappointment. He had wanted so much to see the girl alone.

Long Hungry looked down at the arrows and then at Pedro again. He seemed to feel a sense of obligation for both the gift and the visit. "That tipi is hers." He gestured toward a small tipi tilted slightly backward, standing behind the lodge of his parents. Two encircling stripes of orange were painted entirely around its buff exterior. "Would you like to see it?"

Pedro hesitated. It did not seem proper to go poking into a young girl's living quarters. Long Hungry saw the indecision in his face.

"She's gone. So is Grass Girl, my younger sister. They live in it together." Boldly, the brother entered the girls' tipi.

Pedro found himself following. He had to duck to clear the entrance flap, which faced the rising sun. The flap was covered by an extra pelt, tanned stiff and ingeniously fastened on the windward side with a weight attached to the bottom to make it self-closing.

The minute he stepped inside that lodge, Pedro was overwhelmed with yearning. It was only a small tipi but he knew there was not another like it in the whole Comanche nation. Every cubic foot of it had been lovingly planned by somebody who understood the peace and comfort of a home.

A redolent odor of piñon permeated the place. It came from green sprigs the girl had tastefully fastened with mesquite needles to the buffalo-skin walls. The floor of white river sand had been carefully leveled and swept. Although the firehole in the center was planted so deep that the small buffalo-chip blaze smoldering in it was almost hidden from sight, the lodge had a pleasant warmth. It was not smoky, an achievement the girl had managed by manipulation of two buffalo-skin flaps over the smokehole at the top, each of which could be opened or closed by a pole attached on the outside to keep out the rain and funnel off the smoke.

Pedro marveled at the girl's cleverness. Fresh air was admitted at the bottom of the lodge by raising one wall flap an inch off the ground but the draft was not permitted to blow directly on the people inside. A second wall of buffalo skin, extending entirely around the inside perimeter of the lodge and reaching to the floor, diverted the outside air upward. This second skin wall hung from the tipi poles at a height of five feet. Falling to the floor all around, it was tucked neatly under the outside edge of the beds.

The two beds at the back of the lodge were elevated half a foot off the ground by rawhide slats laid across two short logs of cedar. Warm robes were spread over each and Pedro saw two rabbitskin pillows stuffed with grass. There was a water vessel made from a whole deer skin, a buffalo-horn drinking cup, and four wooden bowls. Several small deerhorn spoons hung in orderly fashion from one of the lodge poles. The lodge's walls were so tightly insulated that they would shut out the fiercest heat, cold, wind, or rain. The whole thing could be set up in fifteen minutes or dismantled in ten. Everything was scrupulously clean.

Pedro sighed. He was not surprised to discover Willow Girl's domestic skill. Although Comanche women were notoriously slovenly housekeepers, Cheyenne women were just the opposite, and Willow Girl was half Cheyenne. She seemed good at anything she undertook.

Depression overwhelmed him. He felt sure that he would never live in this tipi and would never take to wife the girl who had so wisely arranged it.

Long Hungry stepped to the girl's bed and raised the lid of a parfleche box banded with rows of brilliant beading. Curious, Pedro peeked within.

"This is her toilet case." Long Hungry enjoyed his dual role of host and guide. "She keeps her paints in it, mostly red and yellow for her face." One by one, he picked up various objects, glibly explaining their function. "This is a hair parter used to paint the part yellow or red. This is a porcupine hairbrush.

Those are her earrings and bracelets. With this twig she cleans her teeth."

Long Hungry raised the lid of a parfleche trunk near the bed and lifted out a neatly folded buckskin blouse. A quantity of sweet-smelling cottonwood leaves fell out of it onto the floor. Breathing in the scent of Willow Girl's perfume, Pedro sighed again.

"She always keeps a supply of these leaves on hand," Long Hungry ran on. "She packs them among her clothing, puts some in her pillows, and even ties a bunch of them on her necklace beads. Sometimes she and my other sister gather black seeds from a certain kind of weed growing in the swamps along the river. They pound them until they are very fine. Then they sop them and use them to perfume their clothing or their hair. They also use this on the manes and tails of their favorite ponies."

Long Hungry sat down on one of the beds as his tongue wagged on and on. "My mother and all my aunts are always lecturing my sister about her behavior. They tell her not to glance around in public places, not to laugh out loud, not to peep at young men when they come near her tipi, and most of all not to respond to the flashes of mirrors held by young men at a distance, as this would govern a young man's opinion of her character."

"Doesn't she ever go anywhere without her mother?" Pedro asked.

Long Hungry shook his black head. "No. My mother watches her strictly all the time. She even accompanies my sisters when they go to the brush to attend to nature's demands for fear some young man might molest them."

Voices sounded outside. The door flap parted and Willow Girl thrust her head inside. Pedro saw that in the sun her hair was black as the prairie after a burnoff. Parted in the middle, it was smoothed away from her brow and fell in thick profusion about a face that registered astonishment, then embarrassment, and finally annoyance. With a gasp of displeasure, she backed out of the doorway and disappeared.

Long Hungry whooped in alarm and dove beneath the lodge skins, vanishing from sight. Pedro was trapped.

The girl's mother entered, her face black as a thundercloud. She scolded Pedro, fiercely and volubly, in mingled Comanche and Cheyenne.

Pedro did not run. Arms folded, he stood looking coldly down at her. He had never liked noisy females, and he had additional reasons for not liking this one, even if she was the wife of a Yamparika chief.

"Your son invited me in," he informed her haughtily when she paused for breath. "He was only being hospitable. I thought hospitality was a Comanche virtue. And a Cheyenne virtue, too."

Abuse poured from her lips in a fresh torrent. Again he waited until she ran out of breath. His prospects were so poor that he might as well meet the situation boldly, he decided.

"I am here to become better acquainted with you and your family," he announced. "I am considering marrying your daughter."

This infuriated her even more. "You are neither Comanche or Cheyenne. You're just a Mexican. Your blood is like gypsum water. Why should my daughter marry so far beneath herself?"

Pedro felt his temper rising. How could this coarse-mannered woman have mothered such a nice girl? Arms still folded, he drew himself up proudly.

"I am no more Mexican than you are. I am Spanish. My people came to this country in great ships hundreds of years ago. We conquered you easily. In those days your people were dog Indians. You harnessed dogs to your travois poles and had to walk everywhere. We introduced horses to this country. After we defeated you, we made the mistake of ignoring you and letting you have some of our horses. That's the only reason you are here today."

He walked slowly and disdainfully past her, out the entrance. With a yank at his mule's jaw rope, he mounted and rode off, furious with himself. Now he had alienated both the girl and her mother. Why had he let that babbling brother of hers talk him into entering her tipi?

Two days later the weather turned frosty. A light snow fell and the icy north wind cut through everything except the thickest robes. The river froze over. Buffalo and antelope flew before the freezing gale, seeking protection in the canyons and arroyos.

"Fresh meat all gone," Creek Water's squaws announced. Pedro and Old Sore decided to go hunting soon as the wind subsided. Pedro welcomed the challenge of the hunt. For a day or two he would forget his discouraging courtship.

The next night the wind died and the stars came out. Two hours before sunup, Pedro felt Old Sore's rough hand on his shoulder.

"Get up," the old man barked gruffly. "Today we hunt turkey. Turkeys can smell you as far off as elk. We'll have to hunt against the wind."

Four hours later they had the good fortune to find a flock feeding in a patch of wild sunflowers. With a yell, Old Sore rode into them at full gallop, driving them out onto a section of prairie devoid of sage or mesquite. Crowded together and gobbling with alarm, the big black birds ran a few steps. Then with a great whistling of wings, they rose and flew into the open.

"Stay after them! Keep them flying! Don't let them rest!" Old Sore yelled as he flogged his pony with the end of the jaw rope. Pedro's mule was close behind.

They rode furiously in pursuit, and since the birds flew only five hundred yards before setting, it was no trouble to flush them again. This time, the flock flew only a hundred and fifty yards and the huntsmen rode upon them faster. After a third winging, shorter still, the weary birds began to run on the ground, trying to dodge their pursuers.

This was what the old man wanted. He used his bow as a club and rode right up on them. As the exhausted gobblers swerved to escape the horse, Old Sore rapped them smartly across the head, and leaving the dead ones lying on the prairie, rode ahead for others. Pedro followed the old man's example. When they tired of their sport and turned back to recover the kill, they picked up twelve of the heavy birds. Old Sore showed Pedro how to remove the viscera and leave the feathers on. They tied the dead birds together by the feet in pairs, slung them over the backs of their mounts, and took them to camp.

It was Porcupine Woman, Creek Water's oldest wife, who suggested that Pedro take one of the dressed turkeys to Wallowing Bear's tipi as a peace offering to Willow Girl and her mother. She explained that turkey meat was a delicacy that a whole family might enjoy.

When Pedro rode up to Wallowing Bear's lodge, Grass Girl came out. The turkey he handed to her was so heavy that she had to hug it to her bosom with both hands.

"Thank you, friend," she said, "thank you for the turkey."

"Tell your mother and your sister that I am sorry I trespassed in your tipi," Pedro said. He hated having to eat crow but the apologizing was not so hard with only Grass Girl there.

"I'll tell them, friend."

"I would like very much to apologize in person to your sister. I would like to see her a moment."

Grass Girl looked at him strangely, but went obediently inside the tipi, and soon came back out.

"My sister says she does not want to see you." A trace of sympathy came into her expressive eyes and Pedro knew that she must have seen the misery in his face. "It isn't permitted," she explained.

That afternoon the sky became heavily overcast again, the north wind freshened, and a light sleet began salting the sandy ground. Old Sore went outside to close the smokehole flap. Pedro laid another buffalo chip on the fire.

"This is a good day to do our winter bathing," the old man said. "A winter bath is always good for a man in love, *español*. It shocks all the passion out of him."

His mind still in upheaval over the failure of his courtship, Pedro followed the old man. Each wore a buffalo robe as they rode off, and Old Sore carried his stone warclub and some antelope skins. What odd accessories for a gentleman's bath, thought Pedro. However, he had long ago learned that Old Sore always had a reason for everything he did, although it often was motivated by fear of the supernatural.

Old Sore led the way along the river until they were a mile above the camp. Here he dismounted and hobbled his horse. Pedro staked out the mule, walked to the river bank, and stared absently at the solid sheet of ice covering the stream.

Without a moment's hesitation the old man dropped his robe, unwound his breechclout, and stepped out of his moccasins. Stark naked in the high country chill, he gazed pontifically over the landscape. Big softly falling snowflakes dissolved against his skeletal ribs and withering shanks, but he seemed to ignore them. To Pedro, he looked like a spectral totem pole.

Stone warclub in hand, Old Sore walked barefoot to the edge of the water. He began to swing the club, breaking up ice near the bank. Soon he had cleared a spot six feet in diameter.

Then the old man hurled the club up to the bank behind him and strode into the open water. Snug and warm in his blanket, Pedro gasped as the icy water rose above the old man's bony knees. He watched Old Sore scoop up the broken pieces of ice in his bare hands, toss them up on the bank behind him, and then sit down in the river as the water rose to his chin.

"Ahh-woooooooooooo!" His bull-like roar reverberated off the nearby bluffs. He completed his skin-tingling toilet by entirely submerging his head. On the bank, Pedro felt his own blood congealing.

Slowly Old Sore came up out of the water, first the top of his head showing, then his eyes, then his nose. Small particles of ice crusted his white hair. Old Sore shook his head vigorously, then whipped the sleet out of his shaggy mane with his hands.

Slowly he walked out of the river. He snorted a couple of times to blow the water out of his nose and sat down in the sand. After putting on his moccasins and antelope leg wrappings, he wound himself into his breechclout. Then, folding himself in his robe, he looked expectantly at Pedro.

Pedro did not hesitate. These were going to be the coldest twenty seconds of his life and he wanted to get them over with as fast as possible. He threw off his robe, breechclout, and moccasins, ran shivering to the bank, steeled himself, and jumped. Holding his breath, he lay down in the water and ducked his head, scalplock, braids, and all, beneath the surface.

To his surprise, his skin burned and stung as if the water were boiling hot. He leaped up and fled to the bank. Now he felt no discomfort, only an intense warmth. He brushed the tiny icicles from his body and out of his hair with the flats of his hands, then dressed quickly, astonished at how vibrantly alive he felt. His whole body tingled and he pulsed with energy and well-being.

"That bath will do you good, *español*," Old Sore barked over his shoulder as they rode back to the village. "That bath will get your mind off love potions, courting flutes, and that girl. It will get your mind back onto war and hunting where it belongs. You won't need another bath until next summer."

Summer almost arrived next day, the weather doing a complete turnabout. It started in the morning with the red birds whistling cheerfully from the bare branches of the elms and tall cedars. By noon the thin crust of snow had melted, revealing an occasional dandelion amid green grass. The air became warm and dry. What a peculiar climate exists in these southwest prairies, thought Pedro. The seasons keep intruding on each other.

The next afternoon Pedro walked in the sunshine to the river to fill their empty waterskin. The day was as clear and mild as Málaga in May. As he straightened up with the filled skin in his hand, he breathed his lungs full of the intoxicating air. Across the river he saw the spherical crowns of the sage, the color of which always blended so beautifully with the landscape, no matter what the season. Just now the sage was gray and brown. God's ways of adorning his world were beyond all human understanding.

While he stood there, he heard a woman calling from the nearby brush. Her voice was low, as if she feared someone might hear her. There was no mistaking the urgency in her tones.

It was Cedar, half hidden in a small thicket of sumac. She held a bundle in her arms. Her face was haggard and worn, her body thin, her hair scraggly. She smelled of burned sage.

"Take it!" she cried, and thrust her bundle toward Pedro. Her voice was hoarse with fear. "If he finds out it's a girl, he will kill it. He's hunting for us now." She kept looking behind her as if expecting to see Belt Whip.

Pedro found himself holding something small and warm and wrapped in rabbit skins. The mother backed reluctantly away. "Give it away to someone," she implored. "She's only a few hours old. Twin girls were born. Belt Whip wanted a boy. If he finds out there were two girls, he will try to kill both. But if I

give one away and don't tell him there were two, he might accept one." She threw another look of terror over her shoulder.
"Don't give it to any of Creek Water's wives. One of them is
related to Belt Whip. She might tell him."

A soft cooing came from the tiny parcel in Pedro's arms. He
looked down at it wonderingly. When he glanced up, Cedar
was gone.

What beasts some of these Comanche fathers were, wanting
to destroy their own children. Pedro lifted the baby a few
inches. How light it was. A human life depended upon him for
survival. And he knew nothing at all about caring for it. If he
could not give it to Creek Water's wives, what woman could he
trust?

His thoughts flashed back to that first afternoon on the
Quitaque when an Indian girl had comforted the newly
orphaned white children as gently as any white mother who
ever lived. Willow Girl would know what to do. If only he
could manage to see her alone.

Desperate, he hurried through the brush along the river.
From a thicket of tamarisk near her father's tipi, he peered
out. Blue smoke drifted from the top of the lodge but there was
no one in sight and he could hear no voices.

A scraping noise came from the river bank ahead, and there
he saw Willow Girl's brother Long Hungry whittling a stick of
mulberry. Pedro hid the baby beneath a clump of sage and
walked up behind him.

"Good afternoon, brother. Where's your sister?"

Long Hungry, busy with his whittling and weary of being
questioned by all his sisters' suitors as to her whereabouts, did
not even look up. "She's gone with the other women hunting
for honey."

"In what direction did they go?"

"That way, brother." Long Hungry pointed to a trail leading into the woods at his right and went on whittling. Before he

left, Pedro carefully studied Willow Girl's moccasined footprint in the sand before her tipi, memorizing every detail.

When he went back for the baby, he was alarmed to find that all the sage clumps looked alike. He was not at all sure which one concealed the baby. To his relief he heard a weak wail come from the same vicinity where a dog was sniffing about. He drove off the dog and found the rabbitskin bundle, picked it up, and began to walk. The baby stopped crying immediately.

He had no trouble following the women's trail. Of all the skills Old Sore had taught him, Pedro liked trailing the best. At a fast walk he followed the women's tracks. The trail could not have been easier to trace if they had scattered confetti along the route. Other trails occasionally cut across it but Pedro was not diverted. The women's moccasins had long fringes along the heel seams that left small brushmarks in the sand. Also he found marks left by people resting with both their legs and feet tucked nearly to one side under them. When men rested, they crossed their feet.

Pedro carried the baby carefully. "Holiest Virgin," he prayed, "with all my heart I venerate thee above all the angels and saints in paradise. Turn then, most gracious Advocate, thine eyes of mercy toward this child. Keep it alive that it may be made worthy of all the promises of Christ."

At a small stream, Pedro put down the baby and knelt to drink. The air was sweet under the trees. As he scooped the water into his mouth, he heard a series of queer, suckling noises that seemed to come from directly over his head. He peered above him into the recesses of a dogwood and gasped at what he saw.

Five cradleboards, ornamented with beads, were lashed to the tree limbs. A Comanche baby was tucked snugly and warmly in each. The cradleboards swung slowly in the wind. The babies, staring and blinking at one another, seemed per-

fectly content. Their Comanche mothers were not in sight but
Pedro knew they must be nearby.

As he stepped closer, one by one the babies caught sight of
him and began to cry. Instantly their mothers came crashing
through the underbrush,

Snatching up Cedar's infant, and hidden by the bushes, he
managed to avoid the squaws. After he had put considerable
distance between himself and the Indian women, he heard
ahead the familiar jingle of the tiny bells that Willow Girl had
sewn to her moccasins. When his nostrils caught her sweet
scent he knew she was directly upwind and close by.

Then he saw her. She was standing in a patch of tamarisk,
looking anxiously in the direction her companions had run.
She wore a tight-fitting deerskin that had a certain elegance in
spite of the fact that its sleeve fringes were worn thin and some
beads were missing from the design on front. A red blanket
hung loosely over her shoulders.

Her mother was not with her.

Surprise and fear came into Willow Girl's face when she saw
Pedro walking toward her with the bundle in his arms. She
turned as though to flee and Pedro remembered what Old Sore
had once told him about Cheyenne women being the most
chaste of all the Indian women on the plains. Whether married
or single, they never permitted themselves to be found alone by
a man. Because of the disturbance at the creekside, Willow
Girl had nobody with her now. Apparently, her mother had
gone with the other squaws.

"Wait," Pedro pleaded, "I have to talk to you a moment. I
have to talk to you about what I am holding here." He nodded
toward the bundle in his arms and stood still, to avoid frightening her away.

Still poised to run, Willow Girl looked at him distrustfully.
Then, as Pedro came no closer, her look of panic disappeared.
Proudly she lifted her chin.

"Why do you keep following me?" she demanded. "You know that a young woman may not be seen talking to a young man without losing her reputation."

"A human life is at stake," Pedro said quickly. "You are the only person I can go to for help." As he looked into her ginger-brown eyes, he realized that he was deeply and irretrievably in love with her. Creek Water's ultimatum had nothing to do with it.

At that moment a tiny mewing cry came from the rabbitskin in Pedro's arms.

Willow Girl forgot about flight or reputation. Gasping, she dropped her blanket and looked at the bundle, her face aglow with such tenderness and compassion that Pedro's heart thrummed liked a plucked guitar string. With a cry of pleasure, she came closer and flipped the blanket from the baby's face.

The infant peered up at them helplessly, blinking its black eyes in the sunlight. Then it began to cry and Willow Girl talked to it, her low, consoling voice mingling oddly with the tiny wailing. Pedro told her how Cedar had given him the baby and why she feared for its life.

Willow Girl took the baby from him. Her hand brushed against his as she made the exchange and Pedro felt a shock of pleasure.

Gently she began to rock the baby in her arms, humming as she did. Yet it was not exactly humming, Pedro thought. Rather it was a strange soothing sound, like the soughing of the south wind through the sage. Pedro marveled as the baby instantly hushed.

"The baby must be suckled quickly or it will die," he said. "What will you do?"

She looked at him pityingly. "Men know very little of these things. A baby isn't allowed to nurse its own mother until four days after birth. It takes that long for the medicine woman to free the mother's breast from harmful secretions. During that time, the mother is given doses of the milk medicine to induce a free flow of milk. I will ask some other woman who has a child to nurse it until I can find a home for it. There are five such women in our party here."

Pedro blushed, remembering the five papoose boards swinging in the breeze back at the creek. He told her about disturbing them and she laughed.

"They probably thought you were a bear." Still lightly rocking the infant she confessed, "I always wanted a child myself." The Comanche syllables, sonorous and flowing, rolled beautifully off her tongue.

Pedro watched her a moment. Then he said quietly, "I'm sorry I went with your brother into your tipi. I did not know it was not allowed. I haven't learned all your customs. It was a nice tipi, much the nicest I've ever seen since your people captured me years ago."

She looked at him strangely, but Pedro hurried on. As he talked, he felt surer of himself. This might be the last chance he would have to talk to her. He must make as much of it as he could. "I don't like some Comanche customs. I don't like the one that keeps me from seeing you oftener. I like you very much. I want to marry you. I want it more than I ever wanted anything in my life."

She cuddled the baby closer, staring at him curiously.

"Comanche girls are not promised to young men who have not been to war," she informed him. "My people do not consider a young man grown until he has taken an enemy scalp in battle or at least stolen horses in a raid."

"I know," he said bitterly. "I have no ponies to give your father. In my country, we do not buy our wives like vegetables in the marketplace. When a young man finds the girl he loves, he goes with his parents to visit her home and to ask her father

and mother for the honor of her hand. After that, they are engaged and permitted to speak to each other daily for a time.
The girl sits behind the iron railing of her window and the boy
stands outside."

Her chin went up again. "Offering ponies to a girl's father
for her hand is a great honor for the girl. If a young man risks
his life to steal horses so that he can offer them as her price, it
shows how much he values her."

Thoughtfully, Pedro brushed a gnat off his wrist. He had to
acknowledge that if he were a young man with horses he had
captured at great risk, he could think of no finer way of spend-
ing them than to offer them for this girl's hand. He would not
dream of offering them for a young woman who was not chaste
or competent.

But he had no respect for the obstacles that were put in a
young man's way. "And what's the good of standing outside
her tipi half the night blowing a flute that plays only two
notes?" he scoffed. "Even the dogs dislike it and bark at it."

Willow Girl's brown eyes flashed. "It's the sweetest music in
the world to a girl. Sometimes that flute music is the only kindness she ever gets from a husband."

Pedro looked at her with new respect. This girl knew the
hard facts about Comanche marriage. Judging from what he
had seen and heard about the subject, she was right. And yet
he could not imagine any husband mistreating a girl as lovely
as this.

He acknowledged that his great mistake was trying to woo
her in her own country by applying his Spanish courting code.
If he was going to win her against such enormous odds, it
would have to be done the Comanche way, with stolen ponies
and a battle reputation. But there was not time for that.

Carefully she shifted the baby to her other shoulder, and at
the same time she gave Pedro a searching look. "Where did
you live before we captured you?" A cautious hostility crept

into her voice. "Do your horsemen carry long knives on their rifles and wear blue coats? Are their skins white?"

Pedro shook his head. With quiet pride he explained that he belonged to the Spanish nobility, that his nation lay two months' sailing distance over a wide ocean, and that Spain had no blue-coated cavalry.

She seemed satisfied. "When I was a little girl, the Blue Coats massacred us," she said. "My aunt and I were visiting our Cheyenne relatives at Sand Creek. The head men of the Blue Coats invited us to bring our families under the protection of the fort. There were five hundred of us, mostly women and children, under Black Kettle. The white commander even gave Black Kettle his flag. One morning, the Blue Coats surrounded us and began to shoot us. Black Kettle raised their flag with the stars and the red and white bands on it. He also raised a white flag. They payed no attention to either flag. We ran up the dry bottom of Sand Creek and hid in the hollow banks but they dragged us out and killed us. All manner of outrages were inflicted on our persons. They clubbed the little children with their guns and dashed out their brains. Using their knives, they ripped open the stomachs of our women. My aunt was killed and her stomach cut open but I got away."

Indians aren't the only savages, Pedro thought soberly. No wonder all Indians hate the white soldiers.

With one hand, the girl brushed a strand of hair out of her eyes. Behind her, the wind blew up softly through a clump of willows. The breeze quietly stirred the long, slim leaves and the musty smell of the bark, the leaves and, the water came pleasurably to Pedro's nostrils.

"Thank you for taking the baby," he said, realizing only now how much trouble she would have before she found a mother for the child.

She glanced anxiously toward the creek. "They're coming back. I have to go."

Her face was close and her lips the color of sumac in the fall. Pedro leaned over and kissed her tenderly on the mouth. Wide-eyed and beautiful, she looked at him.

He tried to kiss her again but she pushed him away, holding the baby in one arm. He who could have had his choice of any number of girls in Spain realized that this dark Comanche beauty would be no easy conquest. He could not even tell whether she liked him.

"Wait for me," he pleaded. "I'll go to war. I'll steal the horses. But it will take time." He thought of Creek Water's ultimatum.

Buckskin skirt swished softly as she retreated a step. "My father won't wait. He may decide tomorrow. I don't know what young man he will select. If I refuse the one he chooses, I could be killed. Any father has a legal right to kill a daughter who won't accept the husband he chooses for her."

Pedro flushed. "I think I could kill any man who got you and was not your choice. I think I could kill him even if he was your choice. I don't think I could bear to see you married to anybody else."

Willow Girl stared at him with wonder.

Voices sounded from the creek. The squaws were returning. Willow Girl stooped to pick up her blanket, and still carrying the baby, ran toward them. She did not look back.

Pedro watched her vanish into the brush, listening to the jinglets on her moccasins sounding fainter until finally he could hear them no more. The sun seemed less brilliant, the willows uglier, and the afternoon insufferably dull.

He expelled his breath in a low whistle of disappointment. He was so much in love with her that he had almost promised to revert to savagery if she would wait for him.

But she couldn't wait.

Bitterly he swung back toward the village.

13 · The Marriage

"I hear that Wallowing Bear will choose Willow Girl's husband tomorrow," Coby warned that night. "Whatever you are going to do, you had better do fast." He had stopped by on his way home from hunting. The carcass of a freshly killed blacktail deer hung across his horse. There was still dried blood on his hands from dressing it.

Pedro felt a chill settling around his heart. The girl had been right when she had told him in the tamarisk thicket that her father would not wait.

"Thank you, brother," he mumbled.

Coby's wide brow wrinkled pensively and his face looked more lonely than ever. "What are you going to do?"

Pedro shook his head. He did not know what he was going to do. Coby sat looking down on him a moment, then rode slowly off, the eagle feather in his scalplock dangling dejectedly.

Next morning Pedro arose early and began to wipe the dried mud and scurf from his mule with double handfuls of gramma grass. His hands shook as he worked. He tried to plan ahead. If he succeeded in winning the girl, they would need a place to live. He had a tipi, although Old Sore shared it. There would be no trouble providing food and clothing. He had found hunting so fascinating that he was now killing most of the meat for Creek Water's household. Kildee had told him that the girl's family was not obliged to furnish any housekeeping necessities but they would make out somehow. The most important thing was to win the bride.

Coby rode up on his cream warhorse. As he watched Pedro doggedly groom the mule, he tugged at his scalplock.

"Brother, I don't think you ought to count on getting that girl. I don't think her father will let you have her. Everybody is after her. Most of them have warrior reputations. They have all got a better bride price to give than you. All you have to give is that mule."

Pedro looked somber and went on with the grooming. He tried to think clearly, but his emotions kept interfering. He could not abide the thought of her marrying anybody else. He realized Coby was probably right. But he had to keep on trying no matter how poor his chances seemed.

Coby slid off the cream, reached down for a double handful of grass, and began to help Pedro clean the mule. The mule looked around at Coby with hostility, one long ear cocked forward, the other toward the rear. He began to quiver all over and lifted one hind foot, as if resenting Coby's low opinion of him. Coby moved out of range, and walking around to the front, began to work on him there.

"Brother," he told Pedro, "last night I prayed to my Guardian Spirits about this. I asked if they would help us."

Pedro went on rubbing. All he could think of was how smoky black Willow Girl's hair had shone yesterday in the sunlight filtering through the trees.

Coby's resonant voice grew quieter and more confidential. "Later in the night, after the moon was down, my Guardian Spirits replied to me in a dream. They said that conditions for achieving this were not good now but that they might be good later. They said I could tell you about this. But you must never reveal it to anybody or the *nenapi* will not like it."

Pedro lifted the mule's right hind foot and began to scratch the mud off it with a twig. Politely, he asked, "Who are the *nenapi,* brother?"

Coby leaned closer, his voice sinking to an awed whisper.

"They are the little men. They stand only a foot tall but they have great power. Their shields are no bigger than a leaf and they carry little bows and arrows. Their lances are so small that the points of them look no bigger than cactus spines. But they are sure killers, these *nenapi!* They kill every time they shoot. Their medicine is so powerful that it's dangerous. A man might kill somebody he does not want to kill. I always ask them to help me before I go into battle. This is the first time I have ever asked their help for any other reason."

Pedro was moved. Coby wanted to share his power with him and had disclosed its source. He knew that the source of a man's medicine was a life-and-death secret. It could be revealed only with the power's consent.

Pedro said, "Thank you, brother, for helping me with your power." But his mind was not on what Coby had told him. This was the day he might lose his love forever. He would know in a few short hours.

As he leaned against the mule and watched Coby ride off he felt fear twisting his insides again. The only thing that might be in his favor was the opinion of the girl herself. Coby had said that it was always best to win the love of the girl, if possible. It seemed to him that he had made a start in that direction, but how could he be sure?

Nervously, he glanced at the sun. It was time to get himself ready. Inside the tipi, he began to comb his hair and put on his paint. He had adorned both cheeks before he noticed that he was splashing on Old Sore's red instead of the purple he had planned for himself. Angrily, he began to scrape it off.

Halfway to Wallowing Bear's lodge, Pedro saw Two-in-a-Blanket going in the same direction. A flood of jealousy swept through him. The dandy was escorting a spread of twelve immaculately groomed pintos, riding the lead animal himself. Their tails were braided. All of them had bits of blue cloth tied in their carefully combed manes. They were surefooted, clear-eyed, and easy-gaited. Pedro felt a flash of foreboding when he saw them. How could he compete against a gift like this?

Two-in-a-Blanket looked as flawlessly groomed as his animals. Daubed all over his brown body from his waist to his chin were innumerable small circles of olive green. He was as colorfully speckled as a trout.

When he saw Pedro leading his mule, Two-in-a-Blanket covered his mouth with his hand in amusement. He turned away to draw his yucca brush through his glossy hair. He kept tossing his long black braids over his shoulder with sudden twists of his head. To Pedro, the gesture seemed almost a sneer.

They arrived together at Wallowing Bear's lodge. Two-in-a-Blanket slid off the front horse, hobbled them all, and disengaged a cocklebur from the tail of one of the animals. As he moved about, he was careful to keep the embroidered buckskin flaps that trailed a foot behind his moccasins from dragging in the dusty grass.

Pedro staked out his mule and sat down several feet away from his rival. Other suitors appeared. After hobbling their strings of ponies near the lodge entrance, they squatted unsociably on the grass. None of them spoke.

Now Wallowing Bear, the Yamparika father of the girl, came out of his tipi. He wore a blue blanket about his shoulders. Walking slowly among the horses, he examined their hocks, looked into their mouths, picked up their feet. He reminded Pedro of a shopkeeper thumping and smelling the wares of several peddlers before deciding what basket of melons he wished to buy. Pedro's mule, however, he ignored completely.

Hoofbeats sounded from the adjacent river valley, and there was a smell of dust in the air. A great splashing came from the river, accompanied by a multiple snorting, stamping, nickering, and tail swishing. Pedro turned to watch, amazed at the great number of horses filling the river and swarming over both banks. Somebody must be moving a herd to a new grazing area.

He had never seen such a variety of colors. There were sorrels, creams, iron grays, buckskins, bays. Clean-limbed and nervous, these horses had small feet, delicate limbs, and wicked eyes. Their manes tumbled, wild and unruly, down over their sharp noses and high nostrils. Their long tails dragged in the shallows of the river or swept the sandy ground. Obviously, they were newly captured from some wild herd and freshly subdued.

Then their hoofbeats slowed and they milled gently about as the many Indian herdsmen riding on both flanks stopped them, skillfully holding them. Restless and suspicious, the splendid animals raised and lowered their heads, wiggled their ears, and looked about them with mingled curiosity and fright. Some grazed briefly, moving from grass clump to grass clump. Others bumped into each other and reared, whistling shrilly and clicking their teeth belligerently. But why had they stopped?

A travois, drawn by a big, shaggy-maned piebald, pulled into view. The butt ends of its two supporting poles dragged heavily in the sand. Pedro stared at it. Crimson stripes had been painted down the piebald's withers; gaudy fragments of red flannel and calico streamed from the cedar shafts.

In the travois sat an extraordinarily large, fat man. He weighted down the vehicle so heavily that when it ascended the river bank his broad buttocks left a smooth, double furrow in the sand. His cold, acquisitive little eyes darted about him as though he enjoyed the furore he was causing. Then Pedro recognized him.

It was Paunch, the wealthy chief who had beaten the woman so brutally the day he and Creek Water had gone to the hunting dance. Paunch, the Comanche Midas who owned nearly two thousand horses but was so fat himself that he could not ride a single one.

The strange rig stopped in front of Wallowing Bear's tipi. Paunch lifted one fleshy, brown leg over the nearest travois pole and rolled out, bending the pole almost to the breaking point. Then he scrambled to his feet. His huge leggings, large as hogsheads, were ornamented with beads and glass, and he wore a headpiece of brightly colored plumes.

Quickly, as if trying to conceal his obesity, he wrapped himself in a black bearskin robe. Wallowing Bear came out and embraced Paunch, then escorted him inside his lodge. The portly chief had difficulty in wedging his body through the entrance flap.

Two-in-a-Blanket dropped his yucca brush.

"Brothers, that's it," he mumbled through stiff lips. Moving with leaden feet among his pintos, he began taking off their hobbles.

Wallowing Bear came out of the lodge alone. Pedro watched him. Wallowing Bear first helped Two-in-a-Blanket untie the rest of his pintos. The favorite had been rejected first.

Then Wallowing Bear began to liberate the clusters of animals offered by the other suitors. But he went nowhere near Pedro's mule. Deep inside Pedro, a spark of hope began to glow. He smothered it ruthlessly, determined not to look forward to a prize he could not win. He watched Wallowing Bear free additional horses while the mule grazed on, undisturbed, stretching its rope tether taut as it pushed out its lips for the nearby shrubbery.

Still afraid to hope, Pedro marveled at the miracle unfolding before him. As Wallowing Bear continued to release gift horses, the little prickle of fire inside Pedro crackled into flame, lighting his expectations. Pedro still tried to smudge it out, refusing to let himself believe what he saw. As he continued staring and the proof persisted, the flame within him flared into a mighty conflagration. A wild triumphant roaring sounded in his ears.

Only when the Yamparika chief cut the hobbles on the last of the gift horses, a pair of buckskin mares owned by a Tenawa with a single black feather in his scalplock, did Pedro stop fighting himself. His heart gave an exultant leap. He thanked the Holy Mother for the astonishing gift.

Wallowing Bear halted at his tipi door, seeming to see the mule and its stake rope for the first time. Grunting, he reached inside his blue blanket. A knife flashed in his hand. Pedro felt a cold, chilling breeze blow through him.

Wallowing Bear ambled laboriously toward Pedro's mule. Like all dismounted Comanches, he looked slovenly and clumsy on the ground. When he reached the mule he grasped the stake rope with his left hand and slashed upright with his right. The rope fell in two strands, cleanly severed.

The defeated suitors arose, one by one, preparing to go. Stunned, they walked like wooden men.

"The chiefs always take the youngest and prettiest ones and leave nothing for us except the hags," one complained.

"That's right," said another. "When I finally get married my wife will be so old that people will think I'm leading my grandmother around."

"Paunch desires her now," snorted the Tenawa. "But he would gladly trade her and all his other wives for the Tafoya herd. That's what he really wants."

Two-in-a-Blanket stood, listening to the celebration in Wallowing Bear's tipi. "I gave that chattering brother of hers six ponies," he mused. He drew a long breath and slowly expelled it. "I know where I can steal that many more tomorrow night."

They all moved off. Bitterly he watched the girl's male relatives dividing up the horses Paunch had brought from his massive herd. Already Wallowing Bear had begun to give so many to this uncle, so many to that nephew and cousin. The men were laughing and exulting over the plenitude of the animals to be distributed. Inside the tipi Pedro could hear the women gossiping as they served food for the wedding feast to which Paunch's relatives had also been invited.

But Pedro would not leave. He sat on the grass, waiting.

Soon he heard the sound he had been listening for, a small jingle of tinkle bells. Willow Girl came slowly out of her father's lodge. In her bridal dress of deerskin she was lovely beyond all belief. Medallions of blue-and-yellow beads were sewn geometrically across the front of her blouse. At her waist clusters of round beads sparkled in the sunshine. A luxurious fringe lined the hem of her skirt. Her moccasins and leggings were highly ornamented. She looked resigned, dispirited, and lonely.

Paunch came out of the tipi, too, and behind him Wallowing Bear and all the relatives on both sides. Their gay chatter filled the air. Willow Girl's mother stood near her, trying to cheer her, but the girl turned away, staring into the distance of sand and sage.

Other maidens, friends of Willow Girl, had walked up to see the leavetaking. They looked at her enviously, for Paunch was the richest man on the prairies. Pedro stared at them. Compared to her, the other girls looked like grimy, stiffly moving puppets. But they were free and she was not.

Paunch grunted a command, waddled to his travois, and clambered aboard, ignoring the girl. A gray pony had been provided for his bride. Willow Girl mounted the pony that would take her away from her home tipi forever. Paunch picked up the long jaw rope and the piebald moved off, the ends of the Travois pole dragging noiselessly through the white river sand. The girl followed on the pony, head down, like a captive.

Rage slashed through Pedro. Twice this girl's age and already with three wives! Why did he need a fourth? Paunch's travois passed so closely that Pedro could see the sensuous curve of the fat chief's mouth and smell the greasy texture of his skin. His glance shifted to the girl.

Tense and rigid, she stared straight ahead until she drew even with him. Then she gave Pedro a look of such tenderness and despair that for a moment he nearly lost his reason.

Her own people had sold her and deserted her. In her heart-sickness she was reaching out to him.

With a gall-swallowing effort he controlled himself and let her ride past without raising his hand. There was nothing he could do. She was married to Paunch.

He picked up the mule's tether and began walking back to camp.

All day long Pedro was tormented by sweet memories of Willow Girl. The sibilance of her speech, the curious graceful-ness of her walk, her fresh leaf odor. The whisper of her feet as she carried Cedar's baby and ran from him in the tamarisk to join the squaws.

Pedro knew that remembering was senseless. Love was an aching heart, an arrow through the guts. He thought of the legend about Cupid, the beautiful winged boy, sharpening his arrows on a grindstone he had wet with the blood from the hearts of his victims. Pedro had smiled at the legend as a boy but he understood it now as a man.

Coby stayed with him all afternoon. Just before evening they took a walk together upon the prairie. Pedro's mind was in ferment.

"Brother, you need to go out with a war party," Coby said to him. "That might make you forget your troubles."

Pedro waited until his friend left him. Then he packed a small parfleche with dried meat and left the village. His fury drove him almost at a trot. He had to liberate the girl at once.

His knife would find an artery somewhere in that huge mountain of suet and then, riding double on the mule, he and the girl would travel by night and hide by day, heading north-east until they found the Cheyennes, her mother's people. He doubted if the Comanches would look so soon for them there.

On foot, he led the mule in a circuitous route until he came in view of the largest of Paunch's tipis. He had just staked out the mule in the dark when he felt a firm hand on his wrist. A familiar voice spoke at his elbow.

"Brother, killing him is no good. You would be killed in turn by his relatives and it would be a legal act. I could not help you. Creek Water could not help you. Not only would you cast a lifetime stigma on the girl but after they found and killed you, one of Paunch's brothers would get her. That's the law. A woman losing her husband by death is inherited by a brother of her husband. You would not get her. You would only dishonor her and lose your own life."

Pedro tried to pull away but Coby restrained him, talking quietly and persuasively. Finally Pedro stopped struggling. With one last look at Paunch's tipi, he gave up. Sobs shook him. He covered his face with his hands.

Coby took him home, leading the mule. Inside the lodge, Pedro sat on the floor, his back to the door. Coby quietly left.

Pedro flung himself on his robe, burying his head in his arms. For the first time in months he wished for his guitar. A *copla* kept running through his mind:

I do not wish you further hurt.
No greater hurt could be,
Than lying beside another man
When still you think of me.

He thought of escape, the goal toward which he had worked so hard until he fell in love with Willow Girl. He had lost all interest in escape. He had excluded everything from his mind except the necessity of winning her. Now that he had lost her, an emotional fatigue drained his energy. He did not know what he wanted to do.

And then, he recalled that the spring moon was now only two short months away. Unless he took a wife of his own choosing, Creek Water would select one for him.

Pedro turned on his back, staring bitterly at the little patch of stars visible through the smokehole in the top of the tipi. Time, like a horse galloping downhill, was closing in upon him.

14 · War Trail Reunion

Pedro rode ahead, scanning the green flatness on all sides for movement. His heart was sore and his belly empty but he endured silently as Old Sore had taught him, never murmuring or complaining. He could hear the arrows moving and settling in the quiver behind his shoulder and feel the bow and shield slung along his back. It was strange to be going to war against an enemy he had never seen.

Beneath the mule's plodding hooves, small bunches of new gramma grass sprouted amid the tall brown tufts of last year. Masses of tiny blue-and-yellow flowers with striped petals grew close to the earth. Pedro was saddened by the brevity of their lives. He knew that they sometimes appeared before the last late snowfall and would die before the coming of the hot spring winds.

He rode the big mule and led the yellow warhorse that Creek Water had given him for the expedition. The spirited animal moved at a light trot, its long hip muscles rippling beautifully. A thick black mane tumbled in wild profusion over its face and neck. Its long black tail swept the ground. It was tethered to the mule by a grass rope.

"My son, I will give you a trained horse to ride into battle against our enemies," Creek Water had told him. "But you must respect him. You must never ride him except in battle. I will give you a strong mule to ride on the trail and a second horse to rest the mule. But never ride the yellow horse until the fighting starts."

The war party advanced slowly, grazing their horses at every opportunity, so they would have the strength to run strongly coming back.

Coby trotted quietly at Pedro's side. He wore a black buffalo robe thrown carelessly over his shoulders like a cape. It always appeared to be falling off. He too rode a mule and led his cream-colored warhorse. His friendship for Pedro was like the affection of one brother for another. When Pedro spoke to him, Coby's lonely face lit up with pleasure but to all others he seemed gloomy and reserved. In camp he always sat apart, his body still as the stones, allowing only his eyes to wander about.

They kept passing buffalo skulls on the prairie. Coby would ride up to them, and bending far off his mule without dismounting, turn the skulls until they faced back toward the home camp.

"Why do you do that?" asked Pedro.

"My Guardian Spirit will send the herds in the direction the skulls are pointing," Coby explained. "Then our people will have good hunting while we're gone."

"Did you ever see a spirit, brother?"

"Yes. In visions. Evil spirits have no pity. I am afraid of them. In daytime I do not like to go into my lodge alone. If I come home, I call to my wife. If she is not there, I sit outside until she comes. I do not fear any man if he is alive and can move. But spirits are different."

Pedro could not help being secretly amused at Coby's belief in the supernatural. Coby always wore little amulets on his arms or tied charms in his hair to ward off this or that. When Pedro made a remark about the little wildflowers passing beneath their mules' hooves, Coby turned his melancholy eyes full upon him.

"Don't ever pick them," he warned. "The Great Spirit put them there for the little men."

The party was accompanied over much of its route by large flocks of what Coby called buffalo birds. These birds seemed unafraid of the horses and mules, lighting on the grass immediately in front of them or perching composedly on the animals' heads and ears and scrutinizing the grass on all sides for insects kicked up by the horses. Pedro was amused at their antics as they caught grasshoppers flushed out of the grass by the caravan. They would somersault in the air and throw themselves about in the most comical manner while trying to seize the flying hoppers in their bills. Coby told Pedro that these birds were very useful in destroying insects which would have annoyed the horses.

The warriors talked very little as they rode, giving Pedro opportunity for much thought. Although war parties went out from the village every day, Pedro had never before been permitted to accompany one. He wondered why they let him go this time? Had Coby used his influence to bring it about? Three years earlier Pedro would have greeted with the wildest joy this chance to enlarge his knowledge of Comanche geography in order to hasten the day of his escape. Now he welcomed it for different reasons.

He leaned forward, his eye following the indentations made by the Apache horses. It was a gray, foggy morning which matched his own mood. He had accepted Coby's suggestion that they accompany Horse Whipper's war party on the expedition against the Lipan Apaches who had massacred a small Comanche village, slaughtering the women and children as well as the men. He welcomed the chance to go for he was still trying to forget the loss of Willow Girl and not succeeding at all.

Perhaps a battle would help take his mind off her. Also the spring moon would rise in a few days and he had visions of

Creek Water coming around the corner of the tipi with another revolting female. The longer he delayed that, the better. He was tired, too, of forever being taunted about his want of Comanche blood.

This and his lack of a reputation as a warrior were the reasons he had failed to win Willow Girl. This had wounded his pride and now he was determined to do something about it. Since war honors constituted the principal basis of social prestige among these people, the quicker he tried himself in battle, the better.

He slapped the end of the grass rope resolutely across the mule's flank. The Comanches called themselves the Snakes. The term had first been applied by a Comanche chief leading his band across the mountains to a better hunting ground. His followers became dissatisfied with the cold climate and could not be persuaded to go on. The chief, in disgust, likened them to a snake backing up in its tracks. But their courage in battle was boundless.

Pedro had never seen or heard of people who loved fighting as well as the Comanches. Old Sore had told him the tribe got its name from their enemies the Utes, who called them and the sprawling domain they occupied the "Komantcia." In Ute that meant "enemy," or translated more fully, "anyone who wants to fight me all the time."

Pedro had now lived long enough among them to know that they believed war the noblest pursuit of all. Everyone in the tribe—men, women, and children—heaped adulation on successful warriors. And a man killed in battle was similarly regarded. In fact, many warriors openly risked death with a spectacular act of bravery against the enemy.

The more Pedro pondered this, the less he understood it. In his mind's eye he could still see Old Sore standing in the sage as they were getting ready to ride off, his bony face ablaze with passion. With a poignant gesture of helplessness, the old man had thrust up his long, shriveled arms and his clawlike hands. "I wish I were going with you but I am too old. It is awful to be old, *español!* Nobody remembers your war deeds. Your name dies but you live on. You cannot fight or hunt. Your teeth fall out and you cannot enjoy your food. In winter, you sit on the cold side of the tipi wearing discarded lodge skins for clothing. You grow so feeble and worn out and useless that nobody cares about you and finally your own children leave you on the prairie for the wolves to devour. Death in battle saves a man the miseries of old age. Fight hard, *español!* Don't think of dying; think only of killing. A brave man dies young."

As he steered the mule around a swale, Pedro remembered what Creek Water had told him just before the war party left. "I shall not grieve if you are killed in battle. That is what makes a man, to fight and to be brave. I should be sorry to see you die from sickness. If you are killed, I would rather you die in the open air, so that the birds will eat your flesh and the wind will breathe on you and blow over your bones. It is better to be killed in the open air than to be smothered in the earth. Love your friend and never desert him. If you see him surrounded by the enemy, do not run away. Go to him and if you cannot save him, be killed with him and let your bones lie side by side."

It was all part of a philosophy Cedar had once expressed. Pedro had asked her why Belt Whip's son was seldom punished or scolded or made to do any labor about the camp.

"Because he is going to be a warrior and he may die young in battle," Cedar answered. It seemed to Pedro a stupid explanation. Pedro could not accept that part of the Comanche philosophy even if Creek Water, Old Sore, and the whole nation believed it. Why be born just to die again, like the little flowers that hugged the earth in early spring? It was far better to distinguish oneself in war and live than to die. He aimed to put off death as long as possible.

At the moment, Pedro thought that he was more likely to die of starvation than from a battle wound. They had not eaten for two full days. All other creatures seemed to be eating—birds, rabbits, lizards, ants. That morning he had even seen a deer feeding on the crimson blossoms of a flat Petaya cactus, spreading its lips carefully to avoid the surrounding spines. The sight had made Pedro ravenous. Comanches on the war trail starved themselves relentlessly.

Old Sore had explained why this was best. "If you get an arrow or a lance thrust through the bowels, the bowels will heal quicker if they aren't full of food."

For the hundredth time, Pedro looked into the tannish, greenish distance on all sides, trying to identify every speck and blur as Old Sore had taught him. Now he saw several small, black dots against the endless reaches of prairie on his right. He focused his eyes to evaluate the dots.

Then he rode alongside Horse Whipper, the leader of the raid, and told him what he had seen. Horse Whipper stared into the distance. "Buffalo!" he grunted.

He dispatched Pedro and Two-in-a-Blanket, Pedro's erstwhile rival for Willow Girl's hand, to shoot a buffalo calf or a young cow so they could have fresh meat. Pedro's appetite was so savage that he cared not who his companion was. He changed to his second horse and they galloped off together, riding along the backbone of a small ridge to keep out of sight as long as possible.

As they rode along, Two-in-a-Blanket began to advise Pedro. "Don't kill more meat than your horse can carry. It will just lie on the prairie and rot. Besides, we haven't time to skin more than one animal."

Annoyance spread through Pedro. Just because he had not been born a Comanche everybody assumed he knew nothing. He had already been on one buffalo hunt, killed four bulls, and had been given the fourth roasted tongue at the Buffalo

Tongue Dance afterward. What had Two-in-a-Blanket done to match that?

Two-in-a-Blanket continued to offer his unsolicited counsel. "If a bull starts after you, let your horse have his head. He will carry you to safety."

Pedro kicked his horse in the ribs and spurred ahead, but he could not outrun the dandy's annoying words. Two-in-a-Blanket spoke as if he had taken charge of the hunt and Pedro was his vassal.

"We'll pick out a nice fat cow. Point your horse at the cow you mean to shoot. Then let him go. He'll get you close to the cow. Remember, your horse knows more about hunting buffalo than you do."

Pedro looked at him sharply. "Why don't you do the same as your horse and remain silent? Why don't you stop giving so much advice? Your horse knows lots more about being silent than you do."

Two-in-a-Blanket's reply was quick. "At least he's all mine. I'm riding a horse I captured and trained myself. I did not have to borrow him from my adopted father."

The words galled Pedro. He felt anger billowing in his breast. He had come on this raid to demonstrate that he was somebody and disprove insults such as these.

Striving to control himself, he studied the buffalo through the tops of the spiny yucca that grew along the ridge behind which they were riding. Instead of grazing with their heads down, the buffalo stood in a small circle and seemed disturbed about something.

Two-in-a-Blanket stared curiously too. He had fallen silent as if his feelings had been hurt by Pedro's resentment. As they rode slowly forward, Pedro glanced at him out of the corner of his eye. Two-in-a-Blanket had flattened himself along his horse's back, holding his body immovable, making it blend with the rocks and the landscape.

They stopped behind a small knoll and looked at the buffalo three hundred yards away.

Pedro quickly saw what worried them. Nine bulls, shaggy and gaunt, formed a ring. Their heads were pointed outward. A larger circle of big gray wolves completely surrounded the ring of bulls. Panting, the wolves squatted patiently on their haunches, their pink tongues quivering.

Still keeping their circle roughly intact, the bulls suddenly began to trot toward the southwest. The wolves followed. Neither group seemed in a hurry. Then Pedro saw a small four-legged figure wobbling feebly in the midst of the bulls—a new-born buffalo calf. It apparently had been born so recently that it hardly had enough strength to run. After traveling a short distance, the calf lay down again. Once more the bulls surrounded it protectively and once again the wolves surrounded the bulls. Everytime a wolf came close, the bull nearest him would cock his tail, paw the turf, shake his huge head and let out a menacing bellow.

But where were the buffalo mothers? A grunt at his shoulder gave the answer. Two-in-a-Blanket motioned up a long ravine. There were the cows, grazing. The mother had run away from her offspring, leaving the responsibility to the bulls.

Pedro and Two-in-a-Blanket backed their mounts and rode cautiously around the small herd so as to approach upwind from the cows. Silently Pedro fitted an arrow to his bow, preparing for a rush and a quick kill.

Two-in-a-Blanket grunted and shook his head. "Waterhole ahead," he whispered, leaning toward Pedro. "Let's drive the meat to camp instead of packing it."

He punched his heels in his horse's sides and charged the cows with Pedro close behind. They separated a fat young female from the others, shouted at it, and waved their blankets, herding it into the trail. With Two-in-a-Blanket on one flank and Pedro on the other, the animal was driven at a run.

Ahead, the sun flashed briefly off the surface of a small
stream. When the fat cow neared the running water, Two-in-a-
Blanket shot it neatly, with one well-planted shaft.

Horse Whipper, Coby, and the rest rode up. They all dismounted, drew their knives, and helped with the skinning. The
cow was peeled as quickly as if it had been a squirrel. While
some of the warriors filled their blankets with wood for fuel,
Pedro joined others in a search for several round rocks. They
kindled a fire and heated the rocks in it. Next, they cut the
paunch out of the buffalo, emptied its contents, and turning it
inside out, made a large container of it. They filled it nearly
full of water and suspended it over the fire from four bows
thrust into the ground.

The heated stones were placed in the paunch to heat the
water and replaced frequently to keep it hot. Fresh meat from
the cow was dropped into the boiling water to cook, and was
promptly devoured by the hungry warriors. It was the first time
Pedro had seen Comanches cook without utensils of any kind.

Although he did not join the others in feasting on the raw
meat or the contents of the intestines, the sight of it no longer
spoiled his appetite for the cooked food. He ate until his stomach felt bloated. Like the Comanches, he could now abstain
from eating for several days, then gorge himself, making up
the deficiency in one feast. Usually when they found meat they
had no water or if they found water they had no meat. Today
they had been fortunate to find both.

They had just packed the remainder of the food for the long
trip when one of their scouts rode in, quirting his pony. As he
whirled to a stop in front of Horse Whipper the gravel from
his pony's sliding hooves spattered those nearby. The pony was
panting in deep gulps.

"War party coming this way."

Instantly they sprang on their ponies and spread out in a
single line, weapons ready. Pedro mounted the yellow war-

horse. He saw its ears go back and its muzzle rise as it sighted the approaching invaders. He felt beneath him the stir of its long, smooth muscles. He moved into line and waited.

The strangers rode within a fourth of a league and halted. The afternoon sun flashed off their lances and shields. Their horses were striped with war paint and the riders' faces were painted red. Far more horses than riders comprised their party, which meant they were returning from a raid.

Horse Whipper rode out in front. He raised his hand, palm foremost, and slowly waved it from right to left, meaning, "I do not know you. Who are you?" The strangers replied by making with their hands a motion like the crawling of a snake. In the sign language of the plains this showed they were Comanches too.

The two parties trotted forward and mingled. Controlling their plunging, snorting mounts, the warriors on each side began to converse. The skin of all the strangers shone like copper. Probably tanned by the Mexican sun, thought Pedro.

The chief of the stranger band wore a headdress of buffalo horns. Pedro looked at his face and wondered why the man should look familiar. Then Pedro's eyes dropped to the man's deep chest and gaunt ribs. The man's upper body was lacerated with old scars circled with green tattooed rings. On his stomach was a tattooed green turtle.

Excitement and elation washed through Pedro. He thought of a beloved face he had not seen in nearly four long years, a face he had at times almost forgotten. If his brother still lived, surely he would be riding with this band.

There were forty of the raiders and they were heavily encumbered with horses. As Pedro moved among them, his eyes eagerly searched each face. He thought of Roberto's tender solicitude the last time they had met, of his brother's anguished look when he discovered the scabs and welts on Pedro's body, of his straight young back passing forlornly from view around the corner of a tipi when they parted. Roberto must now be fifteen years old. What would his brother look like now? What were his interests and what were his thoughts?

Pedro pushed his way through the band. He saw bits of calico, an old kettle, a sombrero, a girl's blue hair ribbon lashed to elm saddles or tied onto the packhorses. Obviously the raid had been successful. But where was Roberto? There was one man in the band who could tell him what he wanted to know.

As Pedro turned his horse to find Green Turtle, he thought he saw a familiar figure. A young warrior sitting a lightish bay gelding in the rear of the raiding group was helping to hold the herd of captured horses. Pedro took a swift inventory of the bold face, the wiry brown body, and the yellow feather that hung from the scalplock.

There was no mistaking the proud, stately lift of the young head on the long, thin neck, or the way the black hair curled in wavy ringlets around the scalplock, or the bulge of the protruding lower lip.

Pedro rode closer. "Roberto!"

Roberto recognized him instantly. "*Ner-tá-me*," he exclaimed. It was the Comanche word for "brother." He spoke in a low, deep voice that Pedro had never heard before.

Tears of joy scalded Pedro's eyes. But there was no evidence in his brother's face of an answering emotion, only a distant reserve. Roberto seemed slightly distainful of Pedro's tears.

He turned with a scowl to growl an order to a poor wretched something seated behind him on the bay.

Two small arms, blue with cold, reached around the black buffalo robe Roberto wore as protection against the chill of the early spring winds on the plains. The small, grimy hands were locked desperately around Roberto's middle.

Then Roberto's horse, prancing and curvetting, swung its rump about. Huddled behind Roberto sat a small Mexican boy, not more than eight or nine years of age. His cowed, terror-stricken face was ringed by a mop of black hair that grew like a bramble patch over eyes, ears, and neck. He seemed half-starved; there were scars from a recent beating on his nearly naked body. His bare feet, swollen by cactus punctures, stuck out helplessly on each side of the horse. Pedro could hear the lad's teeth clicking as he suffered in the chilling wind.

"Stop shaking!" Roberto ordered in Spanish. A bullying, arrogant look swept over his handsome face.

"*Sí, sí.*" Locking his jaws, the boy tried to suppress his shuddering.

Pedro's gaze shifted questioningly toward the child, then back to Roberto. With a flash of his old mischievousness, Roberto gestured contemptuously toward the boy.

"I caught him on the Rio Grande," he said, as though he were speaking of some animal. "We've been raiding in northern Mexico." His voice, though it had deepened into the register of a man's, was still soft, musical, and gay. He spoke glibly in Comanche. "I'm going to make a body servant of him."

Pedro stared from Roberto to the frightened child, then back to Roberto. He felt the fear thicken in his belly.

"Where are his parents?"

"Here they are," laughed Roberto. He reached behind him into a buckskin pouch fastened to his elm saddle and pulled out two scalps, hoisting them triumphantly. The scalps were black and glossy. One was that of a man, the other a woman.

The orphaned boy stared at them. Then, as he recognized them, a look of horror spread over his pinched face. Suddenly he seemed to remember where he was. Stealing a fear-crazed look at Roberto, he clenched his lower lip and tried to conceal his feelings.

Pedro sat grimly on his horse, marveling at how speedily his brother had slipped into savagery. He fought off a sudden attack of nausea and looked about him. Temporarily, at least, they were alone.

Pedro slid off the yellow horse and began to pray beneath his breath. "*Santa Maria, Madre de Dios!* I've got to prevent this disaster. If I'm caught, I may be killed or at least lose all the progress I've made with these people the last four years. But dear God, I have to risk it. I have to impress Roberto, return him to his senses."

Straightening resolutely, he looked up at Roberto. "Get down off your horse!" he commanded thickly.

A fleeting look came into Roberto's face, a look faintly tinged with shame and remorse. Slowly he swung off the right side of his pony and stood uncertainly in front of Pedro.

"Get down on your knees!" ordered Pedro as he knelt himself. Roberto did not kneel. Alone on the horse, the captive boy looked on in wonder.

Through lips gone dry, Pedro closed his eyes. "Behold, O Mother of God, a miserable sinner prostrate at thy feet. He does not deserve even a glance of pity from thee. Yet I have learned from my own sinning that thou art the refuge of sinners, the hope of those in despair, the consolation of those who are forsaken. Only thou knowest how to save him. O come to his assistance for the love of Jesus Christ! Deliver him out of this murderous state of mind and divert him back into God's favor. . . ."

Finishing the prayer, Pedro crossed himself devoutly. So did the freezing child on the horse.

Pedro heard a grunt of displeasure behind him. He spun around to find Green Turtle, astride his black horse, looming over him. In his buffalo-horn headdress, the chief of the Nokonis looked sinister and savage. He looked at first one brother, then the other. His eyes caught Pedro's in a merciless glitter.

"He is younger than you, yet already he has killed on the raid and taken horses and a captive. We are going back to the village now so that I can give a feast for him." He looked contemptuously at Pedro. "How many horses and scalps have you taken? What have you ever done?"

His glance swung back to Roberto. "Come, my son! It is time to return to our village so that you can thank the Great Spirit for providing all these things, and so the women can pitch presents at your feet. It's time to think about the victory dance."

Roberto seemed confused and disturbed. He looked once at Pedro, with misgiving and a trace of affection in his expression. Then his attention fastened on Green Turtle and the proud, arrogant look returned. He reached for his pony's jaw rope and mounted in front of the captive boy.

Without a backward glance, he urged his horse alongside that of Green Turtle, and together they rode off northward at the head of the stranger band. The sound of their horses' hoofbeats grew fainter and fainter and the bobbing backs of the riders smaller and smaller. Soon they were mere specks on the landscape that gradually vanished from sight.

Sick with shock and fear, Pedro stared helplessly after them. He had to do something to save Roberto and he had to do it soon.

15 · Coup on the Cuerno Verde

They had no trouble following the trail of the murderers. Brazen and defiant after the bloody deed, the Prairie Apaches had made no effort to complicate the pursuit by dispersing into individual parties.

Despite his preoccupation with the problem of Roberto, Pedro took his turn with the trailers. He had learned the art so thoroughly from Old Sore that already he was the equal of any young man in the party. Leaning off his mule to memorize peculiarities, he unerringly read the killers' trail in the buffalo grass below. He soon perceived that one of their horses had a nicked left front hoof. Pedro grunted with satisfaction. Cross trails were no problem now. That pony would lead them to the assassins' camp as infallibly as though its rider had dropped bits of colored paper all along the way.

Soon Pedro knew almost as much about that Apache pony as he did about the mule he was riding. He knew that it was black, that it had a long bushy tail, that it limped slightly, and that it was very hungry. Some of its black hair had caught in the bushes as it brushed past. Its tail had occasionally dragged in the sand. The depth of the indentation made by its left front foot disclosed the degree of its lameness. Along the way it had nipped at high, dry weeds that Indian horses seldom ate.

He could tell by the extent of the trail that there had been approximately thirty raiders. They had kept their ponies going at a steady run. They had made no stops apparently. The dung of their ponies was widely scattered along the way. He knew that they had suffered no casualties because he found no dried blood on the grass blades, no graves, no wooden wound plugs, no double tracks of a travois hurriedly rigged to transport the sorely wounded.

What to do about Roberto? All Pedro's own personal problems seemed unimportant compared to this greater one of his younger brother's seduction by the Indians. He wished he could think of some way to spirit Roberto out of the Comanche country but he feared that was impossible. For years he had himself been trying to escape from it with no success. Besides, while Roberto traveled north, Pedro was heading southwest. Would he be able to find Roberto when he came back? Would he himself survive the battle and return?

They rode deeper and deeper into the lands controlled by the Apaches, drawing closer and closer to their enemies. Now they traveled in the midst of danger. Horse Whipper doubled the number of his scouts. They ranged half a day ahead, behind, and on each flank.

Pedro strung his bow and looked to his arrows and shield. There was a risk and suspense about this journey that was far more exhilarating than riding through their own country. Every man in the raiding party seemed to feel this, glorying in the challenge of it. Pedro thought it was best epitomized by Ravisher, a tall, gaunt warrior with coffee-brown skin and eyes unblinking as an owl's. That night when they paused to rest, Ravisher, crouching over his small cooking fire, began to sing in an undertone. His gravelly voice was daring and exultant:

Way out here,
On my enemy's ground,
I have cooked my meal.

Early the next morning the scouts came in, reporting strong Apache sign everywhere. Emulating the warriors around him, Pedro courted the favor of the supernaturals by stripping the cover off his shield. He shook loose its ornaments, held it four times toward the earth, then shook it four times toward the sky and slung it over his left arm.

"They are camped just ahead in an elbow-shaped hill called the Cuerno Verde," Khadot, the medicine man, told them. "Better get all your good horses up. There's going to be a battle." Because of his power, he had come along to decide when it was propitious to start the fighting.

Quickly, Horse Whipper established a temporary camp at which they left guards, extra horses, and most of their food. Two-in-a-Blanket reached in his breechclout for his yucca-stalk brush and dragged it through his neatly groomed hair. That one would find time to preen himself even if they were tying him to the torture pole, thought Pedro.

Coby rode alongside Pedro. They had switched to their war-horses, battle-braided their horses' tails, and painted their own faces black. Coby reached into the tubular bag tied at his waist and drew forth the rawhide band he wore to protect his left wrist from the slap of the bowstring. His lonely face seemed to lose some of its solemnity.

"Now don't get nervous and shoot too fast," he warned. "Stay close to me."

Pedro scarcely heard him. His mind was on Green Turtle's band, probably home now. He could see the fire leap up from the dry grass near the scalp pole and hear the rapid beating of the drum and the high, thin wail of the singers. He could see Roberto, his young face flushed with triumph, pirouetting in the scalp dance.

The trail pointed straight at the Apache village half a mile away, with the riding all downhill. No guards had been posted; they rode right up on the village and were close enough to see the women tanning hides over the firepits.

Horse Whipper dug his heels into his pony's flanks and war-whooped shrilly to start them on the charge. The high, sustained scream raised the hair on Pedro's head, startling him almost as much as it must have startled the enemy.

Figures poured out of the lodges like ants out of a burning log. The Apache women and children scuttled up the hill to the protection of the rocks; the men snatched up their weapons. Some ran to their horses tethered behind the lodges.

With Pedro directly behind him, Coby rode straight into their midst. Both the cream and the yellow horse had been trained to obey the pressure of their masters' knees; Coby and Pedro rode without saddle or jaw rope. Several Apaches were caught on the ground. Coby lanced two through the stomach and slid off the back of his horse. Knife in hand, he tore off the scalps of his victims and thrust them into his breechclout. Then, running swiftly along the ground, his lance still in his hand, he made a phenomenal vault astride the cream's back. All this took place in a matter of seconds.

Pedro, waking to the seriousness of the situation, raised his bow. The fleeing Apache who was his target waved a red blanket in the yellow's face, causing it to lunge to one side.

Suddenly Pedro felt his horse falling and his own body soaring through the air. He was thrown so high that for an instant he saw the crossed poles and smoky top of a nearby Apache lodge framed between his flying feet. Then the ground came up roughly to meet him and he felt himself rolling. He crawled to his knees, slightly stunned. The blanket-waving Apache was running toward him, extracting a war ax from his breechclout as he ran. Pedro shook his head, desperately trying to clear it.

A rush of hooves sounded behind him. Too late, the blanket waver tried to ward off the new menace. A Comanche spear, with the force of an eight-hundred-pound pony behind it, gaffed him neatly through the bowels. His scream of agony shocked Pedro into a state of wide-awake alertness. His savior, he discovered, was Ravisher.

Pedro ran several yards to where his yellow warhorse was

slowly getting up, forefeet first. The animal had stepped into a concealed firehole. Pedro mounted. He examined his shield and bow, and found that he had lost half his arrows. Almost at once he was caught up in the battle waging around the body of the man Ravisher had speared.

Rushing toward the fallen Indian were his Apache comrades, their arrows whistling through the air. Pedro knew why they risked so much. If the wounded man lost his scalp, his body would become as worthless as carrion; he would never reach the spirit world.

Despite the lance thrust through his guts, the fallen man still lived. As he lay on his back he shot his arrows up so fast that they were falling point down among the Comanches. Two-in-a-Blanket, his long braids tossing, rode his pinto into a hail of arrows and killed the wounded man with a single lance thrust. However, the Apache counterattack was so furious that Two-in-a-Blanket had to turn back without taking the dead man's scalp. And he lost his horse. Festooned with Apache arrows and screaming with pain, the pinto sat down. Two-in-a-Blanket slid off and ran in zigzag fashion to escape the arrows, his long braids streaming out behind him as though suspended by a supernatural force. When Coby overran him on the cream, Two-in-a-Blanket mounted behind with a single leap and they got away.

In the action that followed, Pedro lost Coby. Both sides were mounted now and riding around in two big circles that revolved in opposite directions, an Apache circle and a Comanche circle. The fighting erupted along the two front arcs, which approached each other but never came together. Thirty yards apart, the rival warriors slid off into the loops around the necks of their horses on the side away from their enemies. They shot their arrows beneath their horses' necks, screaming insults back and forth as their arrows clanked off each other's shields. Occasionally an Apache and a Comanche would burst from the combat and dash toward each other as if determined to clash in personal combat. But each would whirl at the last minute, call his opponent an insulting name, and rejoin his comrades in the revolving ring.

Suddenly a Comanche yell of dismay rang out. The two circles buckled and the warriors began milling. Pedro, riding on the back arc, craned his neck. On the prairie between the two contending forces lay a Comanche, knocked off his horse. Grimacing with pain and obviously weak, he managed to sit up. Blood stained his hands and breechclout. It was Ravisher.

Howling with elation, the Apaches charged to take his scalp, but Coby and Horse Whipper, in a fierce countercharge, drove them off. Then the two Comanches rode one on each side of the wounded man. Stooping low off their running horses, each grasped an arm and hoisted Ravisher onto Horse Whipper's pony, carrying him to safety and saving his soul. But could they save his life? The Apache arrow had penetrated so deep into his abdomen that the feathered end protruded only three inches. He was put on another pony. Then, riding bent over with a comrade helping him to stay on, he was taken toward the temporary camp.

For Pedro, who was riding in the Comanche circle behind Horse Whipper, the fighting went badly. He threw himself on his horse's side and discharged his arrows from beneath its neck, but so many of them sailed wild that he burned with chagrin. Soon he was out of arrows. Then he had the bad luck to drop his shield.

Comanche raiders never fought a battle to the death unless attacking a very small party, so Pedro knew that the fighting was nearly over. The Comanches preferred to strike when the enemy was not expecting it, obtain hair for the scalp dance, and run for home. This raid had accomplished its purpose. At any moment Horse Whipper would turn them back and Pedro's only trophy would be a bruised shoulder suffered from falling off his horse. Alas for his dreams!

Then he thought of Roberto. Before he could find his brother and communicate freely with him, he had to become someone the Comanches would look up to, someone who had distinguished himself in war and would therefore be permitted to move freely about the Comanche domain. So far he had done nothing but disgrace himself.

"That's enough, friends! Let's go!" Horse Whipper's stentorian bellow carried above the din. The attackers instantly swerved away from the village and started north. Ahead, Pedro saw two Apaches fleeing from the fighting, riding northward toward the open prairie. The Comanches swung in behind them like hounds after a fox, heeling their mounts and whooping shrilly.

Joining the pursuit, Pedro gave his horse its head. It understood the problem instantly. Its breathing became deep and regular. Pedro could feel beneath him the flexing of the long, supple muscles and the release of enormous power. The wind was sweet in his face and so was the sting of the flying mane. This horse had running pride. Exhilarated, Pedro realized what a great gift Creek Water had given him.

One by one, he passed every Comanche horse in the chase, a claybank, three pintos, a dun, a roan-brown. The envious faces of the riders imprinted themselves upon his memory as he sped by and bore down upon the two Apaches.

Desperately the two men ahead lashed their ponies. The horse nearer to Pedro was panting; the sound was almost like sobbing.

They will both have weapons, thought Pedro. My horse can run all right, but he may be running me right into trouble, perhaps into death. I have no shield, no lance, no arrows. Only my knife.

With pressure from his right knee, he steered his horse to the left until he was in a straight line with both fleeing enemies. Now the front man could not shoot arrows at him without endangering his companion. As for the one in the rear, Pedro watched him carefully, ready to slide over to the side of his horse, out of range, if necessary.

With a rush of relief and elation he saw that the quivers of both Apaches dangled empty. However, the closer of the two brandished an old musket. Pedro, clinging to the right side of the yellow horse, rode squarely across its muzzle. He felt a moment of panic until he suddenly remembered Coby's words: "Always go right in."

Now the Apache pulled the trigger. The musket only snapped. With a howl of rage, the man hurled the gun from him onto the prairie.

As the yellow horse drew abreast, Pedro's knife was in his hand. The Apache imitated the Comanche trick of sliding off on the opposite side of his mount, with only his heel showing on his horse's back. Surprised, Pedro wondered where he had learned that. Now he wouldn't be able to knife him.

Infuriated at his bad fortune, Pedro reached over, grasped the man's heel in both hands, and jerked violently upward. As the Apache tumbled off his horse, he clutched his pony around the neck with both arms, while his body flapped helplessly. For a moment, the man's face was close to Pedro's and Pedro saw the glare of hatred in the fierce eyes. Then the weight of the man's body forced the animal's head down. Lurching and plunging out of control, it passed from sight and Pedro heard the Comanche shout of triumph behind him.

One to go! The remaining Apache, an older, leanly muscled man with long arms, was flogging his mount with his bow and mouthing insults at Pedro as he looked back over his shoulder. Stripes of red paint ornamented his face and he wore what looked like a pair of brass earrings. Pedro felt his face tightening with resolution. He had lost the first enemy. He had only unseated him; others had made the kill. This was his last chance. This one would not get away.

As his horse's head came up to the Apache horse's rump,

Pedro saw that a knife gleamed in the Apache's hand. Pedro crowded the yellow war horse into the enemy pony. The Apache slashed at Pedro with a long, right-handed sweep of the knife but Pedro withdrew his body at precisely the right moment. During that second when his adversary leaned toward him, off balance, he seized the man's elbow and wrist and jerked him headfirst off his horse, intending to disarm and knife him. The Apache fell face downward between the two racing animals and disappeared from sight; the soles of his moccasins shone for an instant in the sunshine.

When he looked back, Pedro saw the man roll heavily in the grass and bound to his feet just in time to receive the Comanche pursuit. Another gloating yell pealed out behind him. Pedro felt a fury of disappointment rise in him. He turned and jogged back, just as Two-in-a-Blanket was stuffing the scalp into his breechclout and wiping his bloodied knife on the grass. The Apache's brass earrings adorned his ears. Six other Comanches stood grouped about the corpse, dejected because the dandy had beaten them to it.

Then a faint shout echoed in the distance. Pedro felt his blood freeze. A long line of Apache warriors, blackening the landscape, rode straight at them on their calico-colored horses, their weapons and decorated shields glistening in the sunlight of late afternoon. Pedro saw that the Comanches had attacked only a small camp. Around the crook of the elbow-shaped hill was a much larger encampment. Fresh warriors poured from it now.

Horse Whipper bawled a warning, his voice so hoarse from warwhooping that Pedro could scarcely distinguish the words. But their meaning was plain. "Let's get away from here fast! That's a big war party!"

The slap of Comanche buttocks hitting their ponies' backs rang out almost as one sound. They headed north, driving the captured ponies before them. With full speed, and unimpeded by captured stock, the pursuing Apaches gained steadily. Closer and closer they came until Pedro could hear the thunder of their horses' hooves. Their shrill yammering gradually grew louder. The noise of their howling suddenly swelled in volume and wrath. Pedro risked a look back over his shoulder to see what had infuriated them.

Through the dust he saw a single Comanche warrior riding bareback on a cream gelding and cutting laterally across their advance, riding from right to left. As he rode, he stuck out his tongue, made mocking faces and taunted them with insolent gesticulations. It was Coby. The purpose of his pantomime was clear. He was obviously trying to goad the Apaches into murderous rage, drawing attention from his fleeing tribesmen until they could get all their horses moving at a dead run.

His cream-colored horse ran as though it were completely wild, its blond mane and tail floating out behind. Coby rode as if welded to his mount. He slapped both hands on the cream's back and with a flirt of his hips and legs, reversed his position so that he faced his pursuers. Pedro shuddered. If Coby fell while doing the trick riding, or was shot off his horse, or scraped off by a tree limb, he would very quickly be the deadest Indian on the plains.

But Coby seemed to know what he was doing. With his back to his horse's head, he let the cream choose its course. Facing his enemies, he taunted them with gestures that belittled everything from their ancestry to their inability to make war. The air rang with their shrieks of rage and the futile twang of their bows as they tried to reach him with their arrows. So nicely had Coby calculated the distance between them that their shafts fell just short.

Then Coby hooked his feet around the cream's neck and lying on his stomach along the animal's back, shot arrow after arrow into his pursuers, lofting his shafts so that his enemies rode into them as they fell, while he was riding away from theirs. Then he sat up, placed his hands on his horse's back, and began to pivot, facing front, then rear, then front, then rear again. He was riding the cream from its ears to its tail.

Finally, he faced front to grasp the cream's flowing mane with one hand and the hair-rope cinch with the other. Like a pendulum his body swung off the right side of his horse, then over the animal's back and off on the animal's left side. On each descent, Coby's feet touched the prairie briefly as though he were running with the animal.

Tiring of his sport, he shifted frontward until he was hunched over the cream's withers like a jockey. In this position, he waved a scornful farewell to his enemies. Farewell it was, too. The Apaches fell farther and farther back until the pounding of their hoofbeats and the yawp of their imprecations grew fainter and fainter, finally receding from hearing and from view.

They rode hard all that night and most of the next day, pausing only a moment at their hideaway camp to change to fresh horses. Ravisher was so weak by this time that Pedro and the others took turns holding him on his horse. His wound had been hurriedly packed with grass to check the bleeding. As the band rushed onward, he called piteously for water but there was no water to give him and no time to stop.

Pedro kept thinking about the battle. At each recollection, a cold feeling of frustration stabbed him afresh. He had come so far to fight so little. His own part in the fighting filled him with disgust and he was awed by the bravery and self-sacrifice of the others. Ravisher, whom he scarcely knew, had saved his life.

When they were helping or protecting each other, these people were capable of the most noble feats. And yet their concept of making war was a strange one. The purpose seemed to be to hit a small group of the enemy with a surprise dash, score quickly, and get away. They fought for glory rather than annihilation or conquest.

Pedro rode slumped on his right buttock and let his mind

weave the details in and out. He had been thrown off his horse, missed every shot with his bow and arrow, dropped his shield, and failed to kill either of the mounted Apaches he had overtaken. He had shamed the friends who sponsored him, and worst of all, bungled his opportunity to help Roberto. At the thought of his brother, Pedro felt fear thicken in him again.

He wished he could get his hands on Green Turtle. He would like to twist the little stone knife in his guts.

Late afternoon of the second day they made camp by a small creek and sent out sentinels in all directions. The thirsty horses, their shoulders and jaws lathered with foam, their flanks heaving in and out, waded noisily into the muddy shallows. There they thrust their muzzles into the water up to their eyes and drank deeply. After Ravisher was helped off his horse, Pedro made three trips to the creek to bring him fresh drinking water in his hands. Then they laid the wounded man on the grass.

There was a buffalo doctor with the band, a quick-moving little man whose wizened face was ribbed with orange stripes that had melted almost together in the hot sun. He inspected Ravisher's wound. His first move was to cut the feathers off the end of the embedded shaft. The Apache arrowhead had been driven so deeply into Ravisher's abdomen that Pedro despaired of their ever getting it out.

Hopping about like a cricket, the buffalo doctor cut a green willow stick, split it open, scraped out the pith, and rounded the ends. While stony-faced warriors sat forcibly on Ravisher's arms and legs and held his shoulders down, the buffalo doctor inserted the stiff willow tube over the end of the Apache shaft and forced it down both sides of the arrow into the wound until it reached and covered the barb. Then the buffalo doctor bound it tightly to the shaft. Ravisher lay absolutely still. He had fainted from pain.

From his medicine bag, the buffalo doctor extracted a bone

rattle. Lying on his back in the grass, he began to shake it and sing to himself. The warriors squatted patiently about, quiet as the surrounding rocks. Pedro fumed at what appeared to be a senseless delay.

Finally, the buffalo doctor got up, grasped the visible end of the shaft with both hands, and pulling steadily with all his strength, withdrew the arrow and its bloody willow sheath. Pedro could hardly bear to watch. He felt as if they had wrenched his own heart out of his body with their bare hands. The wound bled afresh and the buffalo doctor bound it with split cactus leaves which he had heated thoroughly after first burning off their thorns. Ravisher gave one anguished groan and lay still again.

He's dying, thought Pedro.

At the bank of the creek they cut two long willow poles and bored holes in the ends so that sinew could be inserted. The poles were then tied behind a pony to form a travois. A buffalo robe was lashed across the poles, hammock fashion, for Ravisher to ride in.

After they had eaten dried meat from the food parfleches, Horse Whipper walked up to Pedro and embraced him. "This young man did a braver thing in the battle than any of us. I honor him ahead of myself," he announced.

Pedro could only stare at him.

Two-in-a-Blanket untied a shield from his pony. "Brother, I think you dropped this during the battle." And he handed it to Pedro.

Pedro felt a warm glow of gratitude flowing through him. He had dreaded facing Old Sore without his shield.

"Thank you for finding it and saving it for me," he said. But he did not understand what Horse Whipper had said. Was the man blind? Had he not seen the blunders Pedro had made?

He and Coby walked to the bank of the small stream to strip and wash. As they sat down in the shallow current, splashing cold water on each other, Pedro winced. His hip was raw. He had scraped the skin from it during his fall.

Coby looked at him with brotherly pride. "I see that you don't understand the important thing you did in the battle. The bravest act of all is to count coup on a living enemy—to touch or strike a living, unhurt man and leave him alive. You did that twice. It's a thing that will be remembered when we return to camp."

Although Pedro had heard of coups, he still didn't understand the high value placed upon them. He explained to Coby that in his opinion the deeds that demanded the most personal courage were Coby's ride on the cream in the very jaws of death, Two-in-a-Blanket's rush into a rain of arrows to dispatch the wounded Apache, and Coby and Horse Whipper's feat of scooping Ravisher off the ground and rescuing him. Each of those things involved a much greater personal sacrifice and risk of death.

Coby stood naked on the bank, whipping the water off his body with his hands. In the shade of the willows the muscles beneath his tawny skin rippled in long ridges, like prairie grass puckering in the wind.

He said, "It takes more bravery to touch an enemy than to kill him at a distance with an arrow, a bullet, or a spear."

Pedro stepped out of the stream and wiped the wet sand off his feet on the grass. The value these people placed upon their war deeds was hard to understand. As he stepped into his moccasins and wrapped his blue breechclout about his crotch, he pondered it. This might be valuable, he thought. Because of it, I may now be permitted to ride freely about the Comanche country. If so, I might find Roberto more quickly.

He picked up his robe and weapons and strode beside Coby back to the horses.

16 · Victory Dance

Horse Whipper timed their return so they would enter the village in the morning. When they heard the faint barking of the village dogs, they paused on a small hill and made their preparations.

Coby showed Pedro how to paint the yellow warhorse. First they rubbed him with grass until his coat shone in the sunshine. Then they inscribed three imprints of a human hand on his neck and side in red pigment to show where the enemy's hand had touched when Pedro had pulled him off his horse. Red dots were daubed about two slight wounds on the animal's body where enemy arrows had nicked him. Red lines streaming from the dots represented blood flowing from a wound. The horse seemed indifferent to this artistry, nibbling hungrily at the new buffalo grass and swishing his tail vigorously to brush off the troublesome flies.

Ravisher had died two days after the enemy arrow was removed. Pedro had helped carry him to a crevice on a small hill. Here they had laid him, covering his body with rocks to keep the wolves from eating it. Now the warriors were painting his horse's head black and shaving its tail so it could be led riderless in the victory parade through the village.

As Pedro smeared on the black paint with Coby's brush, he thought of Ravisher. He had been a savage, but Pedro was deeply in his debt. You rode with a man for four hundred leagues, ate with him, fought beside him, and he saved your life in battle. And then he died in terrible pain and you piled rocks on him and rode away, leaving him lying forever in the soil of an alien land. Coby, Horse Whipper, and the others eulogized Ravisher, saying he had died gloriously. They almost seemed to envy him. But what was glorious about being cut off in the prime of young manhood, Pedro asked himself. What was glorious about rotting in an Apache hill?

After they had painted themselves, Coby reddened Pedro's hands from fingertips to wrists because those hands had touched both Apaches he had unhorsed.

Pedro laughed noiselessly to himself. It would be more appropriate, he thought, if they painted my buttocks red and also my lame shoulder, commemorating the spots on my body where I hit the ground after falling off my horse so ingloriously. Yet he liked the Comanche way of saying exactly what they meant with these symbols. Their art seemed to express the sincerity of a free people.

For himself, Coby selected a modest facial decoration of olive green and adorned his horse in the same hue. He worked carefully, stringing his two scalps to the tip of his lance and fastening a third to the cream's lower lip.

Everyone was anointing himself with paint made from clays, weed, and berry juice. Two-in-a-Blanket had garnished one side of his body black and the other side yellow. His face was streaked with black, his eyelids were painted yellow. Fastened to his horse in prominent display were the first Apache's musket and the knife of the second. Pedro could not resist a half smile. Two-in-a-Blanket looked as gaudy as a Kiowa tipi.

Now a wailing that resembled the mewing of gulls sounded in the distance. Pedro remembered hearing it the first day he had been brought to the village as a captive. Scanning the horizon toward camp, he saw a row of moving dots. The women! There they came, singing songs of victory as they ran to meet the men.

Quickly Pedro adjusted his quiver, picked up his shield, and mounted the yellow horse. With anticipation he watched the women approach in their shambling, headlong gait. How different would be his reception this time!

The warriors donned their battle garb and mounted. Horse Whipper, embellished with blue paint and festooned with weapons, rode up beside Pedro.

"I want this young man to ride with me at the head of the parade. He has earned it."

Horse Whipper led Pedro's horse to the front of the line, alongside Coby and Two-in-a-Blanket. The clamor of the approaching women grew constantly louder and shriller.

Horse Whipper stood in his green willow stirrups and looked proudly at the file of warriors lined up behind him, their painted bodies glistening in the sunlight. The leader was obviously enjoying every minute of it. Pedro enjoyed it, too. The raid had been successful and now they were looking forward to the victory celebration. This was why they had fought, this and the revenge. Having won the battle, it was time to reap the glory.

Ravisher's riderless horse was in the long line, too. So were all the captured horses. Five of these were Pedro's, the two Apache ponies he had touched while counting coup and three more Horse Whipper had given him when he divided the captured stock among the warriors.

"Let's start now." Horse Whipper urged his horse forward. He threw back his shoulders and raised his lance. The Apache scalp fastened to it swung in the wind. The cries of the approaching women grew louder and plainer. Could anything in life be finer than this, Pedro wondered.

Horse Whipper raised his voice in song. "We are coming

home happy. See what we have got!" His pulsing tones rang out strong and clear. He was no longer hoarse.

The warriors hoisted their scalp poles for all to see. Accompanied by the women, they led the procession into the village. Slowly they rode past the great half circle of tipis and the throngs of people standing before them. The tumult was terrific.

Relatives and friends of the raiders trotted behind the parade and along both its flanks. In a frenzy the women shouted and sang, while old men thumped their walking sticks on the ground. Maidens intoned songs of honor and stole shy glances at the young warriors in the procession. The children stood enthralled, clutching their mother's legs. Nothing in an Indian camp breeds as much excitement and bedlam as the return of a successful war party.

As the people surged against them from all sides, Pedro sat his horse very straight, turning his head only enough to see segments of the wild scene. He kept stealing little glances at the women, hoping to see Willow Girl. He had tried to put her out of his mind and concentrate on the parade but now that he was back among familiar surroundings that was impossible.

He thought of the day he had first come to this village as a captive. Then, too, hundreds of eyes had been fixed on him. But today it was different. Today there was enthusiastic approval and admiration in their staring as they wondered what feat this young associate of Creek Water's had performed to win an honored place at Horse Whipper's side. Several times he heard his name mentioned in hero songs as the women swarmed about him.

Ravisher's wife took one look at the riderless horse with its head painted black and its tail shaved off. Then she began to howl most fiercely. She slashed at her breasts and arms and began to hack off her hair. Almost immediately her friends howled in sympathy with her as they ran alongside Ravisher's horse. Quickly the widows of other years joined them, and the wails of the mourners and the yells of the celebrants blended in weird pandemonium.

So deafening was the din that when the parade passed Creek Water's tipi, Pedro was glad to drop out. After the wives had all noisily embraced him, he headed for his tipi. Old Sore sat sunning himself outside. Like an aged dog, the old man rose painfully from the dust and followed Pedro inside.

As Pedro told him about the battle Old Sore sat wrapped in his robe, his watery eyes alert. At the story's end, the old man exhaled a mouthful of smoke, grunted, and nodded twice in approval.

"Falling off your horse wasn't so bad, *español*. Any horse frightened by a blanket waved in its face might step in a hole and fall. But losing your arrows and dropping your shield was careless. It takes many days to make war arrows, many weeks to season them. Those Apaches went back to the battlefield and picked up all those arrows you dropped and the ones Horse Whipper's war party shot. Our arrows are much better than the ones they make themselves. They won't have to make any new arrows for a whole year. But we'll have to start making a great many new ones tomorrow."

Pedro looked down at the tipi floor. Would he ever be able to please Old Sore? Apparently those two nods were all the credit he was going to get from the old man. A little hurt, Pedro went outside, mounted the mule, and rode to the herding grounds to leave the yellow warhorse and the five other animals he had won.

Riding back, he passed lodge after lodge. The village had moved several times while the war party had been away. The present camping spot was farther east than the previous ones. A pungent odor came from the willows along the little stream that meandered in lazy loops through the red-soiled country. The tipis had been erected on both sides of the river. Women were seated outside in their shade, visiting in low, murmuring voices.

Suddenly Pedro saw Willow Girl sitting in front of a tipi with a woman he judged to be another of Paunch's wives. She wore a doeskin skirt and blouse decorated with blue glass beads. She was smiling at something the other woman had said. The line of her mouth tilted upward at the corners, gentle and sweet.

Then she saw Pedro and her firm little chin lifted in surprise. The eagerness in her expressive face was so plain that Pedro could not mistake it.

A shiver of delight passed through him and he sawed the jaw rope to slow the mule. Love for her surged through him with such intensity that he forgot that she was married. He forgot everything except the overpowering need to stop and speak to her.

But Willow Girl rose abruptly and went inside the lodge. The other woman followed. The flap closed tightly behind them.

Willow Girl might as well have given him a slap in the face. Angrily, he flanked the mule forward. Why did she have to behave so maddeningly? But no matter how quickly she had withdrawn, she could not erase the joyful welcome he had seen in her eyes.

Pedro rode on. Try as he would, he could not keep his mind off the girl.

Why am I always in such a ferment over her? he scolded himself. She's just an Indian girl with no education whatever. I could never persuade her to leave this wild existence and return with me to Spain. She would never be happy there. Besides, she's married. Why can't I accept that and forget her?

Back at his tipi he slid wearily off the mule and went inside. Bone-tired from his nine days on a horse, he wrapped his robe about him and lay down.

It was late afternoon when he awoke. Someone was standing over him. It was Creek Water. A faint gleam of pleasure enlivened the chief's usually impassive face. He wanted to hear more about the battle, and Pedro gave him a complete account. "Thank you, father, for the yellow warhorse," he concluded. "Without him, I could not have overtaken the two enemies."

Creek Water nodded gravely. "My son, you will be expected to dance tonight, describing your coups. I hope you will deliberate on this and make suitable preparations." He walked out of the lodge.

Pedro had made suitable preparations, all right. Wild horses couldn't have pulled him away from that dance. After a little more sleep, he walked with Creek Water and his wives to the dancing grounds.

There in the center stood a freshly cut cottonwood pole, black and straight against the dull, red sunset. Dangling from the pole were the scalps that had been taken on the raid. A fire of cottonwood logs crackled nearby. Its pleasant, woodsy fragrance blended with the aroma of the buffalo ribs that were being roasted for the feast. Just smelling those ribs cooking in their own juice made Pedro hungry. The firelight flickered over the faces of the people massed about on all four sides, revealing here and there a bit of beadwork, a flash of teeth, a human face. The whole world was Indian, from the smell to the silence, and Pedro felt an affinity with the land and its people that he had never felt before.

Now a drum began to beat. The throb of it ran through Pedro's senses with a fiery surge. Then the singers started up. Softly the leader intoned an opening phrase, allowing the others to identify the melody and the pitch. He repeated the phrase tentatively until all were sure of it. Then, singing it loudly, they joined him.

The drumbeats became more rapid. A line of male dancers began moving slowly around the scalp pole. The bells on their moccasins and knees tinkled in time to the drum. Pedro felt that he was seeing and hearing all this for the first time. Bedecked in red paint, each man whirled, stamped, postured, and spun in imitation of warriors on a raid, scanning the ground for enemy footprints, then pretending to shoot with arrows and thrust with knives. Some had on war bonnets; others wore rosettes of turkey feathers across their buttocks and strutted about like proud birds.

Then a line of women appeared, shoulder to shoulder, side-stepping with perfect unity and lively grace. The two circles were only a few feet apart, and they moved in opposite directions, facing each other. Slowly the circle of women dancers surrounded that of the men. Long fringes of soft buckskin swung gaily from the women's sleeves and the firelight flashed brightly off the bands of blue beading each wore across her shoulders and down her sleeves.

They advanced smartly to the left, a half step at a time, holding the left knee stiff but bending the right one with a vigorous outward swinging movement. The song rose and fell on the wind as the women's high, shrill voices blended weirdly with the deeper tones of the men. Fiercely triumphant and proudly defiant, the music pealed into the night.

As he listened, Pedro yearned for his guitar. How he would have liked to translate this song into his own medium of stringed chords and harmonizations!

Then the drumbeats changed to quarter notes and Pedro forgot all about his guitar as the bowlegged, war-bonneted chiefs rose to dance. Each remaining in his own place, they flexed their knees and leaned gracefully from right to left as they moved their bodies up and down.

Finally the drums slowed, the singing stopped, and it was time for the individual dancing.

One by one, the warriors who had been on the raid capered into the open space. In fierce pantomime, each defined with bold realism how he had distinguished himself in the battle, detailing each lance thrust given, each wound dealt and received.

Horse Whipper, the popular leader of the raid, skipped into the arena next. Whirling so low that his long war bonnet dragged in the sand, he vividly portrayed his feat to the shouted approval of the audience, who clapped their hands and shook their gourd rattles.

When he sat down, his aged grandmother became so excited that she rose and sang in his honor, her quavery, old voice keening with joy. This spontaneous act was greeted with delighted laughter and tumultuous applause.

Next Two-in-a-Blanket, resplendent in a veneer of green that covered his entire body, burst upon the scene and dashed realistically through the various phases of his daring charge into the rain of arrows to kill the wounded Apache. He retired amid enthusiastic applause. Then his mother, not to be outdone by Horse Whipper's grandmother, sprang to her feet and sang his praises.

Coby bounded vigorously onto the hard sand, jigging and curvetting and twitching his head rhythmically. How did he manage to make the two eagle feathers pinned to his scalplock jiggle backward and forward in such perfect time to the drums, Pedro wondered.

Coby's aversion for self-glorification was almost as well known as his valor in battle. Nevertheless, he chose from his many feats his first one of lancing and scalping the two Apaches on foot, and performed with just enough detail to satisfy the minimum of what was required. He sat down to the most rousing ovation of the night. His wife Kildee, continuing what had now become a custom, stood and sang his praise.

And then it was Pedro's turn.

How different was this scalp dance from his first. He hoped Willow Girl was somewhere in the audience. He would show her what good dancing really was. Then he would forget her. He did not need her anyhow.

He had decided to weave into his introduction elements of a flamenco dance. He had purposely sat away from the fire in order to have ample room for his entrance. Ignoring the drumbeats—which were far too slow—he sprinted from his seat in the dancing area and hurled himself upward in a *farruca,* a series of pirouettes. Furiously he rotated his body. At the top of each ascension his face was only a brown blur as he spun in space. He knew that he must look like one of the small prairie-dust funnels that moved across the land in spring.

Just as it seemed his spiraling might orbit him into the sky, he planted himself suddenly into a *caída,* or fall. The contrast was so startling that it brought surprised gasps and then murmurs of approval and pleasure from the audience.

Then he stomped back into the arena, body leaning, feet chopping, and danced his coups in the Comanche way, using such vigorous, exaggerated movements that the narration was plain to all. He enjoyed himself hugely. As he whirled across the sandy floor, he kept stealing little peeps at the spectators closest to him. He was fully conscious of the envy on the faces of Wolf Milk and the other young bucks who had hazed him, of the ardent glances of the young maidens, and of the pride in the countenances of Coby, Kildee, and Creek Water's wives.

Imagining he was a Comanche, he let himself go completely. *All of me—feet, head, torso, hands—feels so joyful, so alive. It feels so good to be accepted by these people. If I did not have to take Roberto back to civilization I could stay in this exciting place forever. I could revel in a life like this until I died.*

He concluded with another flamenco maneuver, springing into the air and repeatedly crossing his feet while suspended at the height of his vault. As he raced to his seat, he could hear the shouting and the handclapping and the gourdshaking swell behind him. A feeling of fulfillment permeated him. And then he realized that something was lacking.

The drumbeats had stopped and there was silence. No female relatives stood to sing him honor—no grandmother, mother, wife, or aunt. Legally, he was still a captive.

Then a young woman rose from the circle of the female dancers. Her buckskin gown, simple and wifely, swished musically as she walked. Her long black hair, parted down the middle, swung freely around her shoulders. Her back was to the fire and her face in shadow as she moved toward him, but Pedro was aware of her with all his senses, aware of the dignity and grace of her movements, her clean ranginess, her warm sweet smell.

She began to sing. It was the first time he had ever heard her voice raised in melody. Her singing was untrained and commonplace, like that of any other woman of the tribe. It was a harsh, trembling falsetto that trailed downward at the end in a sort of wail. But Pedro thought it was the sweetest singing he had ever heard:

In his first battle,
This young man counted coup twice.
Now that fighting is in his bloodstream,
He will go away again,
Seeking more ponies, more coups.
Father, protect him from danger and from pain.
Father, deliver his enemies into his hands.

Pedro was so overwhelmed with emotion that he did not

stay for the feast of juicy buffalo ribs. His kiss on her mouth came back, his pulse pounded, the old heartache returned. . . .

Morning found him still upset. Two maidens of the village, dressed like warriors, gathered before his tipi to sing songs of praise, but Pedro scarcely noticed them. It was Creek Water who went out, proud of Pedro's exploits, to thank them and give them two horses.

The adoption ceremony that took place two days later was no better. When it was over, Pedro vaguely remembered the pipe being passed around the council ring and all the warriors standing up, placing their right hands over their hearts, and marching around in a circle. He recalled promising to perform the duties of a warrior and obey the chiefs in all things relating to war and peace. He remembered the Comanche name they gave him. Henceforth he would be known as Horseback Fighter.

The next morning he and Coby were watering their horses in the river. Coby seemed impressed by the ceremony. "Brother, you are now a free member of the tribe. You can hunt or fight or move about without asking anybody's permission."

Move about! How far would he have to move to get away from a pair of eyes browner than any he had ever seen before, and lips the color of the sumac that grew along the hollows of the sandhills? With a stab of guilt, he realized he had been thinking so constantly about Willow Girl that he had forgotten his aim of finding Roberto. How could he ask Roberto to give up a way of life that he himself had found so enthralling? How could he persuade Roberto to leave unless both of them left together?

17 · Willow Girl

The day came when Pedro reached a decision. He must sever all ties with Willow Girl and with this village that would always remind him of her. The very next morning he would resume his search for Roberto.

There would be no chance of saying goodbye to Coby, because the warrior had gone with a raiding party to the land of the Utes. It was hard to think of parting with him. And Old Sore. He owed much to the one-eared ancient.

It was strange how a man could become attached to a town that was always on the move. Although Pedro had hated it at first, life within this group had now become quite pleasant. Departure seemed almost like desertion. He could hardly bear to think about it.

His hands shook as he packed his belongings in a deerskin pouch. He had told Creek Water and Old Sore that he was going to visit his brother and they had accepted it, expecting him to return in Tah-tsa, the Comanche summer. But Pedro had other plans. Once he found Roberto they would head straight for northern Chihuahua and Spain. Oddly, the prospect did not excite him as it once had.

Old Sore had told Pedro to start looking first for the Nokonis in the area between the Moobetahehoono, or Walnut Creek, and the Pahsehoonoo.

"But if you don't find them until winter, look in the breaks of the Kweetacooeh country, around the river the whites call the Pease," the old man had counseled. "They like to go there for protection from the freezing winds. You will have trouble finding them anywhere, *español,* because they roam in all directions. The Nokonis really never know where they are going because they always turn back before they get there. Their wives always keep their parfleches packed and their travois loaded. Sometimes in summer they don't even bother to put up tipis. They just sleep on the ground in the open air so they will be ready to start roaming again the following day."

Next morning an hour before sunup, when the meadowlarks were chirping sleepily and the cool dawn wind ran along the ground, Pedro swung the elm saddle onto one of his Apache ponies. It was a pinto, with bright, intelligent eyes. He planned to take the other Apache pony too, riding them in turn. He had combed the feathers and other ornaments out of their manes, tails, and forelocks. The thought of leaving the rest of his little herd made his heart heavy. He wanted Coby to have the yellow warhorse and Old Sore the mule, but he could not let anyone know this or they would realize that he was not coming back.

Singing broke out nearby, strident and joyful. Pedro could tell that the men were getting ready to go somewhere and do something exciting. For weeks, he himself had done nothing at all exciting.

One of the singers was Trotting Wolf, a young man who had gone with Horse Whipper and the others on the war party against the Prairie Apaches.

"Come along with us, Horseback Fighter," Trotting Wolf called. "We're going to hunt buffalo."

It hurt Pedro to have to shake his head in refusal. He had not gone buffalo hunting since the previous autumn. Now he must ride endlessly in the sun while everybody else was doing something enjoyable. It would be the first buffalo hunt of the year. The molting season was over and the hides of the bulls were in their prime.

For a moment, he let his mind dwell on the pleasure of the hunt. He thought of riding with the other young men on the surround, of the singing and the talking and the swimming in the creeks. Then would come the excitement of sighting the herd, the thrill of the chase, the smell of the sweating horses, the joy of the shooting and finally the moment of savoring the first juicy bites of roasted buffalo tongue at the feast that followed.

Pedro twisted helplessly. He must renounce all this, just as he had renounced the girl.

He mounted. The hunters were all around him, their horses rearing and prancing and curvetting with excitement. His own horse began to rear, raising its shoulders and then its rump. Head up and ears thrust forward, the pony began nickering and dancing up and down like all the other horses.

Pedro reined down the frisking, bounding animal. As he did, the singing began again, rising in volume and becoming faster and faster.

Wretchedly, Pedro listened. If I were going with them, he thought, I would not be leaving this place forever. I would not be leaving this girl. She would be here somewhere when we got back. She would not be in my tipi but at least she would be here somewhere. I could see her once more before I leave.

The singing was a strongly braided rope pulling Pedro into the hunting party. He felt a pulsing in his own throat. Before he knew it, he was singing too, his high, clear notes echoing above the tops of the willows and fading in the cool air across the river.

What are a few more days? he asked himself as he rode off with them. This will be the last buffalo hunt of my life. When it's over, I'll be leaving all this forever.

The hunting was good. Pedro shot well. Although the

buffalo were scarcer than before, Old Sore's new arrows flew so straight that Pedro killed three bulls, more than enough for Creek Water's wives. He did not win one of the roasted tongues but he enjoyed himself, and so did his Apache pony.

When they returned to camp Pedro went to the Buffalo Tongue Dance. A fire had been built and the tongues were roasting over the embers. When the dark, red meat was done, the men sat in a big half circle. The women dancers sat back twenty steps from the circle's opening.

Willow Girl was sitting back in the shadows with Paunch's other wives. She seemed strangely subdued.

Pedro's heart seemed to turn over and he looked miserably away, sorry he had come. His mind was made up. That very afternoon, he would set off on his search for Roberto. Never again would he see this girl.

As Pedro took what he intended to be his last look at her, Willow Girl turned and her deerskin gown slipped down across one shoulder. Raw, red welts covered her arms as well as her shoulders.

Pedro reached for his knife. Where was Paunch? If he could have found the fat chief at that moment, he would have cut him into a pile of blubber big enough to feed the coyote population for months. He would have done it in the Comanche way, prolonging the pain without killing the subject. But Paunch was off on a horse-buying expedition, Pedro remembered. His hands shook as he tried to fight down his anger. How quickly he could be seized by these murderous rages!

He looked again at Willow Girl. Her chin was up. She was not dancing but she was not staying home. She was hiding nothing.

Pedro thought he knew why Paunch had beaten her. Another of his expeditions to the far-off piñon country to steal the storied Tafoya horse herd had failed. Two warriors of the many he had sent had lost their lives. Their bodies could never be recovered. A third, shot through the bowels with a rifle ball, had died on the way home. Every night at sundown Pedro could hear all three widows mourning.

The howl of the first widow usually set off the other two and they screeched in chorus until their voices gave out. Pedro could understand why Paunch could not bear this wailing that reminded him of his many failures. Furious because he still did not have the Tafoya horses, he had beaten his wives and then left camp for a few days.

Pedro felt no further interest in the dancing or the feasting. How could he leave on the hunt for Roberto now? He had to help Willow Girl first. It was unthinkable that she should continue to risk these brutal beatings. But how was he going to help her?

Pedro walked into Coby's tipi that night, surprised and elated to find that the warrior had returned. Coby was seated at the front of the lodge, braiding a rope out of hunks of black horsehair. His son sat nearby. The boy was amusing himself with two strings tied to a bone. When he pulled the strings together they made a whirring sound that seemed to delight him. Kildee was stitching the hem of an antelope skin skirt with her awl and sinew thread. The lodge was warm and cozy. Pedro envied them their family tranquillity.

Almost at once he blurted out the news of the lacerations on Willow Girl's shoulders and arms.

Coby looked thoughtful. "He probably beat her with his quirt. That's the way he marks up his other wives."

From the back of the tipi came Kildee's decorous tones. "She must not be pleasing him. A husband has the right to beat his wife if she doesn't please him in all things." She shook her black head and clucked her tongue, making deprecating noises. "It's hard on a young wife. The beatings she receives from her husband are the first she ever experiences. Parents do not beat their children."

"Brmm!" sang the whirrer and the boy chuckled with joy at the distracting noise he had concocted.

Pedro described Paunch whipping one of his wives the day he and Creek Water were riding to the hunting dance. "I was going to leave today and try to find my brother," he confessed. "I thought I could go away any time I wanted to. But I can't. I'll never be able to forget her, I guess. I've tried to but I can't."

Coby put down his rope braiding and looked at Pedro with sympathy and affection.

"All right," he said. "If you still want her, I'll help you steal her. You're not a captive now. You're an adopted citizen. You can go anywhere you want to. Even with another man's wife. If she'll go with you."

"She'll go," Pedro breathed. Filled with new hope, he told them about the look on Willow Girl's face when he had first ridden past her tipi on the day of the victory dance. He did not add that she had suddenly withdrawn into the lodge.

"Paunch won't stop with just one beating." Kildee punched a hole in the antelope hide with her bone awl and drew the sinew thread through with her white teeth. "I'm sure he's taken the skin off her several times. She's probably been packed for a week, waiting for you to steal her."

Coby picked up the hank of horsehair, separated it into strands, and resumed his braiding. "We can leave any night you want." He spoke as if stealing a wife happened all the time. "We can take down this lodge in the dark and quickly be on our way. We would have to ride all day and all night for several days because Paunch would be sure to follow us. He has lots of power. If he caught up with us, he would have the right to kill her, or slit her nose. That's Comanche law."

Coby kept on talking, "He's a chief. He has lots of friends. Even if he slit her nose, there would have to be a property settlement of some kind. He'd want everything you've got. Or he might just want his wife back. But I would be there with you and I don't think he would try to take her back or harm her if I was there."

Pedro felt his palms itching. "He would not take her back if I were there, either. He wouldn't kill her. Or slit her nose."

Coby gazed at him with tolerance. "Brother, that would be no good. If you killed him, you would be killed by his relatives. It would be legal. I could not help you. And you would not get to keep the girl. If Paunch died for any reason, one of his brothers would get her. A woman losing her husband by death is inherited by her husband's brother. That's Comanche law."

Pedro suddenly felt weary and bewildered. He was stunned by the harshness of the law.

Also, another small voice from deep inside him murmured against the plan, a voice he had not listened to for many months. How would his church regard this coveting another man's wife and absconding with her? Even if the absconding were necessary to save the girl from the brutality of a husband who already possessed three other wives?

Pedro knew that his chief motive for intervening was his love for Willow Girl, even if she were married. And that being true, he knew that he should in conscience leave. Then he saw the long, red welts on her again. Undoubtedly they would be multiplied many times in the weeks to come by a husband who loved his horses more than his wives.

Pedro looked again at Coby, Kildee, and their son, and thought of the trouble and sacrifice he would be putting them to. "Isn't there any other way to get her besides stealing her?"

Coby scratched his scalplock and looked thoughtful. "You could buy her. Wives are sold every day. If a wife doesn't have children, her husband sometimes becomes impatient and sells her to another man. Everybody wants children. Or sometimes when a husband is drinking heavily, he sells his wife for a bottle of whisky. Or he might get desperate and put her up in a gambling game if he was losing heavily."

Pedro shook his head despondently. "He'd never sell her. He's already the richest man in the tribe."

"That's right," acknowledged Coby. "And he doesn't drink. He's the best dice-stick player in the band. You could not beat him gambling. We'll just have to steal her and run off so far with her that he won't find us. That's the only way."

"Where would we go?" Pedro asked cheerlessly. The enterprise seemed more and more hopeless every moment.

"We could join the Kwahade band," Coby said. "I've been thinking about joining them for a long time. I like the way they live. They live on the open plains where the antelope and buffalo are always plentiful. And it is the country farthest away from the white strangers. Their country is so hot and treeless that they carry pieces of rawhide on their backs that can be held over their heads for a sunshade. That's what Kwahade means. Sunshades on their backs."

Coby went on. "Brother, stealing her is the only way. Why don't you tell her what we're going to do so she can secretly pack and be ready?"

Pedro could feel his face flush. "She won't let me come within a league of her." He described how she had leaped to her feet and hurried inside her tipi at his approach.

Kildee sniffed and tossed her black head disdainfully. "Cheyenne women are too moral," she observed. "They make too much of never being seen alone."

"I'll send Kildee to talk to her tomorrow," Coby promised. "Come back tomorrow morning. We'll see what she says."

Coby reported promptly the next morning. "She says she won't do it." His sad features looked gloomier than ever. "Kildee talked to her when they both went down to the river to wash. She told Kildee she's not running away from anything. I don't think she likes her marriage but she's not quitting. She's not the quitting kind."

Pedro felt sick. "I don't understand. I know she likes me and I know she dislikes Paunch. I know from the way she looked at me when she rode past me with him after the marriage feast, and from the way she looked at me when I rode past her tipi on the way back from the Apache raid. Both times it showed plainly in her face. And why did she sing in my honor at the victory dance?"

Coby tossed a buffalo chip on the fire and watched it flare up. "Brother, I've changed my mind about her," he said thoughtfully. "She's not like other women. She has a strange, virtuous way of looking at everything, even a poor marriage. I think that whatever is done to break her marriage will have to be legal. It must not break Comanche law, or she won't have anything to do with it."

Pedro blew out his breath in one long, weary exhalation.

Coby offered one final suggestion. "We could steal her against her will."

Pedro shook his head. He wanted no part of any plan that forced her to do anything. There had been too much of that already. Her parents had forced her into one marriage and look what it had brought!

Why do I worry so much about her? he asked himself. Does she really mean this much to me? She's just an Indian girl. I can ride right out of her life and back to my guitar any time I want to and never give her another thought.

But the words had a false ring. In every memory he had of her, she shone as beautifully as gypsum sparkling in the sunshine. Willow Girl was so superior in every way to the Spanish girls he had known that he had long since forgotten all of them.

What a spirit she had! He remembered the proud lift of her

chin that day in the tamarisk when the Comanche syllables had rolled sibilantly off her tongue: "If a young man risks his life to steal horses so he might offer them to the girl's father as her price, it shows how much he values her." He valued her, all right, but he had never shown how much by any act of his own.

Back in his tipi, he kept thinking of those welts on her arm and shoulder. For the hundredth time he told himself, Paunch will keep beating her with that horsewhip. But she won't leave him. He won't sell her. And she won't let me steal her. What am I going to do?

Crumpling his deerskin jacket into a ball, he hurled it against the tipi wall. He couldn't buy her. And he had nothing to trade for her, nothing that Paunch wanted anyway.

It was then that he thought of the horses owned by the trader Tafoya and kept in the stockade near Fort Union.

18 · Wrath of the Thunder Bird

Pedro chewed on a mesquite bean, squinting his eyes against the glare of the afternoon sun. As he and Coby rode west he could feel the sweat trickling down his forehead, his calves, his chest. The hot, dry wind cracked his lips and made his nose dry. His breechclout smelled old and stale.

He kept sweeping his eyes over the rough terrain in search of landmarks. All around him, grassy hummocks, big as tipis and shaped like the top half of an egg, thrust themselves upward; the land seemed endlessly nippled by them. Tumbleweed and green sage grew along the trail.

Below them curved the sand river, the Pahseehoono River, a tan gash in the wilderness of green mesquite. Small islands of tamarisk divided the wide river plain. Beyond the stream the bluffs were bald with sand. This is the wildest, hottest country I've ever seen, thought Pedro. I'm probably the only white man who ever ventured into it and survived.

It surprised him to find how easy it was to follow the landmarks Old Sore had described. Before they had left, the old man had asked them to sit down with him. He had brought a bundle of sticks marked with notches to represent each day of their trip through the unfamiliar country. Sucking on his red clay ceremonial pipe, Old Sore blew smoke on all fourteen sticks and prayed over them.

The first day's journey was represented by a stick with one

notch, the second day's journey by a stick with two notches, and so on. Drawing on his memory of landmarks, the old man had begun with the first stick. In his bellowing voice he defined the streams, hills, waterholes, and valleys they should watch for on all the days that would pass before they arrived at the heavily guarded stockade of the rancher Tafoya.

From the New Mexican traders, shreds of information had sifted in about him. He was small and had an olive complexion, a pointed black beard, and quick, sinister eyes that gave him a vindictive look. Although his manners were polished, he was said to be cruel and false. His father had been a Mexican and his mother an Indian. Incredibly rich, he thought everybody should comply with his wishes. When anybody was caught trying to steal his horses, Suarez Tafoya had him executed on the spot. He had acquired most of his wealth by organizing and outfitting the New Mexican traders for their illegal expeditions into the Indian country. Pedro knew these traders made enormous profits by swapping beads, glass, sugar, coffee, and liquor for the Comanches' valuable buffalo robes and for the herds of cattle the Indians were stealing from the Texans. It was rumored that Tafoya was secretly backed by American officers at the nearby fort.

Blooded saddlehorses were Tafoya's passion. He owned a herd of superior animals that not only Paunch but all the Indians on the Southwestern plains—Kiowas, Comanches, Wichitas, and Utes—had vainly tried to steal. Tafoya employed a heavy guard of sharp-eyed Mexican vaqueros armed with six-shooters and repeating rifles to watch them. The herd grazed close to the corral on a level expanse. Every foot of it could be seen for miles around, and all attempts to steal the herd had failed, although many a buck had died trying. At night the animals were driven into a stockade of adobe and logs which had walls ten feet high and three feet thick. Its only entrance was a gate heavily locked and chained from the outside. Another set of armed guards slept in the daytime and patrolled the stockade at night.

As Pedro gazed bleakly at the scorched landscape, he told himself, "I want that girl so badly that I'm behaving like an utter idiot to get her. But she's worth it!"

It was terrifying to be so wildly and overwhelmingly in love. He felt a great sorrow that no one else could taste such rapture.

In late afternoon of the third day a coyote jumped out of the sage ahead, looked back over its shoulder at them, and ran out of sight around a sand plum thicket. Instantly, Coby jerked his horse to a stop and refused to go farther in that direction that day.

"He's warning us that there's danger ahead," Coby insisted. Pedro chafed at the delay. He did not want to lose the two hours of travel before dusk but he knew there was no arguing with Coby's superstitions. They headed for the top of a nearby hill and camped just behind its ridge where they could watch for the approach of an enemy from their rear.

The hill overlooked a small river that twisted sinuously through thickets of tamarisk and mesquite. They walked their horses down to it and let them plunge their muzzles into the warm water, only inches deep, that seemed barely to wet the purplish sand over which it flowed. They both rolled off to drink.

"What river is this?" Pedro asked.

"The Kweetacooeh," Coby replied. "That's Comanche for 'manure.' Big herds of buffalo range here. Much manure."

Both the name and the place seemed faintly familiar to Pedro. Suddenly it all came back to him. This was the place where the terrified white captives had been separated before passing into oblivion. This was where Roberto had been taken from him. Pedro looked around him. The spot seemed strangely hallowed. He could still hear Roberto calling in his childish treble, *"Adiós, caro* Pedro!" his voice growing fainter and fainter as Green Turtle led him away.

While Pedro filled the waterskin, Coby spied a white buffalo skull half buried in the sand. He walked toward it with long, purposeful strides, his moccasins ankle deep in the short yellow wildflowers that grew everywhere.

Pedro watched him, alternately fascinated and amused. It was a walk that could have but one result: Coby bent over a clump of sandburs, picked up the skull, and carefully turned it to face their home camp. Then he wiped his hands on his breechclout.

"Brother," he announced, "I haven't been doing this often enough. That's why the buffalo have been scarcer this year. My guardian spirit always sends them in the direction the skulls are facing. Not enough of them are facing our home camp."

Coby believed so unwaveringly in all his supernatural beings that there was no use hurrying him while he paused to venerate them. When they passed a bluff or a spring or any phenomenon of nature, Coby always halted and did it reverence, explaining that it might be the residing place of a spirit.

Next morning they rode on, ducking behind their horses' necks to avoid the wet, switchlike boughs of the tamarisk flowering everywhere in white, lavender, and pink. Soon they began to pass square-topped peaks capped with outcroppings of gray rocks. The trail led sharply upward and after a quarter of a league of meandering, they climbed out on top of the grassy tableland. Old Sore had told them the New Mexican traders called it *Llano Estacado.* Coby called it by its Comanche name, *Mah Nohh-hphe,* meaning "It's plateau."

Everything here seemed high and breezy and secluded.

Pedro at once felt refreshed and encouraged. It was as if they had found some secret trysting grounds of the gods. The never-ceasing wind rushed through the dwarf mesquite, hissing softly. It was cool on Pedro's cheek. The grass was short and lacy, blending in light greens and yellows as it rippled in the wind. Although the land was dry, they occasionally passed small swales of dark green sedgegrass growing out of black, moist-looking depressions in the prairie floor.

As they rode, they made plans. Each had carefully questioned the warriors who had returned from all the disastrous raids Paunch had thrown against Tafoya. None could quite explain why they had failed except that Paunch's medicine had been wrong. Pedro, after cautious inquiry, learned that all the raids had hit while the horses were grazing on the open plain. Attempts had been made at several different times of day and many different stratagems used. Yet Tafoya's vaqueros had no trouble rushing the horses inside the stockade while sharp-shooters armed with repeating rifles picked off the luckless raiders or shot their horses out from under them and ran them down on foot, shooting them at will.

On the morning they threw away the stick with seven notches, the land began to stretch smoothly and limitlessly ahead of them like a vast lawn. It was the broadest, flattest country Pedro had ever seen. There was no water and no trees or other vegetation except an occasional bush cactus. The atmosphere was so clear and transparent that it seemed to Pedro that he could see the eagles sailing over the crags of the brown hills thirty miles away.

These hills, rising to the south, loomed so low and flat that Pedro imagined a giant could have sat on one while eating his dinner off another. Grimly, he thought, I'm as fanciful as Coby. Before we're through with this Tafoya and his vaqueros, we'll need all the help we can get from both Coby's Little Men and my giants.

Two days later the land became greener and more rolling. Low hills tufted with herbage appeared ahead of them, and soon they could smell the pungent odor of the piñon pines. Sunflowers and gutierrezia yellowed the landscape. On the evening they threw away the last of Old Sore's fourteen sticks a cloudbank rose over the mountains. On the open plain ahead, illuminated in an oasis of sunshine, appeared the white buildings and corrals of the Rancho Tafoya. It was just as Old Sore had predicted.

Next morning before dawn Pedro crept to the top of a small knoll. With an old fieldglass Creek Water had lent him, he studied the rancho's herd procedure. The glass was good and although Pedro lay hidden miles from the scene, he saw plainly the long, low adobe buildings, neatly whitewashed and roofed with red tile. How like his uncle's rancho in northern Chihuahua this was.

Carefully, Pedro moved the glass about. Hundreds of horses, cattle, and sheep grazed beyond the rancho buildings in green fields that were enclosed by what looked like a palisade of mesquite trees rammed into the ground and connected by strips of raw oxhide. Near the stables stood several Mexican carts with large wooden wheels; Pedro knew they were used by Tafoya to haul the cheap merchandise he sent into the Comanche country.

Then the tall brown walls of an immense corral with its strong gate still shut tightly came into focus. Several large, savage-looking dogs rose lazily from their beds in open kennels outside the corral. Pedro lowered the glass. He had not known about the dogs. No doubt they could smell an intruder two arrowshots away.

Finally the vaqueros appeared. Wearing broad-brimmed hats, they stalked leisurely about the premises as their spurs flashed brightly in the morning sunshine. Pedro scanned them carefully in the glass. They stood on both sides of the gate, shaking out the loops of their riatas, each ready to lasso a horse for the day's herding. One man began to wrestle with the locks. Finally he swung the gate open.

Instantly the horses inside rushed through it, bursting out upon the prairie. Although the animals were too far away to be seen plainly, they moved lightly and gracefully and seemed possessed of boundless spirit. Pedro felt a leaping sensation in his chest. It was his first look at the Tafoya herd.

They were mainly medium-sized bays, grays, chestnuts, and browns and he guessed that they were European purebloods. Since there were no pintos, or creams, or claybanks among them they could not be of Indian lineage. With them the rancho's ordinary saddle stock were stabled, and as they too rushed out, the vaqueros hurled their loops, selecting their mounts for the day. Then they saddled them, picked up their rifles, and drove the herd of thoroughbreds to the nearby pasture, where the herbage had obviously been saved for them.

Two hours before dusk the herd was corralled. Later Pedro and Coby crawled closer and examined the animals' hoofprints. Although the saddle stock ridden by the vaqueros wore thin, flat iron shoes with the heels turned up and doubled back in the Spanish fashion, the hoofs of the fabled Tafoya thoroughbreds showed no shoes or nail marks of any kind. Pedro was puzzled. He had never seen Spanish horses that were not shod.

"What do you think?" he asked Coby.

Coby looked again at the marks. "Brother, I know nothing of this. When our horses grow tenderfooted, we sometimes fit them with rawhide boots soaked in water. But these horses wear nothing. I have never seen horses like these in the pens of the white strangers."

For three days, they took turns watching the vaqueros handle the herd. Tafoya's men were very alert. Their guards, stationed a half mile from the animals, never left their posts to take siestas. Pedro remembered hearing the warriors in Paunch's various expeditions tell of their experiences here. When they had tried to slip past these men on the flat prairie, one guard would fire a pistol shot of warning and the herd would be rushed to safety in a moment.

Pedro frowned. Tafoya's pattern of defense was perfect. A night theft was out of the question unless Pedro could get past all those night guards and fierce dogs and devise some way to jump the herd over the ten-foot walls. He would have to steal the herd in broad daylight, when the odds were a hundred to one against his succeeding. And he had to do it quickly. Back in the village Paunch was probably beating his wives.

On the morning of the fourth day, Pedro and Coby lay side by side on their stomachs atop the knoll, taking one final look at the vaqueros' morning procedure, pondering it point by point. Day after day it never varied. Through the glass, they saw the herders collecting at the gate, shaking out their riatas. After a struggle with the locks, the gate swung open. Eager for the day's exercise and grazing, the herd spilled through. As the rancho stock followed, the vaqueros' ropes leaped out to secure mounts for the day's herdings. After saddling, the vaqueros picked up their rifles and drove the herd out for the morning grazing.

Pedro said, "If we could somehow open that gate at night and get the horses out while everybody was asleep, it would be much easier to steal them."

Coby's obsidian-black eyes regarded Pedro fondly. "Brother, horses stampeded at night are unmanageable and do not run well together. Usually they are lost to the stampeders. It is best to take them in the daytime."

Then he went on quietly: "There's a big pile of fodder near the gate. We might hide in it at night, when they can't see us. After the herd is turned out in the morning, each of us could run out of the fodder, mount a horse as it runs by, stampede the herd and get away."

Pedro considered it carefully. It was risky. If he and Coby failed to catch a horse after exposing themselves, they could expect nothing but swift death. Still, with all the danger involved, this seemed more practical than any other plan.

Pedro stirred uneasily, feeling Coby's warm body next to his in the grass. His Comanche brother's devotion made his eyes mist over and for a moment he had difficulty swallowing. For a venture like this, he could not have had a better companion than cool, daring Coby. No man would be more likely to bring it off. But Pedro hesitated to involve Coby in such a suicidal adventure.

The thought of Kildee and the boy back in the Comanche camp, fourteen riding days distant, filled him with shame. He could picture Kildee gashing herself and hear her wails of mourning. She and the son Coby loved so dearly would become dependent upon the warrior societies for their food and meager living. And Paunch would go on beating Willow Girl.

Yet they had to try something. Or Paunch would go on beating her anyhow.

They decided to make the effort that night.

At the small arroyo where they had concealed their horses, they filled their waterskins and bathed in the small rivulet, carefully washing their bodies, breechclouts, and lassos with mud and water. Horses can detect the slightest odor of horse-flesh on Indians who have eaten it; they will not permit anyone smelling of it to approach. While everything dried in the warm sunshine they rested.

Just before midnight Coby lit his pipe. They each blew puffs of smoke to the moon rising in the east.

"Mother Moon is the guardian of the raid," Coby explained simply. He laid his horsehair rope on the prairie in a big loop.

They sat within it, each praying earnestly in his own way.

"Mother, if it be your will, let this rope take many horses," Coby said aloud.

Silently, Pedro prayed. "Holy Mother, take this enterprise under thy protection. Protect us, O my mother, and obtain for us pardon of our sins, love for Jesus, a good death, and finally heaven." That he had included his Indian friend in his Christian prayer seemed so natural and appropriate that he never gave it a second thought.

As they waited, a cloudbank rose in the west. They un-hoppled their horses and placed them on loose tether for a quick flight eastward. Then they set off on foot for the rancho three miles away. The advancing cloud mass hid the moon and the wind began to freshen. When they had loose-tied the horses, Coby had said, "If we don't come back, our horses can pull loose from the tether and shift for themselves. That way, they won't starve."

If we don't come back. The contemplation of it was gloomy and disquieting.

A fork of lightning slashed the darkness to their left. Thunder rumbled. The air became heavy. Large lukewarm raindrops began to fall, stinging their faces as they walked.

To Pedro's surprise, Coby flinched and looked nervously at the heavens with each flash of the lightning.

"Don't say anything to it," Coby begged, his melodious voice awed. "It's angry. It has no pity."

Pedro was nonplused. "Of whom are you speaking, brother?"

"Of the Thunder Bird. You can see it every time the heavens light up. It's a great bird with red streaks extending from its heart to its tail and wing tips. In its talons, it carries arrows of fire with which to strike its enemies. Its arrows sometimes kill."

Pedro fell silent, surprised that he had finally come upon something Coby feared. All Comanches dreaded death in the dark. They believed that the spirit of a man dying on a black night left his body to wander aimlessly forever, unable to find its way to the afterworld.

Coby went on, "When the great bird becomes angry, it makes lightning by rapidly opening and shutting its flashing eyes. The thunder is caused by the flapping of its great wings. Its shadow is the thundercloud. The rain that follows comes from the lake it carries on its back."

The rain swept across the prairie in filmy sheets, drenching them. Coby's bird must have turned that lake upside down, thought Pedro as they walked on through the wind and downpour, but he welcomed the storm. It would drive the dogs and perhaps also the night guards to cover and they should be able to reach the fodder stack without incident.

He explained this to Coby but Coby was too preoccupied to respond.

Now the heavens opened and the rain descended in a deluge. Pedro could feel the water running down inside his breechclout and into his moccasins. The thunderclaps crashed in salvos, like cannonshots. On all sides, the lightning darted to amazing lengths, running along the ground in fiery balls. The air was charged with electricity and smelled like sulphur.

On they sloshed in their wet moccasins, already about three-quarters of the way to the Rancho Tafoya. Pedro was glad they were finally making the effort. Best to get it over with. They had made their plan and prayed over it. Now it was time for success or failure.

Ahead of them in the violent lightning flashes, the corral walls loomed tall and sinister. The chocolate color of their adobe sides showed plainly with each heavenly conflagration and the green of the prairie was vivid and eerie.

Pedro's heart began to hammer wildly. Within those walls lay the possibility of freedom for Willow Girl and fulfillment of Pedro's dream of marrying her.

Focusing his eyes on a point to the left of the corral, he waited for the next lightning flash to reveal the fodder stack. Just then a terrific bolt of lightning snapped and detonated almost in their faces. Spearing the prairie immediately ahead of them, it exploded deafeningly into a hundred quivering stems. It was as though somebody in the heavens had cracked a gigantic whip of fire.

The whip's molten tip gently caressed the stack of fodder. The fodder glowed for a moment like a clump of fiery coral, then burst in flame, pouring black smoke up into the downpour.

Pedro stood in the rain, gawking with astonishment. The lightning bolt had ignited the haystack, destroying their plan. Like the fodder, their scheme had gone up in smoke.

Stunned, he turned toward Coby. Bitterness was so strong within him that he felt nauseated. Coby calmly stared at the smoldering fodder stack and the storm. He had a look of delighted wonder on his face.

"Waugh!" he grunted in silent admiration as another bolt veined the sky. For a moment he seemed to have forgotten Pedro's presence.

In the dwelling where Tafoya lived, a light came on and shuddered, as if in danger of being blown out by the furious gale. The noise of the storm had awakened the rancho. Soon the whole place would be aroused. What could they do?

Pedro cleared his mind of everything but the problem at hand. They had come too far and sacrificed too much to turn back now. Whirling, he took another look at the corral walls. There was no one in sight. Guards and dogs alike had apparently sought shelter from the storm.

He gripped Coby's bare arm and led him away from the fire. By a circuitous route they came up behind the corral, away from the house and the burning fodder. There was a momentary lull in the storm.

Looking up, Pedro saw in the slate-colored sky a narrow, brassy zone that widened phenomenally as he watched. Then came a fierce rush of wind and a few big hailstones that stung his bare back and clattered off the solid walls of the corral. With each lightning flash, Pedro saw hailstones the size of marbles and white as salt smiting the wet ground and bounding high into the air. The air grew chill and the hail suddenly began hammering down so thickly that it raised blood blisters on their hands and faces. Pedro had to hold his arms over his head to protect it from the pelting stones. Coby huddled down quietly beside him.

Pedro reached out and felt the wall with his hand, then put his mouth to Coby's ear.

"Brother, lend me your gourd rattle." Coby reached into his war bag and handed it over. Pedro again pressed his mouth to his friend's ear. "Let me stand on your shoulders. I'm going to climb over this wall into the corral. When they let the herd out in the morning, I'll try to stampede it. Wait for me out of range of their rifles."

Coby comprehended instantly. Without a word he stooped and raised one hand. Clutching Coby's hand, Pedro climbed lightly upon the warrior's shoulders. Placing his own hands against the wall to balance himself, he felt himself being lifted into the air. When the top of the wall came almost within reach, Coby grasped his left foot and hoisted him higher. Pedro crouched a bit, then sprang upward. His fingers gripped the top of the smooth wall. For a moment he hung suspended in the air, the hail flailing his bare back and legs. Then Coby's hands, held together, grasped one of his feet and pushed him still higher.

Pedro pulled upward and managed to get first one elbow and then the other on top of the wall. Next he swung one leg up, got a toehold, and scrambled atop the parapet.

As he rested for a moment, staring down into the darkness,

he told himself: This might be my death trap. If they catch me in here in the morning, they'll ask no questions. They'll lance me through the belly or hang me to a beam.

There could be no compromise now. Either he would turn back and face unbearable shame and self-loathing, or he would meet the challenge head on.

He let his feet down and dropped quickly to the ground inside the corral, rolling to soften his fall.

19 · The Horses of Tafoya

The splash Pedro made in the mud inside the corral seemed loud enough to warn every man on the rancho. Horses snorted in fright and lunged away. As he stood, lacquered from head to foot with mud, he wondered if any guards or vaqueros slept inside. The hail still beat down but now the wall protected him somewhat. There was a strong odor of wet manure in the air and in the lightning's shimmer he saw scores of horses cowering along the opposite wall. The great size of the enclosure gave an impression of solid security. There was no human habitation of any kind in sight and Pedro decided that he was alone with the herd.

Curious to determine the breed of the fabled animals he was risking so much to acquire, Pedro strained to see them better, but the lightning was less cooperative now. The hail had stopped and the wind had died. Looking up, he saw that the cloudbank had parted, revealing a single star that sparkled through the chilled, washed atmosphere like a beacon of hope.

He walked silently about the corral, the horses moving before him, and found a spring-fed tank of drinking water in which he washed off the mud. In one corner of the corral was a long, wooden feed trough with some hay in it, protected by a thatched roof, a rude shelter redolent with the odor of horses. Here Pedro lay down, covering his body with straw. It was warm and cosy.

While he waited for dawn, he thanked the Holy Mother for

281

bringing him safely thus far and prayed earnestly for a continuation of her divine favor. Why the Virgin Mother kept seeing fit to reward his poor prayers was a constant mystery to him. He knew he was not worthy.

As Pedro lay on his back in the trough, he noticed a curious something bobbing and dancing in the wind from the top of a tall, scraggly pole in the center of the corral. It looked like a constellation of round balls. The night was too dark to permit identification but the mystery intrigued him.

Twice he dozed off. When, after a second siesta, he looked again at the top of the pole, a bird flew out of one of the round objects. It was a gourd, he discovered, green with yellow stripes. There were several and they had been hollowed out to provide a nest for the martins. This was the first time in years that Pedro had seen bird nests fashioned by human beings. Surely he could expect mercy from such a people who had bird nests in their souls.

Suddenly he sat bolt upright. If he could recognize the stripes on the gourds, daylight must be near! The sky above the stockade's eastern walls was tinted pale lemon. The birds were twittering noisily. Inside the corral, objects were gradually taking shape; the inner walls were of adobe, too, with joists of cedar and pine. The horses were all standing near the gate in expectation of their daily freedom.

Of medium size with long, round bodies, these horses were thick-necked, full-loined, and deep through the heart. There was something familiar about their Roman noses and their tails, set low in their sloping rumps, something reminiscent of his native Andalusia. Then Pedro recognized them. They were Barbs, the light, clean-legged Moorish horses that had been brought to the New World by the Spanish explorers.

With mounting excitement, Pedro climbed stiffly out of his comfortable trough to go closer. These Barbs looked like a pure strain. Had Tafoya imported them? In Spain all Barbs were raised in the mountainous regions of southern Andalusia, near the ports of embarkation to the Americas.

As he watched the graceful animals prance and caper, Pedro understood why every Indian in the country had tried to steal them. Awareness of their own beauty and noble descent seemed to show in every lift and turn of their proud heads.

The eastern sky was faintly touched with crimson and pearl as Pedro moved quietly among the horses. Selecting a tawny-colored male, he grasped its mane and leaped astride. The animal's back seemed to grip him fast, as if made for his seat and legs alone. Careful to stay in the rear of the horses milling about the tall, locked gate, he clutched Coby's gourd rattle.

As he waited, he prayed simply: "Protect me, O my Mother, and obtain for me pardon of my sins, love for Jesus, a good death, and finally heaven." He felt strangely calm.

The new day grew clearer and rosier. Voices approached from outside the wall, speaking Spanish. They sounded soft and off guard. Pedro heard the vaqueros murmuring in wonder at the devastation of the storm. Here was a heap of ashes where the fodder stack had stood. There the hail had chewed up the grass and stripped the leaves from a tall cottonwood in the master's yard.

The tantalizing smell of a cigarette made of real tobacco drifted through the chinks of the gate. Crouching low over the withers of his horse, his heart thumping against his ribs, Pedro waited.

At last came the sound he had been waiting for, the rattle and clank of the gate chains as someone outside struggled with the locks. Heads raised, ears up, the horses all around Pedro began to dance and crowd forward. Pedro flattened himself along his animal's neck, burying his face in its mane to keep from being seen. His principal dread was being roped off his horse. He knew that all vaqueros were devilishly accurate with their riatas.

With a great grinding and creaking and wrenching, the gates swung open. Squealing and nickering, the first horses began pouring through. Pedro felt the ground trembling as the animals rushed through the gap, rearing, plunging, crowding, snorting. When nearly all were outside, Pedro, too, shot through the gate. Once outside, he began to yell shrilly and shake his gourd rattle.

Despite their patrician breeding, the Barbs reacted just like any other horses, bolting toward the open range. With them went the rancho's extra saddle stock. Shouts of alarm, angry and frantic, rang out in Spanish, biting through the tumult. Pedro flung a look back over his shoulder, exulting in the confusion he had caused.

The rancho's saddle animals that had just been roped were trying to join the runaways, too. In their terror they jerked the vaqueros off their feet, dragging them along on their stomachs and yanking the riatas out of their hands.

From Tafoya's yard came a piercing neigh. A brown stallion being led to drink by an old man wearing a sombrero threw up its head and pulled loose from its handler. Gracefully jumping a palisade of mesquite trees, it joined the fleeing mass. Some of the vaqueros ran to warn the master, but without mounts there could be no pursuit.

Pedro let the frightened animals run, listening with pride to the thunder of their hooves. They ran as if they did not feel the ground beneath them, breathing deeply and regularly and obviously relishing their freedom. Accustomed to running together, they made little trouble. All Pedro had to do was point them eastward. He thanked the Holy Virgin for her help. The venture was succeeding unbelievably well.

Now Coby rode in at an angle up ahead, leading their extra horses. Soon the stampede was following him. Coby was careful to stay in the lead, conducting the herd over the best ground and in the direction he wished it to take.

Filled with gratitude and high spirits, Pedro remembered a gypsy *copla* about a stolen mule. His voice broke into song:

He picked up a halter.
On the other end of it was a mule.
He did not steal the mule.
The mule just came along of his own accord.

All day long they pushed the herd at an easy, ground-gobbling gallop. Pedro knew Tafoya would quickly organize a pursuit and that it would come hard and fast with every resource of the rascally trader's wealth and influence behind it. But he was no longer worried. He knew what these desert-bred beauties could do. Their ancestors had been desert horses of Berber blood, accustomed to running long distances in the heat on scanty rations and little water. Besides, Tafoya could pursue only to the limits of the Comanche domain. He would not dare enter it very far.

At the first water stop they removed the riatas from the necks of the rancho saddle stock and examined the thoroughbreds. It was no wonder that the blooded animals were unshod; their hoofs were like iron. Now Pedro understood why he had seen no nail marks in their tracks.

When they paused at a tiny creek at midmorning of the second day, Coby gave a surprised grunt and pointed at the horizon behind them. A faint dust haze showed over the trail they had been traveling.

"Tafoya!" Coby spat out the word hatefully.

The trader must be burning horseflesh recklessly, Pedro realized with swift foreboding. He remembered the hundreds of horses grazing in the fields beyond the ranchhouse. Tafoya must have used these to mount his vaqueros. Or perhaps he had organized a pursuit on superior mounts furnished by his officer friends at the fort. Pedro knew that to shake them off, he and Coby would have to run the guts completely out of them.

They quickly set the herd in motion again. "The chasers must be getting pretty tired by now," Coby reasoned before he rode to his position at the head of the herd. "I think they know they have to catch us soon or not at all."

"Remember, brother," Pedro reminded him, "they have rifles. How far behind are they?"

Coby studied the dust, gauging the distance. "Not very far. They must have ridden part of the night to get this close. I don't think they can keep going that fast very long."

Riding in front, Coby did not accelerate the pace despite the gains scored by Tafoya.

The dust film hung on, and as the sun rose higher, the running Barbs began to perspire although they showed no signs of fatigue. The air was very hot and dry. Pedro and Coby kept changing to the backs of fresh mounts. Without slowing down, they ate the remainder of their dried buffalo meat and drank sparingly from their waterskins. All afternoon and into the dusk they kept the herd moving.

Pedro's eyes were blinking. Already he had gone two nights without rest. Coby showed him how to moisten a pinch of tobacco with saliva and rub it into his eyelids in order to stay awake.

They kept going until dark, then turned south for another league until they came to a low range of hills. Here they hid the herd and bedded down. Their tracks would not betray them in the dark.

The respite was only temporary, however. The dust cloud was still visible behind them when, an hour after sunrise, they stopped at a creek heavily fringed by willows. Here they gave the thirsty animals their first drink in almost twenty hours.

Now Coby looked grim. Raising from the creek bank where he had been drinking, he studied the dust haze carefully. After they had filled their waterskins, he untied his lance, adjusted his bow and quiver, and changed to a fresh mount. "Brother," he said, "I think when they arrive at this creek, they will be so thirsty that they will throw themselves off their horses and be very busy drinking. Perhaps they will not bother to secure their horses while they drink. Ride on ahead with the herd. I'll come later." Splashing across the creek, he rode downstream a quarter of a league. There he recrossed and disappeared into the willows.

Pedro pointed the herd east and pressed the horses into a steady run. Tafoya's men had rifles and revolvers; they had the advantage of numbers, too. On his side Coby would have surprise and his Comanche genius for attacking boldly and expertly in a crisis.

Pedro looked apprehensively at the herd. The Barbs still ran smoothly, scattering the miles behind them with easy unconcern. But the dust film behind rose higher and more darkly brown.

Ahead he saw the long line of white cliffs, shaped like stone fortifications, that marked the western boundary of Mah Nohhhphe. They were nearing Comanche territory. The breeze that was cooling his sweating chest and back must be cooling the horses, too. They were going well. Their breathing was still excellent. Their hot odor came back to him in the dry air.

Anxiously, Pedro looked again at the dust pall behind him. He could not understand how his pursuers managed to stay so near. Then suddenly the answer came to him. They had probably exchanged their jaded horses for fresh ones at all the small ranchos along the way.

Pedro looked again at the Barbs loping along, mile after mile. Their pace had been comfortable and sustained. The men pursuing them had probably lashed their horses cruelly all the way. If, by some miracle, Tafoya threatens to overtake us, Pedro thought, I can put these beauties into a dead run. They have the speed, the stamina, and the breeding to go hard all morning in this dry heat.

But he was concerned about Coby. He decided to ease up a moment and rest the herd for the final effort while he scanned the prairie behind with Creek Water's glass.

He swung the glass up and felt the hair rising on his scalp. On the trail behind him appeared several moving specks. Tafoya's men! They were going to try to run him down. Coby had failed and might be dead. Pedro focused the glass again, chancing a final look, and discovered an odd movement in the distant picture.

One horse seemed to be riding sinuously behind the others, from left to right, keeping them bunched and moving. Pedro's spine tensed. The rider certainly knew how to herd horses. Flanking them neatly, he was like a good sheep dog controlling a flock. That could mean but one thing. The other horses must be riderless. Pedro felt his heart leap. It must be Coby!

It was Coby! Driving a dozen horses ahead of him, his friend approached. Each horse wore a big Spanish saddle and almost every saddle had a rifle lashed to it. The horses were panting in strangled sobs; they were foam-flecked and looked dead on their feet.

Pedro sat his horse, waiting. Affection and admiration surged through him as Coby rode up. His arm was bleeding.

"A broken willow limb gashed it," Coby explained. He cleaned the laceration with his tongue, like a dog, and spat the blood spittle on the grass.

"What happened, brother?" Pedro asked.

"They were all on their hands and knees drinking, away from their horses and their weapons."

"Did you run off all their horses?"

Coby's black eyes were inscrutable. "Not quite all, brother. One man mounted and pursued me. He stayed behind."

Pedro stared at him, not understanding.

"But his hair is going with us." Coby reached into his war bag and held up a bushy, black scalp. From its pink underside the blood still seeped.

From then on they rode more slowly, halting for brief periods to rest the herd and let it graze. Soon they reached the upper Kwahade country, safe from all pursuit.

Beside a small pond, they took the saddles off the horses Coby had acquired and changed them to the backs of fresher animals. The Barbs waded into the shallows to drink. Arching their necks gracefully downward and rolling their eyes warily, they plunged their velvety muzzles eye-deep into the gray, muddy water. Their stamina continued to amaze Pedro. Although they had galloped hundreds of leagues, the proud animals remained full of life, impatient of restraint, eager to be off again.

Coby's gaze moved from horse to horse, his usually somber face alight with pleasure.

"Brother," he asked, "are you sure that girl is worth all these beautiful horses? Don't you think you could bring yourself to give her up and choose some other woman so you could keep this wonderful herd?"

Pedro eyed a small, dainty, reddish-yellow mare he planned to give to Willow Girl. The mare had intelligent eyes and legs as slender as a woman's wrist. In the sun's slanting rays, her coat gleamed like polished copper.

He smiled at Coby. "She's worth two herds like this."

Yet the closer they came to the village, the more nervous and apprehensive Pedro became. Willow Girl was peculiar and independent. She might not want him even after he had gone to all this trouble. While they paused to broil an antelope steak two days' traveling distance from the village, he confided his fears to Coby.

With his lean, muscular hands, Coby tore some white meat off the shank he was holding. "If you trade for her, she's yours.

She will surely prefer you to Paunch and his quirt. You'll have to beat her some, of course, but not as much as he beats his wives."

Pedro stared moodily across the fire at the low hills in the distance. "How do you know Paunch will want to trade?"

Coby sank his white teeth into the succulent meat. "He'll trade, all right. He has wanted this herd for years."

Pedro looked about him at the Barbs feeding quietly on the gramma grass that was turning golden yellow now that early autumn had arrived. They swung their soft muzzles backward to sweep biting flies off their flanks and swished their tails. For the time being they were safe from all pursuit, but what if some stranger Comanche band tried to run off the animals? There was much at stake.

"Do you think they'll be safe here?" he asked.

Coby regarded him steadily with unblinking eyes. "Why would they not be? There isn't a white man within ten days riding distance."

Pedro fell silent. He should have known better. Nowhere in the world is Indian property safer than in a camp. He had learned that long ago. If you lost a knife, a pipe, or anything else, you had only to inform the camp crier and a few minutes after he had shouted news of the loss through the village, the article, if found, would be returned.

Soon they began to encounter hunters from their own band, who paused to stare enviously at the celebrated animals. Pedro and Coby sent word by the hunters that they would soon be parading the Tafoya herd through the village. And now, Pedro cut out the little mare with the coppery coat that was intended for Willow Girl.

To Coby he gave a choice of any five animals in the herd. After Coby had selected them, Pedro isolated another fine gelding for Creek Water, and still another for Old Sore. The brown stallion he kept for himself. He was determined to become as skillful a breeder as any buck in the band. By crossing the Barb stallion with the mustang mares he planned to capture from the wild herds, he would strengthen the blood of his own little herd. Besides the sixty animals of the Tafoya herd, they had brought along thirty animals of the rancho work stock. Pedro divided these evenly with Coby. In addition, Coby had the dozen animals he had stampeded while the vaqueros drank at the creek, as well as several saddles, rifles, and riatas. It had been a profitable raid.

They were grooming the animals at a stream five miles outside the camp, rubbing the mud and scurf off their coats and combing out their manes and tails, when they saw a small puff of dust approaching. Soon a heavily laden travois came in sight. It was drawn by a big, shaggy-maned piebald whose driver beat it with a quirt nearly every foot of the way. The odd-looking rig drew alongside. An extraordinarily obese man rolled out of the travois to the ground, scrambled to his feet, and marched toward them. It was Paunch.

For a moment he feasted his cold, greedy eyes upon the captured animals, missing no feature of their sprightly beauty. As he turned to Coby excitement and cupidity struggled for mastery in his greasy face.

"Friend, I would like to purchase all these horses."

Without a word, Coby pointed to Pedro and turned his back. Surprise and irritation showed in Paunch's features. It was obviously hard for him to accept the fact that Creek Water's captive had come into all this property and wealth. He swung around to face Pedro and repeated his question.

"Purchase them?" Pedro feigned surprise. "Why, friend, we just stole them. Now we want to enjoy them. I do not want to sell a single animal." Turning his back, he resumed his grooming.

Paunch's mouth tightened. "I will let you take your choice from my herd of twice their number if you will give them to me."

Pedro could not resist badgering his enemy a little longer. "Friend, what would I do with that many horses? I have always had all I need."

Paunch grew openly insolent. "Until now, you had only seven."

Pedro looked at him coolly, hating him with each breath he drew. This was the fat dog who had beaten Willow Girl, cutting the soft skin on her shoulder and arm.

"Why do you want these when you already have three thousand?" he demanded.

Paunch glared at him, his right hand tightening whitely on the handle of the quirt. "I will let you take your choice from my herd of three times their number."

Pedro said, "Don't talk to me of trading ordinary horses for these horses. These are quality horses. You know that there isn't another herd like them in all of Komantcia. Why should I trade valuable horses like these even if you offer your ordinary horses twenty to one in exchange?"

Paunch was silent.

"What else have you got to trade?" purred Pedro. "I'm a young man starting out in life. I have no hunting arrows, no buffalo robes, no lodge skins, no wives. I might trade later for something besides horses. But right now I don't want to trade for anything. I want to enjoy these horses. I want to parade them through the village." Again he turned his back on Paunch.

For a moment the fat chief stood glaring at Pedro. Then he waddled back to his travois, the ends of his braids swinging angrily like suddenly jerked picket ropes.

He clambered in, sat down heavily, and laid his quirt viciously across the back of the piebald. The frightened beast sprang forward and the strange contrivance moved off toward the village, rising in its wake twin dust funnels of defeat.

Later, after they had decorated the manes and tails of the horses, Pedro and Coby tied the animals together, the tail of one to the lower jaw of another, and led them in triumph through the village, now located in the sunshine along the banks of a sweetwater creek.

As they entered the open side of the camp, all activity ceased. The old men stopped their arrow making, the women laid down their skinning knives, and the children halted their play. Soon every person in the village was staring at the spirited herd so many warriors had died trying to steal.

The captured Barbs seemed conscious of being admired. Necks arched majestically and tails held high, they pranced and pirouetted with their light, elastic tread, rolling their eyes in gentle fright as they shied away from the dogs that howled inhospitably and from the strange sights and smells and voices of hundreds of curious people.

But Pedro saw all this only indirectly. He ignored the adulation of these fierce people who ranked spectacular horse thievery above everything save counting coup on a live enemy.

He scanned each row of faces, each tipi door. He had not seen Willow Girl for several weeks. He was starved for a single look. They had left in the Comanche summer. Now it was autumn.

If he could see her just for an instant, he would be better prepared for his next encounter with Paunch. Any gesture, sign, or look would do. But he searched in vain.

When the parade was over and Pedro drove the horses back to the herding ground, Paunch was waiting for him there. His fleshy fingers opened and closed on the quirt gripped tightly in his hand.

"What do you want for them?" he demanded, his voice hoarse with avarice. "You would not have gone to all this risk if you hadn't wanted something."

Pedro looked at him with loathing, wishing that he could pay back, lash for lash, all the beatings he had given his wives.

"Friend," he said scornfully, "I don't want your horses. What else have you got to trade? The only other chattel property you own are your women and your dogs. Do you think all your wives and dogs together are worth one of these beautiful animals?"

"Take them," Paunch implored. "You can have any of my wives you wish. You can have them all. Just give me the horses."

A chilled sweat prickled the insides of Pedro's palms. Now was his chance to take on this hardy brute.

"I might be willing to trade part of my herd for five hundred of your ponies, fifty buffalo robes, and my pick of all your wives." He spoke casually, as if he were thinking of the barter for the first time. His hands trembled uncontrollably. He put them behind him but he was too late.

Paunch's quick, darting eyes narrowed shrewdly. With a sudden gesture of understanding, he struck the prairie sharply with his quirt.

"So it's Willow Girl you want!" he cried triumphantly. "That's why you went to all that trouble to steal the herd. So you could trade the herd to me for Willow Girl. You were courting her when I won her from you and from the others."

Blood surged into Pedro's head and he felt a premonition of disaster. He tried to hide his feelings but he knew they must show plainly on his face.

Now that he was in command of the situation, Paunch became openly contemptuous. "Friend, I'll trade even. The woman for the whole Tafoya herd."

Pedro shook his head. "The woman for the herd you saw

Coby and me lead through the village this afternoon. I have already cut out nine animals for gifts and sent them to the herding grounds." He was tired of bartering.

Paunch shook his head fiercely, his swinging braids flailing the hot air. "The whole herd or none."

"No."

One of the Barbs nickered. Gentle as a kitten, it walked up to Pedro and nuzzled him. Pedro fondled the animal's ears and the horse yawned contentedly. Paunch watched with greedy fascination, his breathing loud and rapid. His look of greed came back.

"All right, friend. The woman for that part of the herd I saw this afternoon."

"One thing." Pedro came closer. Placing his hand on the shaft of his knife, he looked squarely at Paunch. "If you beat her again before she comes, I'll kill you."

Paunch's eyes went liquid with surprise, as if no woman was worth getting so excited about.

"I'll send her to you tonight, friend."

"Send her without any whip marks on her or I'll come looking for you."

Paunch seemed not to hear the threat. He walked to his travois and drew from it a battered cavalry bugle. The several long toots he blew were a signal for his herdsmen to come and take the Barbs. Then he walked among his new acquisitions and began fondling them with his beefy hands and talking to them in a gentle murmur.

Pedro felt no sense of loss. His hands still shook and his legs felt weak. A familiar feeling of foreboding came over him, knotting his insides. He had waited so long and gone through so much. Would Willow Girl run from him again?

When he reached his tipi two hours before sunset, Pedro did not recognize it. His bedding had been taken out, shaken, and spread in the sun. His cooking utensils, fresh-scrubbed in the creek, were drying. A pile of buffalo chips had been gathered for fuel. His weapons were neatly stacked on a small platform by the door.

As he grasped the door flap he noticed that the torn place had been neatly mended with sinew thread. He lifted the flap and stepped inside. A wild, sweet smell of burning sage permeated the interior. Everything had been put to rights. The sand floor had been swept. The backflaps of the lodge had been raised three inches to let in the fresh air.

Willow Girl looked up from her task of flaking dried buffalo meat into the stew kettle. Her glossy hair swirled about her shoulders in a rich, unbridled fall. This time she did not run. She had had little time to get herself ready but Pedro saw that the ends of her lustrous tresses were wet and that somehow she had contrived to bathe. Her cottonwood-leaf scent was most pleasant.

She shot one startled look at him, her long black eyelashes flaring widely, then dropped her face into her hands and began to cry.

Pedro's eyes were hot and wet. He moved timidly to her side. Putting his arms around her, he comforted her, his voice low and gentle.

His heart began to sing like a thousand meadowlarks splitting their throats. He was the happiest man on earth.

There is one well-documented exception to the tragic cases of Cynthia Ann Parker, John Tanner, Frances Slocum, and other white captives who could never become regenerated after returning to civilization from a life of Indian savagery.

He was Pedro Espinosa, a Mexican boy born in 1810 on the bank of the Rio Grande near Laredo, Texas. When Pedro was nine, his father's rancho was hit by the Comanches and the entire adult population put to death with the usual accompaniment of horror. Pedro and other children were carried into captivity and adopted.

For nineteen years, until he reached age twenty-eight, Espinosa grew up amid the crime and licentiousness of the Comanches. He learned his savage lessons so fast that at age thirteen, only four years after his capture, he accompanied a raiding party against the Tonkawas. At fourteen he became a distinguished warrior. He married and fathered an Indian family. He fought, stole, committed outrages, and participated in the ceremonials of his adopted people. However, he was never permitted to join a raid sent into the Laredo country from which he had been taken.

Espinosa secretly hated the Comanches. He had never forgiven them for the violation and murder of his mother. One night in 1838 he escaped while hunting black bear in the Guadalupe Mountains. Returning to Laredo, he found his white relatives. He married, settled down, became a faithful father, an honest citizen, and a respected member of his community.

He also became a scout for Colonel Richard Irving Dodge, who not only saw military action against the Comanches but wrote books about them. I found out about Espinosa while reading Colonel Dodge's *The Plains of the Great West* (New York, 1877) and *Our Wild Indians* (Hartford, 1882).

Espinosa is a rough prototype of Pedro Pavón, the hero of this narrative. *Komantcia* deals with his life as a Comanche. A second novel will describe his return to his uncle's ranch in northern Mexico.

I should like to acknowledge the aid of four Comanche oral sources, the late Albert Attocknie and his son Joe, Yamparikas of Oklahoma City; Mrs. Mattie Maddische, Yapah from Indianahoma, Oklahoma; and Topay, seventh and last living wife of War Chief Quanah Parker, who lives near Cache, Oklahoma. My main source on the *Llano Estacado* was Albert Attocknie, the Yamparika, who hunted on it as a boy with permission of the tribal Indian agent.

A book I kept constantly in front of me was *The Comanches, Lords of the South Plains,* by Ernest Wallace and E. Adamson Hoebel (Norman: University of Oklahoma Press, 1952). Background suggestions came from Indian captive narratives related by Nelson Lee, the Reverend J. J. Methvin, Clinton and Jeff D. Smith, T. A. "Dot" Babb, and Herman Lehman, as well as from John Cremony, Captain Randolph Marcy, George Catlin, Abbe Emmanuel Domenech, Dr. C. C. Rister, and Captain Robert G. Carter.

Individuals who gave assistance were Professor Dwight V. Swain, associate professor of professional writing at the University of Oklahoma, who read the novel in manuscript; Dr. Ralph Bienfang, professor of pharmacy at the University of Oklahoma and well-known olfactionist; Professor Joseph Taylor, Professor William Burgett, Dr. Norman Boke, and Olive Hawes, all from the university; Dr. Jim Haddock, Norman, Oklahoma, for anatomical advice; and Debbie Reid, Norman, for all sorts of advice concerning horses. Mari Sandoz gave general advice. Addie Lee Barker, my assistant in sports publicity at Oklahoma, oriented my grammar and spelling.

For help on the Catholic phase of the novel I am indebted to Sister Mary Marcellin, B.V.M., Wahlert High School, Dubuque, Iowa; Joseph J. Quinn and Mrs. Quinn of Oklahoma City; James and Helen Driscoll of Key West, Florida; and Father David Monahan, principal of McGuinness High School of Oklahoma City, who read the galleys. My old teacher Dr. E. E. Dale, research professor emeritus of history at the University of Oklahoma, also read the galleys and made valuable suggestions.

I worked parts of seven summers in the Edward Ayers Collection of Indian Captive Literature at Chicago, where I found a valuable depository of manuscript material. The people there who helped most were Doris Welsh, head cataloguer; Therese Bissen, reference librarian; Antonia Matosos, assistant custodian; and Ramiro Chiriboga, page, who did translating for me.

The four people I pestered the most in the University of Oklahoma's William Bennett Bizzell Memorial Library were Sandra Stewart, assistant in the Frank Phillips Collection; Mrs. Vinita Davis, information librarian; Dr. Arrell M. Gibson, curator of the Phillips Collection; and Opal Carr, history-government-geography librarian. I am also grateful to the Faculty Research Fund for photostats.

I am indebted to Virginia, my wife, for again tolerating our lack of social life as I tried to fit the seven-year researching and writing around my duties as University of Oklahoma sports information director.

HAROLD KEITH

University of Oklahoma

ABOUT THE AUTHOR

Harold Keith won the 1958 Newbery Award for *Rifles for Watie*. For seven years, Mr. Keith has been involved in research on all phases of Comanche life, and in the writing of *Komantcia*. He pored over countless private manuscript collections on the lore of the Plains Indians and Indian captives, and he talked to old Comanches still living on the reservation near Lawton, Oklahoma. The remainder of Pedro Pavón's life with the Comanches will be described in another historical novel by Harold Keith, now in preparation.

The author, a native Oklahoman, was educated at Northwestern State Teachers College in Alva, and at the University of Oklahoma. He has been director of sports information at the university for many years.